In A Page Pediatric Signs & Symptoms

Jonathan E. Teitelbaum, MD
Assistant Professor of Pediatrics
Drexel University School of Medicine
Director, Pediatric Gastroenterology and Nutrition
Monmouth Medical Center
Long Branch, New Jersey

Kathleen O. DeAntonis, MD
Faculty, Department of Pediatrics
Mercy Hospital of Pittsburgh
Pittsburgh, Pennsylvania

Scott Kahan, MD
Intern, Franklin Square Hospital
Baltimore, Maryland

Blackwell Publishing

Blackwell Publishing, Inc., 350 Main Street, Malden, Massachusetts 02148-5018, USA
Blackwell Publishing Ltd, 9600 Garsington Road, Oxford OX4 2DQ, UK
Blackwell Science Asia Pty Ltd, 550 Swanston Street, Carlton, Victoria 3053, Australia

04 05 06 07 5 4 3 2 1

ISBN: 1-4051-0427-9

Library of Congress Cataloging-in-Publication Data

In a page. Pediatric signs & symptoms / [edited by] Jonathan E. Teitelbaum, Kathleen O. DeAntonis, Scott Kahan.
p. ; cm.
Includes index.
ISBN 1–4051–0427–9
1. Pediatrics—Handbooks, manuals, etc. 2. Children—Diseases—Diagnosis—Handbooks, manuals, etc. 3. Symptoms—Handbooks, manuals, etc.
[DNLM: 1. Pediatrics—Handbooks. 2. Signs and Symptoms—Handbooks. WS 39 I348 2004] I. Title: Pediatric signs & symptoms. II. Teitelbaum, Jonathan E. III. DeAntonis, Kathleen O. IV. Kahan, Scott.

RJ48.I49 2004
618.92—dc22

2004046279

A catalogue record for this title is available from the British Library

Acquisitions: Bev Copland
Development: Kate Heinle
Production: Debra Murphy
Cover design: Gary Ragaglia
Interior design: Visual Perspectives
Typesetter: TechBooks in New Delhi, India
Printed and bound by Sheridan Books in Ann Arbor, MI

For further information on Blackwell Publishing, visit our website:
www.blackwellmedstudent.com

Notice: The indications and dosages of all drugs in this book have been recommended in the medical literature and conform to the practices of the general community. The medications described and treatment prescriptions suggested do not necessarily have specific approval by the Food and Drug Administration for use in the diseases and dosages for which they are recommended. The package insert for each drug should be consulted for use and dosage as approved by the FDA. Because standards for usage change, it is advisable to keep abreast of revised recommendations, particularly those concerning new drugs. This book is intended solely as a review book for medical students and residents. It is not written as a guide for the intricate clinical management of medical patients. The publisher and editor cannot accept any legal responsibility for the content contained within this book nor any omitted information.

Table of Contents

Table of Contents

Table of Contents

Table of Contents

Table of Contents

Attributions

Larry J. Alexander, OD, FAAO
29. Diplopia, 31. Flashes of Light & Floaters, 32. Leukocoria, 34. Papilledema (Optic Disc Swelling), 36. Proptosis/Exophthalmos, 37. Ptosis, 38. Retinal Hemorrhage, 39. Scleral Injection (Red Eye), 41. Vision Loss

David H. Chi, MD
50. Cleft Lip/Palate, 51. Drooling, 52. Dysphagia, 53. Halitosis, 54. Hoarseness, 56. Salivary Gland Enlargement, 57. Snoring, 58. Sore Throat, 74. Stridor

Irini Daskalaki, MD
10. Fever – Acute, 11. Fever – Cyclic, 12. Fever – Recurrent, 13. Fever – Unknown Origin, 15. Hypothermia

Kathleen O. DeAntonis, MD
30. Eye Discharge, 33. Nystagmus, 35. Periorbital Edema, 40. Strabismus, 47. Chronic Rhinitis, 55. Macroglossia, 59. Stomatitis, 62. Torticollis, 98. Back Pain, 120. Limp, 155. Hallucinations

Fatma Dedeoglu, MD
113. Arthritis – Multiple Joints, 114. Arthritis – Single Joint, 115. Asymmetric Limbs, 123. Raynaud Phenomenon

Katherine MacRae Dell, MD
103. Dysuria, 104. Enuresis, 105. Hematuria, 107. Proteinuria, 109. Pyuria, 138. Edema, 159. Hyperkalemia, 160. Hypernatremia, 163. Hypokalemia, 164. Hyponatremia, 166. Metabolic Acidosis

Kari A. Draper, MD
22. Abnormal Head Shape, 112. Vaginal Discharge

Shannon Fourtner, MD
71. Gynecomastia

Sarah Friebert, MD
4. Lymphadenopathy, 78. Abdominal Masses, 91. Splenomegaly, 146. Pallor, 156. Anemia, 165. Leukocytosis, 167. Neutropenia, 168. Thrombocytopenia

Adda Grimberg, MD
6. Polydipsia, 7. Polyphagia, 18. Obesity, 19. Short Stature, 20. Tall Stature, 71. Gynecomastia, 99. Abnormal Vaginal Bleeding, 100. Amenorrhea – Primary, 101. Amenorrhea – Secondary, 106. Precocious Puberty, 108. Pubertal Delay, 157. Hypercalcemia, 158. Hyperglycemia, 161. Hypocalcemia, 162. Hypoglycemia

Maria J. Henwood, DO, FAAP
157. Hypercalcemia, 161. Hypocalcemia

Francis M. Hoe, MD
158. Hyperglycemia, 162. Hypoglycemia

Vlad D. Ianuş, MD, MPH
117. Clubbing, 135. Alopecia, 136. Annular Rashes, 139. Hand & Foot Rashes

Attributions

Tomislav Ivsic, MD
148. Pigmented Lesions, 149. Pruritus, 150. Purpura, 151. Urticaria, 152. Vesicular Rashes

Douglas A. Jacobstein, MD
1. Anorexia, 17. Failure to Thrive, 21. Weight Loss, 79. Abdominal Pain, 89. Hematemesis, 90. Hepatomegaly, 95. Vomiting, 96. Vomiting – Projectile, 143. Jaundice in Infants – Direct, 144. Jaundice in Infants - Indirect

Heather Kasten, MD
140. Hirsutism, 141. Hyperhidrosis (Excessive Sweating), 142. Hypopigmented Lesions, 145. Morbilliform Rashes, 147. Petechiae

David J. Kay, MD, MPH
24. Facial Paralysis, 42. Hearing Loss – Acquired, 43. Hearing Loss – Congenital, 44. Otalgia (Ear Pain), 45. Otorrhea (Ear Discharge), 48. Epistaxis (Nosebleed), 49. Nasal Obstruction & Rhinorrhea, 50. Cleft Lip/Palate, 53. Halitosis, 60. Neck Masses

Roy J. Kim, MD, MPH
100. Amenorrhea – Primary, 101. Amenorrhea – Secondary

Don Lujan, MD, MS
98. Scoliosis, 116. Genu Varum (Bowed Legs), 118. Hip Pain, 119. Knee Pain, 124. Toeing In, 125. Toeing Out

Sheela N. Magge, MD
6. Polydipsia

C. Becket Mahnke, MD
16. Tachycardia/Palpitations, 65. Chest Pain, 70. Abnormal Heart Sounds, 72. Heart Failure, 137. Cyanotic Newborn

Christina Lin Master, MD
92. Umbilicus – Delayed Separation, 93. Umbilicus – Herniation, 94. Umbilicus – Single Umbilical Artery

Timothy D. Murphy, MD
64. Apnea, 66. Cough – Acute, 67. Cough – Chronic, 68. Crackles/Rales, 69. Cyanosis, 70. Dyspnea, 73. Hemoptysis, 75. Tachypnea, 76. Wheezing

Bankole Osuntokun, MD
77. Abdominal Distension, 80. Ascites, 82. Bowel Sounds – Increased, 84. Diarrhea – Acute, 85. Diarrhea – Chronic, no Blood or Weight Loss, 86. Diarrhea – Chronic, with Weight Loss, 87. Encopresis, 88. Hematochezia

Asim R. Piracha, MD
29. Diplopia, 31. Flashes of Light & Floaters, 32. Leukocoria, 34. Papilledema (Optic Disc Swelling), 36. Proptosis/Exophthalmos, 37. Ptosis, 38. Retinal Hemorrhage, 39. Scleral Injection (Red Eye), 41. Vision Loss

Attributions

Mustafa Sahin, MD, PhD
3. Irritability, 8. Syncope, 23. Enlarged Anterior Fontanelle, 25. Headache, 26. Increased Intracranial Pressure, 27. Macrocephaly, 28. Microcephaly, 61. Nuchal Rigidity, 121. Muscle Weakness – Distal, 122. Muscle Weakness – Proximal, 126. Ataxia, 127. Chorea, 128. Hyperreflexia, 129. Hyporeflexia, 130. Hypotonia, 131. Paresthesias, 132. Seizures – Neonatal, 133. Seizures – Childhood, 134. Vertigo, 153. Coma

Nader Shaikh, MD, MPH
105. Congenital Penile Anomalies, 114. Scrotal Pain, 115. Scrotal Swelling

Jonathan E. Teitelbaum, MD
2. Fatigue, 81. Bowel Sounds – Decreased, 83. Constipation, 154. Delirium

Nicole J. Ullrich, MD, PhD
61. Nuchal Rigidity, 121. Muscle Weakness – Distal, 128. Hyperreflexia, 129. Hyporeflexia, 131. Paresthesias, 134. Vertigo

Ronald Williams, MD, FAAP, FACP
9. Bradycardia, 14. Hypertension, 46. Tinnitus

Weizhen Xu, MD
19. Short Stature, 20. Tall Stature

Abbreviations

5ASA 5-aminosalicylic acid
6MP 6-mercaptopurine
AAT alpha-1 antitrypsin
ABCs airway, breathing, circulation
ABG arterial blood gas
ACE angiotensin converting enzyme
ACTH adrenocorticotropin hormone
AD autosomal dominant
ADEK vitamins A, D, E, and K
ADEM acute disseminated encephalomyelitis
ADH antidiuretic hormone (vasopressin)
AG anion gap
AIDS acquired immunodeficiency syndrome
ALT alanine aminotransferase
ALTE acute life-threatening event
AMN acquired melanocytic nevi
ANA antinuclear antibody
ANC absolute neutrophil count
ANCA antinuclear cytoplasmic antibody
AP anterior-posterior
APSGN acute poststreptococcal glomerulonephritis
aPTT activated partial thromboplastin time
AR autosomal recessive
ARDS acute respiratory distress syndrome
ARF acute rheumatic fever
ASD atrial septal defect
ASO antistreptolysin-O
AST aspartate aminotransferase
ATN acute tubular necrosis
AV atrioventricular
AVED ataxia with vitamin E deficiency
AVM arteriovenous malformation
BALT bronchus-associated lymphoid tissue
BE barium enema
BiPAP bilevel positive airway pressure
BL bilateral
BMI body mass index
BP blood pressure
BP bullous pemphigoid
BPPV benign paroxysmal positional vertigo
BRBPR bright red blood per rectum
BRE benign rolandic epilepsy
BS bowel sounds
BUN blood urea nitrogen
C3 complement 3
C5 fifth cervical vertebra
C6 sixth cervical vertebra
C7 seventh cervical vertebra
Ca calcium
CA cancer
Ca^{++} calcium ion
CAH congenital adrenal hyperplasia
CBC complete blood count
CBG capillary blood gas
CCAM congenital cystic adenomatoid malformation
CCHD congenital cyanotic heart disease
CCHS congenital central hypoventilation syndrome
CD celiac disease
CF cystic fibrosis
CHARGE coloboma, heart defect, choanal atresia, genital hypoplasia, ear anomalies
CHD congenital heart disease
CHF congestive heart failure
CHL conductive hearing loss
CI clubbing index
CIDP chronic inflammatory demyelinating polyradiculoneuropathy
CK creatine kinase
Cl^- chloride ion
CLE congenital lobar emphysema
CML chronic myelogenous leukemia
CMN congenital melanocytic nevi
CMT Charcot-Marie-Tooth
CMV cytomegalovirus
CN III cranial nerve three
CN VI cranial nerve six
CN VII cranial nerve seven
CN XII cranial nerve twelve
CNS central nervous system
CO carbon monoxide
CO_2 carbon dioxide
COPD chronic obstructive pulmonary disease
CPA cerebellopontine angle
CPAP continuous positive airway pressure
CPEO chronic progressive external ophthalmoplegia
CPK creatine phosphokinase
CPP cerebral perfusion pressure
CPR cardiopulmonary resuscitation
Cr creatinine
CREST calcinosis, Raynaud, esophageal hypomotility, sclerodactyly, telangiectasia
CRP C-reactive protein
CSF cerebrospinal fluid

Abbreviations

CT	computerized tomography
CULLP	congenital unilateral lower lip palsy
CVA	costovertebral angle
CVAT	costovertebral angle tenderness
CXR	chest X-ray
D5W	5% dextrose in water
DDAVP	desmopressin (1-deamino-8-D-arginine vasopressin)
DDH	developmental dysplasia of the hip
DH	dermatitis herpetiformis
DHEA-s	dehydroepiandrostenedione sulfate
DI	diabetes insipidus
DIC	disseminated intravascular coagulopathy
DIDMOAD	diabetes insipidus, diabetes mellitus, optic atrophy, and deafness
DKA	diabetic ketoacidosis
dL	deciliter
DLB	direct laryngoscopy and bronchoscopy
DM	diabetes mellitus
DMARD	disease-modifying antirheumatic drug
DMSA	dimercaptosuccinic acid
DNA	deoxyribonucleic acid
dsDNA	double-stranded DNA
DTRs	deep tendon reflexes
DUB	dysfunctional uterine bleeding
EB	epidermolysis bullosa
EBV	Epstein-Barr virus
ECG	electrocardiogram
Echo	echocardiogram
EEG	electroencephalogram
EEMG	evoked electromyography
EIA	exercise-induced asthma
ELISA	enzyme-linked immunosorbent assay
EM	electron microscopy
EMG	electromyography
ENT	ear, nose, and throat
EOM	extraocular muscles
ESR	erythrocyte sedimentation rate
ET	endotracheal
ETS	environmental tobacco smoke
F IX	factor nine
F VIII	factor eight
FAMMM	familial atypical multiple mole melanoma
FB	foreign body
FDP	fibrin degradation product
FEES	functional endoscopic evaluation of swallow
$FEF_{25\text{-}75\%}$	forced mid-expiratory flow between 25% and 75%
FEV_1	forced expiratory volume in 1 second
FHH	familial hypocalciuric hypercalcemia
FI	febrile illness
FISH	fluorescence *in situ* hybridization
FK506	immunosuppressant tacrolimus
FNA	fine-needle aspiration
FOH	functional ovarian hyperandrogenism
Fr	French scale
FSGS	focal segmental glomerulosclerosis
FTA-ABS	fluorescent treponemal antibody absorption test
FTT	failure to thrive
FUO	fever of unknown origin
g	gram
G6PD	glucose-6-phosphate dehydrogenase
GBS	Guillain-Barré syndrome
GBS	group B streptococcus
GC	gonococcus
GCSF	granulocyte colony stimulating factor
GER	gastroesophageal reflux
GERD	gastroesophageal reflux disease
GGT	gamma-glutamyltransferase
GH	growth hormone
GI	gastrointestinal
GM2	G_{M2} gangliosidosis
GN	glomerulonephritis
GnRH	gonadotropin-releasing hormone
H&P	history and physical exam
H2	histamine-2
HA	headache
HAV	hepatitis A virus
HBV	hepatitis B virus
HC	head circumference
hCG	human chorionic gonadotropin
HCM	hypertrophic cardiomyopathy
HCO_3	bicarbonate
hct	hematocrit
HCV	hepatitis C virus
HEENT	head, eyes, ears, nose, throat
HELLP	hemolysis, elevated liver enzymes, low platelets
HFMD	hand-foot-and-mouth disease
Hb_{A1c}	glycosylated hemoglobin
HIDA	hepatic immunodiacetic acid

Abbreviations

HIDS	hyper-IgD and periodic fever syndrome
HIV	human immunodeficiency virus
HLA	human leukocyte antigen
HMD	hyaline membrane disease
HMG CoA	3-hydroxy-3-methylglutaryl-coenzyme A
HPI	history of present illness
HPS	hypertrophic pyloric stenosis
HR	heart rate
HSP	Henoch-Schönlein purpura
HSV	herpes simplex virus
HSV-2	herpes simplex virus type 2
HUS	hemolytic uremic syndrome
I&D	incision and drainage
IBD	inflammatory bowel disease
ICP	intracranial pressure
ICS	inhaled corticosteroids
ICU	intensive care unit
IgA	immunoglobulin A
IgD	immunoglobulin D
IgE	immunoglobulin E
IGF-1	insulin growth factor-1
IGFBP-3	insulin growth factor binding protein-3
IM	intramuscular
INO	inner nuclear ophthalmoplegia
INR	international normalized ratio
IO	intraosseous
IQ	intelligence quotient
ITP	idiopathic thrombocytic purpura
IV	intravenous
IVF	intravenous fluid
IVH	intraventricular hemorrhage
IVIG	intravenous immunoglobulin
JAS	juvenile ankylosing spondylitis
JME	juvenile myoclonic epilepsy
JRA	juvenile rheumatoid arthritis
JVD	jugular venous distension
K	potassium
kg	kilogram(s)
KOH	potassium hydroxide
KUB	kidneys, ureters, bladder (abdominal X-ray)
L	liter(s)
L to R	left to right
L4	fourth lumbar vertebra
LAD I/II	leukocyte adhesion defect I/II
LCP	Legg-Calvé-Perthes
LDH	lactate dehydrogenase
LES	lower esophageal sphincter
LE	lower extremity
LFT	liver function test
LH	luteinizing hormone
LLSB	left lower sternal border
LMM	leptomeningeal melanosis
LP	lumbar puncture
LSD	lysergic acid diethylamide
LUQ	left upper quadrant
LUSB	left upper sternal border
MCAD	medium-chain acyl-CoA dehydrogenase
MCNS	minimal change nephrotic syndrome
MCT	medium-chain triglyceride
MCV	mean corpuscular volume
MD	muscular dystrophy
MECP-2	methyl-CpG-binding protein-2
MEE	middle ear effusion
MELAS	mitochondrial myopathy, encephalopathy, lactic acidosis, and stroke-like episodes
MEN	multiple endocrine neoplasia
mEq	milliequivalents
MERRF	myoclonus, epilepsy, and ragged red fibers
Mg	magnesium
mg	milligram(s)
Mg^{+++}	magnesium ion
mL	milliliter(s)
MM	malignant melanoma
mmHg	millimeter(s) of mercury
mmol	millimole(s)
MODY	maturity onset diabetes of the young
mOsm	milliosmoles
MRA	magnetic resonance angiography
MRI	magnetic resonance imaging
MS	multiple sclerosis
MSUD	maple syrup urine disease
Na^+	sodium ion
NaCl	sodium chloride
$NaHCO_3$	sodium bicarbonate
NARP	neurogenic weakness, ataxia, and retinitis pigmentosa
NAT	non-accidental trauma
NDI	nephrogenic diabetes insipidus
NEC	necrotizing enterocolitis
NF	neurofibromatosis
NF1	neurofibromatosis type 1
ng	nanogram(s)
NG	nasogastric
NHANES	National Health and Nutrition Examination Survey
NICU	neonatal intensive care unit
NMJ	neuromuscular junction
NPO	nil per os (nothing by mouth)

Abbreviations

NRDS	newborn respiratory distress syndrome
NS	nephrotic syndrome
NSAIDs	nonsteroidal anti-inflammatory drugs
NTBC 2	(2-nitro-4-trifluoromethylbenzoyl)-1,3-cyclohexanedione
O_2	oxygen
O&P	ova and parasites
OAV	oculoauriculovertebral
OCP	oral contraceptive pill
OCR	ossicular chain reconstruction
OM	otitis media
OSA	obstructive sleep apnea
OSAS	obstructive sleep apnea syndrome
OSD	Osgood-Schlatter disease
osm	osmole(s)
OT	occupational therapy
OTC	over the counter
PaO_2	partial pressure of oxygen, arterial
$PaCO_2$	partial pressure of carbon dioxide, arterial
PAN	polyarteritis nodosa
PCD	primary ciliary dyskinesia
PCKD	polycystic kidney disease
PCOS	polycystic ovarian syndrome
PCP	phencyclidine
PCR	polymerase chain reaction
PE	physical examination
PEPCK	phosphoenolpyruvate carboxykinase
PFAPA	periodic fever, aphthous stomatitis, pharyngitis, and adenitis
PFIC	progressive familial intrahepatic cholestasis
PFT	pulmonary function tests
pH	potential hydrogen
Ph^{+++}	phosphorus ion
PHP	pseudohypoparathyroidism
PHPV	persistent hyperplastic primary vitreous
PI	pancreatic insufficiency
PID	pelvic inflammatory disease
PKD	polycystic kidney disease
PKU	phenylketonuria
PLF	perilymphatic fistula
PMH	past medical history
PO	per os (by mouth)
PPD	purified protein derivative
PPS	peripheral pulmonary stenosis
P-R	the distance between the P and R on an ECG
PRL	prolactin
prn	pro re nata (according to need)
PSH	past surgical history
PT	physical therapy
PT	prothrombin time
PTH	parathyroid hormone
PTHrP	parathyroid releasing protein
PTT	partial thromboplastin time
PUD	peptic ulcer disease
PUVA	psoralen and ultraviolet light A irradiation
PV	pemphigus vulgaris
PVD	posterior vitreous detachment
PVM	pulmonary vascular markings
PVR	pulmonary vascular resistance
RAST	radioallergosorbent test
RBC	red blood cell
RDW	red cell volume distribution width
RF	rheumatoid factor
RLQ	right lower quadrant
RMSF	Rocky Mountain spotted fever
ROM	range of motion
ROP	retinopathy of prematurity
ROS	review of systems
RPR	rapid plasma reagin
RR	respiratory rate
RSD	reflex sympathetic dystrophy
RSV	respiratory syncytial virus
RTA	renal tubular acidosis
RVH	right ventricular hypertrophy
S_1	first heart sound
S1	first sacral vertebra
S_2	second heart sound
S_3	third heart sound
S3–4	third to fourth sacral vertebra
S3–5	third to fifth sacral vertebra
S_4	fourth heart sound
SaO_2	oxygen saturation, arterial
SBE	spontaneous bacterial endocarditis
SBI	serious bacterial infections
SCA	spinocerebellar ataxia
SCFE	slipped capital femoral epiphysis
SCM	sternocleidomastoid
SD	standard deviation
SG	specific gravity
SI	sacroiliac
SIADH	syndrome of inappropriate antidiuretic hormone secretion
SJS	Stevens-Johnson syndrome
SLE	systemic lupus erythematosus
SLO	Smith-Lemli-Opitz
SMA	superior mesenteric artery
SNHL	sensorineural hearing loss
SpA	spondyloarthropathies

Abbreviations

SSSS	staphylococcal scalded skin syndrome
STD	sexually transmitted disease
SUA	single umbilical artery
SVT	supraventricular tachycardia
T3	tri-iodothyronine
T4	thyroxine
TAPVR	total anomalous pulmonary venous return
TAR	thrombocytopenia absent radius
TB	tuberculosis
TCPP	true central precocious puberty
TEF	tracheoesophageal fistula
TEN	toxic epidermal necrolysis
TFT	thyroid function tests
TGA	transposition of the great arteries
TIA	transient ischemic attack
TIPSS	transjugular intrahepatic portosystemic shunt
TM	tympanic membrane
TMB	transient monocular blindness
TMJ	temporal-mandibular joint
TNF	tumor necrosis factor
TOF	tetralogy of Fallot
TORCH	toxoplasmosis, other, rubella, cytomegalovirus, herpes simplex virus
TPN	total parenteral nutrition
TRAPS	TNF receptor-associated periodic syndrome
TS	tuberous sclerosis
TSH	thyroid stimulating hormone
TSS	toxic shock syndrome
UA	uric acid
U/A	urinalysis
UGI/SBF	upper GI/small bowel follow through
UL	unilateral
URI	upper respiratory infection
US	ultrasound
UTI	urinary tract infection
UV	ultraviolet
V/Q	ventilation/perfusion
VCD	vocal cord dysfunction
VCUG	voiding cystourethrogram
V_e	minute ventilation
VF	visual field
V-fib	ventricular fibrillation
VMA	vanillylmandelic acid
VSD	ventricular septal defect
V_t	tidal volume
V-tach	ventricular tachycardia
vWD	von Willebrand disease
vWF	von Willebrand factor
VZV	varicella-zoster virus
WBC	white blood cell
WG	Wegener granulomatosis
WHO	World Health Organization
XL	X-linked

Contributors

Larry J. Alexander, OD, FAAO
Adjunct Clinical Assistant Professor
Indiana University School of Optometry
Bloomington, Indiana

David H. Chi, MD
Fellow, Department of Pediatric Otolaryngology
Children's Hospital of Pittsburgh
Pittsburgh, Pennsylvania

Irini Daskalaki, MD
Clinical Instructor, Department of Pediatrics
Drexel University College of Medicine
Fellow, Pediatric Infectious Diseases
St. Christopher's Hospital for Children
Philadelphia, Pennsylvania

Fatma Dedeoglu, MD
Instructor, Pediatrics
Harvard Medical School
Attending, Immunology
Children's Hospital Boston
Boston, Massachusetts

Katherine MacRae Dell, MD
Assistant Professor, Pediatrics
Case Western Reserve University
Attending Pediatric Nephrologist
Division of Pediatric Nephrology
Rainbow Babies and Children's Hospital
Cleveland, Ohio

Kari A. Draper, MD
Clinical Assistant Professor, Pediatrics
University of Pennsylvania School of Medicine
Attending Physician, Primary Care Center
Children's Hospital of Philadelphia
Philadelphia, Pennsylvania

Shannon Fourtner, MD
Fellow, Pediatric Endocrinology
Children's Hospital of Philadelphia
Philadelphia, Pennsylvania

Sarah Friebert, MD
Assistant Professor, Pediatrics
Northeastern Ohio University College of Medicine
Rookstown, Ohio
Director, Division of Pediatric Palliative Care
Pediatric Hematologist/Oncologist
Children's Hospital Medical Center of Akron
Akron, Ohio

Contributors

Adda Grimberg, MD
Assistant Professor, Pediatrics
University of Pennsylvania School of Medicine
Attending Physician, Pediatric Endocrinology
Children's Hospital of Philadelphia
Philadelphia, Pennsylvania

Maria J. Henwood, DO, FAAP
Instructor, Pediatrics
University of Pennsylvania
Fellow, Endocrinology and Diabetes
Children's Hospital of Philadelphia
Philadelphia, Pennsylvania

Francis M. Hoe, MD
Fellow, Pediatric Endocrinology
Children's Hospital of Philadelphia
Philadelphia, Pennsylvania

Vlad D. Ianuş, MD, MPH
Instructor in Pediatrics
Brown Medical School
Fellow in Neonatology,
Women and Infants Hospital
Providence, Rhode Island

Tomislav Ivsic, MD
Chief Resident
Department of Pediatrics
Monmouth Medical Center
Long Branch, New Jersey

Douglas A. Jacobstein, MD
Fellow, Division of Gastroenterology and Nutrition
The Children's Hospital of Philadelphia
University of Pennsylvania School of Medicine
Philadelphia, Pennsylvania

Heather Kasten, MD
Resident, Department of Pediatrics
Children's Hospital of Pittsburgh
Pittsburgh, Pennsylvania

David J. Kay, MD, MPH
Department of Otolaryngology
University of Pittsburgh School of Medicine
Department of Pediatric Otolaryngology
Children's Hospital of Pittsburgh
Pittsburgh, Pennsylvania

Contributors

Roy J. Kim, MD, MPH
Fellow, Division of Pediatric Endocrinology
University of Pennsylvania School of Medicine
Children's Hospital of Philadelphia
Philadelphia, Pennsylvania

Don Lujan, MD, MS
Resident, Orthopedic Surgery
University of New Mexico
Albuquerque, New Mexico
University of Pittsburgh Medical Center
Pittsburgh, Pennsylvania

Sheela N. Magge, MD
Instructor
University of Pennsylvania
Fellow, Pediatric Endocrinology
Children's Hospital of Philadelphia
Philadelphia, Pennsylvania

C. Becket Mahnke, MD
Major, Medical Corps, US Army
Department of Pediatrics
Tripler Army Medical Center
Honolulu, Hawaii

Christina Lin Master, MD
Clinical Assistant Professor
University of Pennsylvania School of Medicine
Assistant Director, Pediatric Residency Program
The Children's Hospital of Philadelphia
Philadelphia, Pennsylvania

Timothy D. Murphy, MD
Assistant Professor of Pediatrics
University of Pittsburgh School of Medicine
Children's Hospital of Pittsburgh
Pittsburgh, Pennsylvania

Bankole Osuntokun, MD
Clinical Fellow, Division of Gastroenterology, Hepatology, and Nutrition
Cincinnati Children's Hospital Medical Center
Cincinnati, Ohio

Asim R. Piracha, MD
Clinical Instructor in Ophthalmology and Visual Sciences
University of Louisville
Louisville, Kentucky
Cornea, Refractive, and Anterior Segment Surgery
John Kenyon Eye Center
Jeffersonville, Indiana

Contributors

Mustafa Sahin, MD, PhD
Instructor, Neurology
Harvard Medical School
Assistant, Neurology
Children's Hospital Boston
Boston, Massachusetts

Nader Shaikh, MD, MPH
Clinical Instructor, Department of Pediatrics
University of Pittsburgh School of Medicine
Division of General Academic Pediatrics
Children's Hospital of Pittsburgh
Pittsburgh, Pennsylvania

Nicole J. Ullrich, MD, PhD
Instructor in Neurology
Department of Neurology
Children's Hospital Boston
Boston, Massachusetts

Ronald Williams, MD, FAAP, FACP
Associate Professor, Pediatrics
Assistant Professor of Internal Medicine
Director, Combined Internal Medicine/Pediatrics
Residency Program
Pennsylvania State University
Milton S. Hershey Medical Center
Hershey, Pennsylvania

Weizhen Xu, MD
Attending Physician, Pediatric Endocrinology
Cooper Health System
Assistant Professor
University of Medicine and Dentistry New Jersey
Camden, New Jersey

Preface

The *In A Page* series was designed to streamline the vast amount of material that saturates the study of medicine, providing students, residents, and health professionals a high-yield, big-picture overview of the most important clinical medical topics. We expect this book to be especially useful for medical students, residents, physician assistants, nurse practitioners, and other health professionals.

In A Page Pediatric Signs & Symptoms is the seventh handbook of this series. Whereas previous books have been organized by a disease-per-page, this book is organized by a sign- or symptom-per-page. Thus, it is essentially a handbook of differential diagnoses. The format we use is especially effective for use in clinical settings, where knowledge of a quick, thorough list of differential diagnoses and a simple diagnostic scheme are necessary to work up the patient.

As in the initial books of the series, we were constrained by the size of the template and the need to keep each sign or symptom within a single page. We had to be quite succinct in our explanations and descriptions and we sacrificed details in some cases, such as drug dosages. Furthermore, we abbreviated liberally.

We are certain that the final product will be a very effective resource. Our contributors include some of the foremost pediatric specialists from the top children's hospitals in the country, Children's Hospital of Philadelphia and Children's Hospital of Boston. Reviews from medical students and residents have been very positive. We anticipate that this book will be a valuable tool in clinical settings, as board review, and for independent study. We welcome any comments, questions, or suggestions – please address correspondence to drkahan@yahoo.com.

Acknowledgments

I would like to thank my friends and colleagues who gave their time and expertise in contributing to this book. I would also like to thank my mentors at the Children's Hospital of Philadelphia and the Children's Hospital of Boston whose many pearls of wisdom I continue to cherish. Mostly I would like to thank my parents and my family. To my wife and best friend, Michelle, for her unconditional love, support, and encouragement and my daughters, Gillian and Marissa, who brighten my every day.

—Jonathan

I would like to acknowledge my husband, Joe DeAntonis, and my sister, Andrea Richard, for their support in writing this book. Their loving encouragement and belief in this book's contribution sustained me. I would also like to thank Dr. Bradley Bradford for his mentorship and devotion to medical education, as well as the many students and residents who inspired me by their enthusiasm for learning and their expressions of gratitude for the *In A Page* learning tool.

—Kate

All my thanks to Jonathan and Kate for the hard work and dedication to this project. We must thank all the contributors in this book for taking the time and effort to share their expertise. And thanks to the staff of Blackwell publishing, especially Kate Heinle, Deb Murphy, Bev Copland, and Laura DeYoung.

—Scott

Section 1

General Topics

IRINI DASKALAKI, MD
SARAH FRIEBERT, MD
ADDA GRIMBERG, MD
DOUGLAS A. JACOBSTEIN, MD
SHEELA N. MAGEE, MD
MUSTAFA SAHIN, MD, PhD
JONATHAN E. TEITELBAUM, MD

1. Anorexia

Anorexia refers to a loss of appetite. The hypothalamus is thought to be the center of appetite control, but the stimuli that influence this control are poorly understood. Prolonged anorexia accompanied by weight loss or poor weight gain usually denotes a serious underlying organic or psychological disorder.

Differential Diagnosis

- Psychosocial/psychiatric
  - Unrealistic parental expectations of what child should eat leads to pressure and causes food refusal
  - Anorexia nervosa: Common among adolescents, particularly females
  - Depression
- Infectious
  - Gastroenteritis: *Salmonella, Shigella, E. coli,* Norwalk agent
  - HIV
  - Hepatitis A, B, C
  - Pyelonephritis
  - *Mycobacterium tuberculosis*
- GI disorders
  - Gastroesophageal reflux disease
  - Constipation
  - Appendicitis
  - Celiac disease
  - Pancreatitis
  - Crohn disease
  - Achalasia
  - Esophageal foreign body
  - Liver failure
- Metabolic/endocrine disorders
  - Hypothyroidism
  - Hypercalcemia
  - Panhypopituitarism
  - Addison disease
  - Diabetes insipidus
  - Lead poisoning
- Nutritional disorders
  - Zinc deficiency
  - B12 deficiency
  - Iron deficiency
  - Dietary chloride deficiency
  - Hypervitaminosis A
- Cardiopulmonary disease
  - Congestive heart failure
  - Cystic fibrosis
- Drug toxicity
  - Illicit drugs
  - Antihistamines
  - Methylphenidate
  - Ephedrine
  - Digitalis
- Rheumatic disorders
  - Systemic lupus erythematosus
  - Juvenile rheumatoid arthritis
- Pregnancy

Workup and Diagnosis

- History
  - Nausea, vomiting, weight loss, diarrhea, hematochezia, melena, abdominal pain, pica
  - Fever, sick contacts, recent travel, headache, rashes, diaphoresis, dysuria, cough, rashes, joint complaints, insomnia, activity level
  - Medications: Prescription and over-the-counter
  - Dietary history: Quantity and types of food
  - Social history: Changes in home environment, abuse, drug use, alcohol use, tobacco use, changes in grades in school, changes in activities/interests
- Physical exam
  - Height and weight, pulse, blood pressure
  - Scleral icteris, jaundice, abdominal pain/distension, hepatosplenomegaly
  - Dentition, mucous membranes, murmurs, lung sounds, joint tenderness, skin turgor, rashes, neurology exam including funduscopy
- Labs/studies
  - Electrolytes and CBC with differential
  - Consider LFTs, amylase and lipase, thyroid tests
  - Stool for blood, stool culture, urinalysis with culture
  - Vitamin levels, lead level, HIV test, hepatitis panels
  - Pregnancy testing
- Consider upper endoscopy/colonoscopy
- Consider chest X-ray
- Consider upper GI with small bowel follow through

Treatment

- Treatment geared toward specific causes
- Maintain hydration status and correct any electrolyte and vitamin imbalances
- Treat infectious causes if indicated
- Counseling for psychiatric causes
- May require NG feeds to maintain nutrition
- Remove toxic agents
- Lower esophageal dilation or myomectomy for achalasia
- Parental education regarding expectations
- Treat depression

2. Fatigue

Complaints of fatigue indicate a general state of decreased endurance for, or interest in, activities. It is typically associated with tiredness and sleepiness. Depression as a cause of fatigue in adolescents frequently goes undiagnosed.

Differential Diagnosis

- Inadequate rest
- Excessive exercise
- Insufficient caloric intake
- Depression
- Infectious mononucleosis: Common in adolescence, typically due to EBV or CMV
- Anemia
- Hepatitis
  - –Viral (e.g., HAV, HBV, HCV)
  - –Consider autoimmune in adolescent girls
- Drugs
  - –Antihistamines, anticonvulsants, opiates
- Obesity
  - –Rapid fatigue with exertion
  - –Somnolence with elevated $PaCO_2$ is termed Pickwickian syndrome
- Tonsillar-adenoidal hypertrophy
  - –Impaired air exchange while sleeping
  - –Associated with restless sleeping
- Chronic fatigue syndrome
  - –Controversial diagnosis
  - –Underlying depression is common
- Polycythemia in neonates can be associated with cyanosis and feeding problems
- Encephalitis/meningitis
- Tuberculosis
- Brucellosis: Weight loss, low-grade fever, back pain
- Hypothyroidism
- Adrenocortical insufficiency: Often with hyperpigmentation and weakness
- Hypoglycemia
- Inflammatory bowel disease
- Juvenile rheumatoid arthritis
- Systemic lupus erythematosus
- Intussusception
- Dermatomyositis: Often with muscle weakness and pain
- Congestive heart failure: With tachypnea and dyspnea on exertion
- Pericarditis: Fatigue and dyspnea may precede friction rub
- Renal tubular acidosis
- Uremia
- Myasthenia gravis
- Malignancy

Workup and Diagnosis

- History
  - –Duration of complaint
  - –Sleeping habits (length of sleep, restfulness, snoring)
  - –Eating habits (number of meals per day, caloric intake)
  - –Psychosocial stressors
  - –Associated signs and symptoms (weight change, fever, muscle aches, breathing difficulty, diarrhea, vomiting, sore throat)
  - –Medications, including over-the-counter drugs
- Physical exam
  - –Vital signs and weight
  - –Oral exam for tonsillar hypertrophy, exudates, erythema
  - –Palpable lymph nodes
  - –Hepatomegaly with tenderness
  - –Splenomegaly (seen with EBV, CMV, lymphoma)
  - –Skin pallor, jaundice, cyanosis
  - –Increased work of breathing, wheezes, rales
  - –Cardiac exam for rubs, murmurs
  - –Psychological assessment of mood and affect
- Labs
  - –Consider screening CBC for anemia
  - –WBC differential for atypical lymphocytes (in EBV, CMV) or blasts (in leukemia)
  - –Viral serology for EBV or CMV
  - –ALT and AST for hepatitis
  - –TSH and free T4 for hypothyroidism
  - –BUN and Cr for renal dysfunction
  - –Other specific testing based on history, physical exam

Treatment

- Behavioral modifications based on cause
  - –Increase duration of sleep
  - –Ensure three calorically adequate meals per day
- Correction of anemia
  - –Iron supplementation
  - –Blood transfusion if hemodynamically unstable
- Depression
  - –Psychological counseling and antidepressants
- Infectious mononucleosis
  - –Rest if fatigue is severe
  - –No contact sports with significant splenomegaly
- Anti-inflammatory drugs for inflammatory causes
- Chronic fatigue syndrome
  - –Emotional support
  - –Psychological treatment if indicated
  - –Modification of schedule as needed
  - –Various medications have been attempted, however no clear consensus, high rate of placebo effect

3. Irritability

The differential diagnosis for irritability is large and varied. In young children irritability may be the only presenting complaint for life-threatening disease states. A careful history and physical exam are needed to narrow the differential so that only indicated tests are performed.

Differential Diagnosis

- General/nutritional
  - –Colic
  - –Teething
  - –Malnutrition/hunger
  - –Atopic dermatitis
- Infectious
  - –Otitis media
  - –Meningitis, encephalitis
  - –Stomatitis
  - –Gastroenteritis
  - –Osteomyelitis, diskitis, septic arthritis
- Trauma
  - –Abuse/shaken-baby syndrome
  - –Fracture
  - –Hair tourniquet (e.g., on digit or penis)
  - –Corneal abrasion or foreign body in eye
- Gastrointestinal
  - –Constipation
  - –Gastroesophageal reflux
  - –Anal fissures
  - –Milk protein allergy, celiac disease
- Surgical
  - –Testicular torsion
  - –Incarcerated hernia
  - –Intussusception
- Metabolic
  - –Electrolyte disturbances
  - –Hypoglycemia
- Medications/drugs
  - –Narcotic withdrawal, fetal alcohol syndrome
  - –Medications (e.g., URI preparations)
  - –Lead or mercury poisoning
- Hematologic
  - –Leukemia
  - –Iron deficiency anemia
  - –Sickle cell with vaso-occlusive crisis
- Cardiac/respiratory
  - –Myocarditis, pericarditis, arrhythmias
  - –Congestive heart failure
  - –Respiratory failure, hypoxia
  - –Carbon monoxide poisoning
- Neurological
  - –Increased intracranial pressure
  - –Subdural hematoma
  - –Migraines
- Other
  - –Psychosocial
  - –Urinary retention
  - –Glaucoma

Workup and Diagnosis

- History
  - –Medications, past medical history
  - –Duration of symptoms, time of day child is irritable
  - –Anything that makes the irritability better or worse
  - –Feeding difficulties
  - –History of trauma
  - –Associated symptoms (e.g., URI, vomiting, diarrhea)
  - –Psychosocial stressors in the family
- Physical exam
  - –Vital signs
  - –Signs of abuse or infection
  - –Hair tourniquets
  - –Fluorescein the eyes for corneal abrasion
- Labs/studies (based on clinical suspicion)
  - –CBC with differential, blood culture, urinalysis and urine culture, lumbar puncture, sedimentation rate and C-reactive protein for infectious cause
  - –X-rays for possible fracture
  - –Brain MRI or CT scan for tumors or hematomas
  - –Bone scan for osteomyelitis and diskitis
  - –Joint aspiration and culture for septic arthritis
  - –Electrolytes, including glucose
  - –Echocardiogram/ECG for cardiac defect
  - –Abdominal X-rays or ultrasound for surgical abdomen
  - –Air or contrast enema for intussusception
  - –Drug screen, lead, or carboxyhemoglobin level
- Consult ophthalmology to look for retinal hemorrhages in shaken-baby syndrome

Treatment

- Stabilize the patient (ABCs)
- Pain can be treated with acetaminophen or ibuprofen; in more severe cases, a narcotic may be required
- Treat infections with the appropriate antibiotics
- Consult subspecialists, such as hematology, surgery, orthopedics, or neurosurgery, as needed
- Correct electrolyte disturbances
- Discontinuation of causative medications or toxins
- Educate the family about colic and teething, treatments, and natural history
- Social work involvement as needed

4. Lymphadenopathy

Lymphadenopathy, both localized and systemic, is an extremely common presenting symptom encountered by practicing pediatricians. To be considered enlarged, nodes must be at least 1 cm in cervical and axillary regions and 1.5 cm in the inguinal region. Most children have shotty adenopathy, usually due to uncomplicated infections that are transient and self-limited. Stepwise management (obtain clues from history, physical examination, and less invasive testing) will aid in selecting appropriate patients for further workup.

Differential Diagnosis

- Infectious
  - –Viral (URI, varicella, EBV, CMV, HIV, rubella, mumps, measles)
  - –Bacterial (strep, staph, mycobacterium, atypical mycobacterium, brucellosis, tularemia, syphilis, chlamydia)
  - –Fungal (histoplasmosis, coccidioidomycosis)
  - –Protozoal (toxoplasmosis, malaria)
  - –Scalp infection
- Allergy
  - –Seasonal or individual
- Inflammatory
  - –Kawasaki disease
  - –Sarcoidosis
  - –Cat-scratch disease (*Bartonella henselae*)
  - –Drug-induced (phenytoin, isoniazid, hydralazine, dapsone, procainamide, allopurinol)
- Malignancy
  - –Leukemia
  - –Hodgkin disease
  - –Non-Hodgkin lymphoma
  - –Neuroblastoma
  - –Rhabdomyosarcoma
  - –Histiocytic disorder
- Collagen vascular disease or systemic illness
  - –Rheumatoid arthritis
  - –Systemic lupus erythematosus
  - –Serum sickness
  - –Autoimmune hemolytic anemia
  - –Cystic fibrosis
- Immunodeficiency
- Storage diseases
  - –Gaucher disease
  - –Niemann-Pick disease
- Non-lymph node masses simulating lympadenopathy
  - –Thyroglossal duct cysts
  - –Branchial cleft cysts
  - –Cystic hygroma
  - –Hemangioma
  - –Teratoma
  - –Thymoma
  - –Inguinal hernia

Workup and Diagnosis

- History
  - –Duration, fever, weight loss, night sweats
  - –Sore throat, rash, limp, joint swelling/pain, bone pain
  - –Sexual history and HIV risk factors
  - –Exposures: Food contamination, pets (e.g., kittens)
  - –Immunizations, recurrent infections, meds, allergies
  - –Long-standing or unexplained skin rash, transfusions
  - –Family history of autoimmune/inflammatory diseases
- Physical exam
  - –All lymph node chains: Size, tenderness, fluctuance, consistency, warmth, surrounding erythema
  - –Splenomegaly, hepatomegaly
  - –Trauma or animal/insect bites along lymph drainage
  - –Rash, including "eczema," lesions, petechiae, purpura
  - –Signs of respiratory compromise
  - –Scalp for signs of infection
  - –Genitalia for signs of sexually transmitted disease
- Labs
  - –Common: CBC/peripheral smear, ESR, LDH, electrolytes, BUN, Cr, LFT, uric acid, EBV, CMV, *B. henselae* titers, PPD, throat culture
  - –Less common: ANA, ACE level, anti-dsDNA, specific infection titers, immunodeficiency workup
- Studies
  - –Chest X-ray; bone marrow exam; biopsy or I&D of node, echo/ECG, biopsy of rash

Treatment

- Mild adenopathy with associated viral/URI symptoms
  - –Observation and recheck in 1–2 weeks
  - –Malignancy-associated adenopathy can sometimes wax and wane (especially Hodgkin disease) and appear to improve with antibiotics
  - –TB nodes may be firm, matted, fixed, and nontender
- Erythematous, warm, tender nodes
  - –Trial of oral antibiotics for staph/strep
- Inflamed/fluctuant lesions: Referral for I&D
- Refer to pediatric hematologist/oncologist
  - –Nodes that fail to resolve over 6 weeks
  - –Nodes that increase in size over 2 weeks
  - –Firm, matted nodes
  - –Supraclavicular nodes
  - –Nodes that generalize to two or more noncontiguous groups or more than two contiguous groups
- CBC with differential, CXR before biopsy

5. Night Sweats

Night sweats are an often-underreported symptom that consist of profuse sweating during the night. They may or may not be accompanied by excessive sweating during the daytime, and they can be confused with hot flashes or flushing. They are among the "constitutional" symptoms (fever, malaise, weight loss, etc.), and their frequency is difficult to determine because they are rarely reported spontaneously by patients, even when the amount of sweating is so excessive that it requires changing of bedclothes.

Differential Diagnosis

- Environmental
  - High room temperature, excessive wrapping or too many bed covers may be the most common cause (young children cannot control their environment)
- Tuberculosis
  - The disease most commonly associated with night sweats in the medical literature
- Malignancy
  - Hodgkin lymphoma is the malignancy most commonly associated with night sweats; night sweats are among the "B" symptoms in staging, but their presence does not adversely affect prognosis
  - Leukemia and solid tumors may also cause night sweats
- Alcohol or spicy food ingestion
- Drugs
  - Antidepressants, cholinergics, antitussives, antipyretics, decongestants, insulin, sulfonylurea agents
- Other infections
  - Indolent chronic infections: Subacute endocarditis, osteomyelitis, abscesses often present with fever, night sweats
  - HIV
  - Histoplasmosis
- Endocrinologic disorders
  - Nocturnal hypoglycemia
  - Hyperthyroidism
  - Diabetes insipidus
  - Pheochromocytoma
- Anxiety disorder/panic attacks
- Sleep disorders
  - Obstructive sleep apnea
  - Nightmares
- Drug abuse
- GERD
- Neurologic disease
  - Hypothalamic lesions
  - Head injury
  - Cerebral palsy
  - Familial dysautonomia
- Pregnancy
- Obesity
- Autoimmune diseases
- Mercury poisoning

Workup and Diagnosis

- History
  - Bedroom temperature, sleep habits
  - Fever, weight loss
  - Fatigue, sleepiness at school
  - Other symptoms: Heartburn, cough, flushing, polydipsia, polyuria
  - Nightmares, palpitations, panic attacks
  - Past medical history and medications
- Physical exam
  - Vital signs, growth parameters
  - Lymphadenopathy, pallor, petechiae
  - Skin exam (heat rash, erythema nodosum)
  - Hypertrophic tonsils
  - New-onset murmur
- Labs
  - CBC, ESR if hematologic malignancy or chronic infection is suspected
  - Fasting blood sugar
  - Electrolyte abnormalities for DI
  - Urine VMA for pheochromocytoma
- Radiology
  - Chest X-ray may show lesions consistent with TB or mediastinal widening due to lymphoma
- Studies
  - PPD to test exposure to tuberculosis
  - Sleep study if sleep apnea is suspected
  - pH probe if confirmation of GERD is necessary

Treatment

- Reassurance of the parents
- Education concerning "normal" temperature and bed clothing in children's rooms
- Pulmonary TB is treated with 6 months of isoniazid and rifampin supplemented with 2 months of pyrazinamide initially
- Chemotherapy for Hodgkin or other malignancies
- Discontinuation of offending drugs if possible
- Treatment or control of endocrinologic disorders
- BiPAP or surgery for obstructive sleep apnea
- Treatment of specific infections
- Treatment of GERD with acid blockade and/or prokinetics
- Behavioral therapy for anxiety disorders

6. Polydipsia

Polydipsia is fluid drinking in excess of 2 L/m^2/day. In normal older children, water intake must surpass 10 L/m^2/day to cause hyponatremia. In contrast, neonates and small infants cannot dilute urine to the same extent. These infants are prone to develop hyponatremia at water intake in excess of 4 L/m^2/day.

Differential Diagnosis

- Diabetes mellitus (type I and type II)
  - –Hyperglycemia drives an osmotic diuresis that causes polyuria, which then leads to dehydration, increased thirst, and polydipsia
- Diabetes insipidus
  - –Abnormal water balance due to vasopressin (ADH) deficiency or resistance, causing excretion of large amounts of dilute urine
- Central or neurogenic diabetes insipidus (vasopressin deficiency)
  - –Congenital
  - –Familial (autosomal dominant)
  - –Acquired: Neurosurgery, tumor (e.g., craniopharyngioma), head trauma, infiltrative/inflammatory, infectious
- Nephrogenic diabetes insipidus (decreased responsiveness of the kidneys to vasopressin)
  - –Familial (X-linked dominant and recessive forms)
  - –Acquired: Renal disease, obstructive uropathy, hypercalcemia/hypercalciuria
  - –Hypokalemia, drug-induced (e.g., lithium, diuretics, ethanol, cisplatin)
  - –Gestational DI: Increased clearance of ADH by placental vasopressinase, lower osmolar threshold for thirst and ADH release
- Primary polydipsia
  - –Compulsive water drinking
  - –Dipsogenic DI
- Primary hyperaldosteronism
- Diabetes insipidus, diabetes mellitus, optic atrophy, and deafness (DIDMOAD) syndrome
- Bartter syndrome
- Hypertension (e.g., pheochomocytoma)
- Neuroblastoma
- Cystinosis
- Congestive heart failure

Workup and Diagnosis

- History: Quantification of fluid intake and urine output, drinking overnight, polyphagia, polyuria, nocturia, enuresis, psychosocial factors, interference with normal activities, growth progression, weight loss, weakness, fatigue, leg cramps/muscle aches, neurologic symptoms (headaches, visual changes)
- Physical exam: Vital signs (HR, BP), weight, height, hydration assessment (mucous membranes, capillary refill, extremities' temperature, skin turgor), neurologic exam (optic discs, EOM), energy level, muscle pain
- Initial labs
  - –Serum electrolytes, BUN, creatinine, glucose, calcium
  - –Urinalysis with specific gravity, glucose and ketones
  - –Simultaneous serum and urine osmolality (mOsm/kg)
  - –Serum osm >300 and urine osm <300 = DI
  - –If serum osm <270 and urine osm >600 DI unlikely
- Further diagnostic workup
  - –Water deprivation test in case of ambiguous history and labs (patient deprived of water, then ability to concentrate urine is assessed)
  - –Differentiates between DI and water intoxication, and between central DI and nephrogenic DI (by response to a dose of vasopressin administered at the end of the study)
- MRI of brain with special attention to the pituitary
- Imaging of adrenal glands if hyperaldoterone suspected

Treatment

- Insulin and/or oral medications for DM
- Central DI
  - –Desmopressin treatment for older children
  - –Not in immediate post-op period
  - –Free water replacement
  - –Desmopressin may lead to hyponatremia in infants and in postoperative cases that may also involve SIADH
- Nephrogenic DI
  - –Thiazide diuretics
  - –Mild salt depletion
  - –Prostaglandin synthesis inhibitors
- Behavioral modification for compulsive water drinking
- Surgical intervention for tumor
- Strict measurement of input and output
- Must assess presence or absence of intact thirst mechanism for central DI

7. Polyphagia

Polyphagia, or hyperphagia, refers to the excessive consumption of food or display of food-seeking behavior. Obesity does not necessarily occur.

Differential Diagnosis

- Exogenous obesity
- Bulimia
- Depression
- Anxiety
- Diabetes mellitus
- Hypoglycemia
- Diabetes insipidus in infants
  - –On breast milk or formula diet, excessive drinking is misinterpreted as excessive eating
- Hyperthyroidism or Graves disease
  - –Increased metabolic rate, increased appetite, and increased oral intake as well as increased stool output
- Medications
  - –Corticosteroids
  - –Cyproheptadine
  - –Tricyclic antidepressants
  - –Valproic acid
  - –Tetrahydrocannabinol
  - –Neuroleptics
- Hypothalamic lesions (hypothalamic dysfunction stimulates drive to eat)
  - –Tumors (e.g., craniopharyngioma)
  - –Inflammation/autoimmune
  - –Central nervous system infection
  - –Head trauma
- Genetic syndromes
  - –Prader-Willi syndrome
  - –Laurence-Moon-Bardet-Biedl syndrome
  - –Kleine-Levin syndrome
- Cystic fibrosis
  - –Malabsorption results in chronic malnutrition, especially of fat

Workup and Diagnosis

- History
  - –Nutritional history/diet recall for 24–72 hour
  - –Onset (age, life events) of change in eating behaviors
  - –Symptoms of depression, anxiety, eating disorders, or other psychiatric illness
  - –Symptoms of diabetes: Polyuria, polydipsia, wt loss
  - –Symptoms of hyperthyroidism or Graves disease: Palpitations, proximal muscle weakness, heat intolerance, ocular symptoms, difficulty concentrating, tremulousness
  - –Past medical history, medications
  - –Symptoms of brain tumor or infection/injury to CNS: Headaches, visual changes, fever, trauma, mental status changes
  - –A history of poor feeding and hypotonia at birth, developmental delay, hypogonadism, and hyperphagia with subsequent obesity suggests Prader-Willi syndrome
- Physical exam: Height and weight, visual fields, optic disks, visual acuity (brain tumor), proptosis, goiter, lid lag (Graves), syndromic features
- Labs/studies: Blood glucose; TSH, T4, T3, thyroid stimulating immunoglobulin; genetic testing for Prader-Willi or Laurence-Moon-Bardet-Biedl syndrome; simultaneous serum and urine osmolalities may indicate DI; often requires formal water deprivation test
- MRI of the brain and pituitary

Treatment

- Insulin therapy for diabetes mellitus
- Graves disease is treated with antithyroid medication, thyroid radioablation, or surgical thyroidectomy
- Stop offending medications or substances if possible
- Psychiatric conditions require treatment directed at the specific cause
- Lesions of the hypothalamus require treatment directed to the specific cause
- Syndromes such as Prader-Willi and Laurence-Moon-Bardet-Biedl require multidisciplinary treatment from endocrinology, nutrition, and other subspecialities
- Diabetes insipidus
  - –Free water replacement while on formula
  - –DDAVP when older

8. Syncope

Syncope is temporary loss of consciousness and muscle tone due to decreased cerebral blood flow. It is otherwise known as fainting or blackout. Syncope is a common pediatric problem that, in contrast to that in adults, usually has a benign etiology. However, it can be a sign of a serious underlying disorder, so a complete H&P is critical.

Differential Diagnosis

- Vasovagal
  - –Most common etiology (more than 50%)
  - –Also known as neurocardiogenic or vasodepressor syncope
  - –Typical in adolescents; greater in females
  - –Occurs after prolonged standing in a warm place; with emotional upset, pain, hunger, the sight of blood; crowded places
- Postural/orthostatic hypotension
  - –Occurs when standing up quickly
- Micturition syncope (a rare form)
- Breath-holding spells
  - –Usually at ages 1–5 years
  - –Two types: Cyanotic (80%) vs pale (20%)
  - –Cyanotic spells start with crying
  - –Provoked by anger, frustration, or pain, or used as an attention-getting behavior
  - –May have generalized clonic jerks
- Cardiac etiologies (less common)
  - –Arrhythmias
  - –Supraventricular tachycardia is the most common cause
  - –Long QT syndrome (QTc >0.44 seconds): Causes ventricular arrhythmias, Romano-Ward (autosomal dominant), Jervell and Lange-Nielsen (autosomal recessive with deafness)
  - –Medications (e.g., cisapride)
  - –Sinus node dysfunction and atrioventricular block may lead to bradyarrhythmias
  - –Post-op congenital lesions and dilated cardiomyopathy lead to arrhythmias
  - –Structural cardiac disease
  - –Severe obstructive lesions (e.g., hypertrophic obstructive cardiomyopathy, aortic stenosis, pulmonic stenosis, atrial myxomas, and pulmonary hypertension)
- Hysterical fainting
- Migraine
- Hyperventilation
- Pregnancy
- Anemia or hypovolemia
- Hypoglycemia
- Carbon monoxide poisoning
- Medications and drugs of abuse
- Electrolyte abnormalities
- Intracranial hypertension
- Epilepsy may mimic syncope
- Adrenal insufficiency

Workup and Diagnosis

- History: Most important aspect to guide diagnostic workup
  - –Vasovagal syncope: Prodromal symptoms (e.g., cold, clammy skin; pallor; nausea; blurry vision; yawning; dizziness; lightheadedness; palpitations; hyperventilation)
  - –Duration: Vasovagal syncope is short (seconds to minutes)
  - –Inciting situations
  - –Lightheadedness: In orthostatic hypotension Syncope at rest or recumbent in seizure or arrhythmia; syncope without prodrome or with exercise/exertion in cardiac etiology
  - –Auras in migraine headaches
  - –Seizures may have incontinent or post-ictal state or generalized tonic-clonic movements
  - –Family history: Sudden or unexplained deaths, cardiac abnormalities, seizures, or deafness
- Physical exam
  - –Orthostatic blood pressures and pulse
  - –Perform a thorough cardiac and neurologic exam
- Extensive laboratory workup is not usually needed
  - –Most clinicians would do an ECG
  - –Tilt-table testing to diagnose vasovagal syncope is controversial as it is not very reproducible
  - –Labs might include CBC, glucose, electrolytes, drug screen, carboxyhemoglobin, EEG, or head CT as guided by history; if cardiac abnormalities are suspected, may get a chest X-ray, Holter monitoring, or exercise testing

Treatment

- Vasovagal syncope
  - –Educate family and patient to recognize precipitating factors and to avoid hypovolemia
  - –Have patient lie in a recumbent position until the symptoms subside
  - –Reassurance
- If severe, β-blockers can be used for recurrent vasovagal syncope
- For breath-holding spells, education is also imperative
- Iron has also been advocated in patients who are found to be iron-deficient
- Cardiac abnormalities are treated on an individual basis
  - –Structural lesions will require repair
  - –Arrhythmias may require medication or pacing
  - –Prolonged QT is treated with β-blockers, left cardiac sympathetic denervation, or demand cardiac pacing

Section 2

Vitals

IRINI DASKALAKI, MD
C. BECKET MAHNKE, MD
RONALD J. WILLIAMS, MD, FAAP, FACP

9. Bradycardia

Bradycardia is a slow pulse (<90 in infants and <60 in children and adolescents). Causes range from the benign (athletic heart) to the life threatening (sepsis, severe heart block). Assessing the child's ABCs is the first priority.

Differential Diagnosis

- Vasovagal response
  - Defecation, yawning, rectal stimulation, placement of nasogastric tube, sight of blood, etc.
- Drug reaction
  - β-blockers, calcium channel blockers (diltiazem, verapamil), carbamates, clonidine, digoxin, opiates, organophosphates, gamma-hydroxybutyrate ("date rape" drug), and plants (lily of the valley, foxglove, oleander)
- Healthy athlete
  - Sinus bradycardia
- Hypothermia
- GER (in infants, especially premature)
- Low birth weight infants: Sinus bradycardia (great variations in sinus rate, can have junctional escape beats)
- Congenital complete heart block: Associated with maternal SLE
- Congenital heart disease
- Sepsis
- Obstructive sleep apnea
  - Seen in children with obesity, tonsillar or adenoid hypertrophy, craniofacial anomalies, neuromuscular diseases
  - Hypoxia and hypercapnia lead to pulmonary hypertension and arrhythmia
- Electrolyte abnormalities can lead to dysrhythmias
- Anorexia nervosa
  - Prolonged QT syndrome and junctional arrhythmia
  - Associated hypokalemia may also cause ECG changes and life-threatening dysrhythmias
- AV node blocks (second- and third-degree)
- Idioventricular rhythm
- Hypothyroidism (myxedema)
- Allergic reaction/anaphylaxis
- Increased intracranial pressure (IVH, extradural hemorrhage, trauma, etc.)
- Sick sinus syndrome (tachy-brady syndrome)
- Psittacosis, typhoid fever, Lassa fever
- Myocardial infarction

Workup and Diagnosis

- History
  - For acute patients, history of present illness, associated symptoms
  - Birth history, PMH, and review of systems
  - Medications, medications around the house, alternative medicines/herbs
- Physical exam
  - Vital signs, growth parameters, nutritional status, physical fitness
  - Craniofacial and ENT exam
  - Complete cardiac exam: Evaluate cardiovascular stability, BP, pulse, perfusion, mental status, tachypnea, as well as heart sounds, murmurs, distal pulses
- Labs
  - ECG: Look for block, prolonged QTc, abnormal P wave, or QRS complex
  - Electrolytes (include potassium, calcium, magnesium)
  - CBC: Look for infection
  - Consider drug screen: Look for toxic ingestion
- Studies
  - Consider upper GI series, pH probe, or pneumogram (if suspect apnea as well) to look for GER
  - Consider 24-hour Holter monitor if episodic bradycardia
  - Consider echocardiogram to rule out congenital heart disease

Treatment

- Stabilize the patient with attention to ABCs
- If bradycardia is symptomatic or life threatening, consider using:
  - Epinephrine: 0.01 mg/kg (maximum: 10 mL/dose) every 3–5 minutes IV, IO; or 0.1 mg/kg (0.1 mL; 1:1,000)/kg/dose ET
  - Atropine 0.01–0.03 mg/kg/dose every 5 minutes prn via IV, endotracheal, or interosseous
- Keep the patient in a monitored setting when appropriate (heart monitor to follow the bradycardia)
- Treat the underlying cause when possible: Stop causative medications; treat sepsis, hypothermia, increased intracranial pressure, and electrolyte abnormalities emergently; intensive therapy for eating disorders; synthroid for hypothyroidism
- Cardiac surgery for CHD may not resolve arrhythmias
- Cardiac pacing (transcutaneous or implanted may be needed)

10. Fever – Acute

Fever is an elevation of body temperature over the normal daily range for a specific individual in response to different insults. It occurs when the thermoregulatory center in the hypothalamus is reset to higher temperature because of exogenous and endogenous pyrogens. It should be distinguished from hyperthermia, which describes the inability of the body to maintain the temperature that is set centrally because of environmental or internal factors. Fever is the primary complaint for 30% of patients seen by a pediatrician.

Differential Diagnosis

- Viral infections
  - Account for the majority of febrile illnesses (FI) in infancy and childhood
  - Upper respiratory infections (e.g., parainfluenza virus)
  - Lower respiratory infections (e.g., RSV)
  - Non-bacterial gastroenteritis (e.g., rotavirus)
  - Aseptic meningitis (e.g., enterovirus)
- Bacterial infections
  - UTIs account for 1.7% of FI in children <5 years and 7.5% in infants <8 weeks
  - Pneumonia (e.g., group A streptococcus)
  - Bacteremia (2% of FI in all children, highest rates seen in younger infants)
  - Meningitis (0.8% of FI in all children)
  - In febrile neonates, the overall rate of serious bacterial infections (SBI) is ~13%
- Vaccine reaction
- Collagen vascular diseases
  - Kawasaki disease: 3,000 cases per year in the U.S., rates higher in Asia, 80% of cases occur in children <5 years
  - Henoch-Schönlein purpura: Low-grade fever is present in 50% of cases
  - Juvenile rheumatoid arthritis: Incidence 1/10,000
  - SLE
  - Acute rheumatic fever
- Malignancy
  - Leukemia: Most common childhood malignancy; early symptoms include fever, fatigue, pallor, anemia, bone pain
  - Lymphoma
  - Solid tumors (neuroblastoma, sarcoma)
- Inflammatory bowel disease
  - Diarrhea, pain, fever, blood loss
  - Crohn disease, ulcerative colitis
- Tissue injury (trauma, hematoma, burns)
- Drug reaction
- Biologic agents (blood products, gamma-globulin)
- Endocrinologic disorders
  - Thyrotoxicosis
  - Pheochromocytoma
- Genetic diseases
  - Familial Mediterranean fever
- Factitious fever

Workup and Diagnosis

- History
  - Rash, vomiting, diarrhea
  - Cough, nasal or eye discharge
  - Myalgias, arthralgias, bone pain
  - Bleeding, weight loss
  - Sick contacts, daycare attendance
  - Birth history (prematurity, neonatal complications)
  - Travel, animal and insect exposure
  - Medications, recent antibiotic use; immunizations, last date received
  - Immunodeficiency, chronic illnesses
- Physical exam
  - Temperature: Rectal preferred for infants <3 months
  - Vitals: Relative brady- or tachycardia, tachypnea
  - Growth parameters especially if frequent febrile episodes/infections (immunodeficiency)
  - Appearance, irritability, quality of cry, consolability
  - Skin (color, rash, desquamation), conjunctivitis, ocular or nasal discharge, mouth lesions, throat and ear exam
  - Lymphadenopathy, abdominal exam, neuro exam
  - Joint exam (arthritis), muscle tenderness
- Labs
  - Febrile neonates (<28 days) should have sepsis evaluation (CBC; blood, urine, CSF culture)
  - Febrile young infants are evaluated according to general appearance and/or focus of fever by exam
- Immunologic workup and/or bone marrow for prolonged fever and/or other clinical evidence

Treatment

- Treating febrile episodes is common despite substantial evidence that fever is more beneficial than harmful; exception is patient with history of febrile seizures
- Antipyretics are relatively safe drugs that inhibit prostaglandin synthesis and reduce hypothalamic set point to normal
- Acetaminophen is safest antipyretic for young children
- Aspirin must be avoided (risk of Reye syndrome)
- NSAIDs are potent antipyretics and have anti-inflammatory effects
- Physical methods (cooling blankets, lukewarm baths) may be counterproductive if not combined with an antipyretic; alcohol baths are not recommended
- Most viral syndromes are self-limited, requiring only anti-pyretics and increased fluid intake for risk of dehydration
- Empiric treatment with antibiotics and hospitalization recommended only in neonates and critically ill patients

11. Fever – Cyclic

Cyclic or periodic fever is an unexplained fever that recurs after fever-free periods at almost predictably fixed intervals. True cyclic fever is rather uncommon in childhood; it should be differentiated from recurrent fever, which refers to fever prone to relapse at unpredictable and irregular intervals. Often, infections that recur with some regularity are misinterpreted as periodic fever. Thorough interviewing may identify a new source of infectious exposure, such as starting day care.

Differential Diagnosis

- PFAPA, or Marshall syndrome
  - –Periodic fever (usually high, 104°F [40°C]), aphthous stomatitis, pharyngitis, and adenitis
  - –Most common diagnosis for true cyclic fever, usually in children <5 years
  - –Recurs every 3–4 weeks
- Cyclic neutropenia
  - –Periodic fever, average cycle of 21 days
  - –Pharyngitis, mouth ulcers, and lymphadenopathy are also noted
  - –May not be associated with infection
- Infectious diseases
  - –Relapsing fever due to *Borrelia recurrentis*, relapses every 10–14 days
  - –EBV may occur at 6–8 week intervals
- Familial Mediterranean fever
  - –Brief attacks of fever and serositis
  - –Autosomal recessive disease
  - –Sephardic Jews, Arabs, Turks, and Armenians commonly affected
  - –50% have onset before 10 years of age
  - –May occur in regular 7–28-day intervals
  - –Amyloidosis is a possible complication
- Hyper-IgD and periodic fever syndrome (HIDS)
  - –High fevers, abdominal pain, cervical lymphadenopathy, sometimes diarrhea and arthritis, in early infancy
  - –Autosomal recessive, most patients from Western Europe (French, Dutch)
  - –Cycles may be regular every 14–28 days
- TNF-receptor-associated periodic syndrome (TRAPS) or Hibernian fever
  - –Fever, myalgias with migratory pattern, conjunctivitis and rash
  - –Autosomal dominant
  - –first described in Irish/Scottish individuals but other ethnic groups involved
  - –Amyloidosis is a possible complication (25% of untreated individuals)
- Familial cold autoinflammatory syndrome or familial cold urticaria
  - –Rash, fever, arthralgia, and conjunctivitis
  - –Precipitated by exposure to cold
- Factitious fever

Workup and Diagnosis

- History
  - –Age of onset, duration of episodes, duration of symptom-free periods, associated symptoms (pharyngitis, aphthous ulcers)
  - –Lymphadenopathy, abdominal pain
  - –Family history of cyclic fever, ethnicity
  - –Exposure to ticks (woods, camping), travel history
- Physical exam (during fever episode)
  - –Mouth ulcers, pharyngitis, lymphadenitis, conjunctivitis
  - –Abdominal tenderness, hepatosplenomegaly
  - –Arthritis, rash
  - –Pericardial friction, pleurisy
- Physical exam (during fever-free interval)
  - –Growth parameters
  - –Neurologic exam (ataxia, retardation)
  - –Heart murmur
  - –Hepatosplenomegaly, lymphadenopathy
- CBC with differential, diagnostic for cyclic neutropenia
- Immunoglobulins IgA and IgD (elevated in HIDS)
- Dark-field microscopy examination of wet peripheral blood for *Borrelia recurrentis*
- Familial Mediterranean fever
  - –Major and minor diagnostic criteria are available
  - –Confirmed by gene analysis
- Low levels of serum type 1 TNF receptor in TRAPS
- Documentation of fever in the office should exclude factitious fever

Treatment

- PFAPA
  - –Single dose prednisone with the onset of symptoms
  - –Prophylactic cimetidine and tonsillectomy have been tried to prevent recurrences
- Cyclic neutropenia
  - –Life-long therapy with GCSF decreases risk of infection
- Familial Mediterranean fever
  - –Daily colchicine to prevent attacks and amyloidosis
- Hyper-IgD
  - –Prednisone and colchicine have been used
  - –Even without treatment, attacks decrease with age
- TRAPS
  - –Prednisone and etanercept have been reported to be effective

12. Fever – Recurrent

Recurrent or relapsing fever is a cluster of febrile episodes that occur over a period of time, with documented fever-free intervals and without an apparent medical cause for each episode. It should be differentiated from cyclic fever, which refers to febrile episodes with periodicity, and from fever of unknown origin, which refers to prolonged daily fever with no fever-free intervals.

Differential Diagnosis

- Repeated viral infections
  - Most common cause of recurrent febrile episodes in childhood
  - Start of day care or change of geographic location may be related
- Urinary tract infection (UTI)
  - May be self-limited but recur especially if underlying anomaly exists
- Epstein-Barr virus (EBV)
  - May present with recurrent febrile episodes due to one initial infection
- Other specific viral syndromes
  - Parvovirus B19
  - CMV
- Immunodeficiency
  - Repeated bacterial infections should lead to investigation of immune status
- Dental abscess (non-dental abscesses typically present with prolonged daily fever)
- Chronic meningococcemia
- Acute rheumatic fever
- Inflammatory bowel disease (IBD)
- Juvenile rheumatoid arthritis (JRA)
- Behçet disease
- Tumor necrosis factor receptor-associated periodic syndrome (TRAPS) or Hibernian Fever
  - Autosomal dominant disease with fever, myalgias with migratory pattern, conjunctivitis and rash
- Familial cold autoinflammatory syndrome or familial cold urticaria
  - Rash, fever, arthralgia, and conjunctivitis
  - Precipitated by exposure to cold
- Muckle-Wells syndrome
  - Similar presentation to familial cold urticaria
  - Symptoms not triggered by cold
- Brucellosis
  - Most prevalent around the Mediterranean and Arabic countries, also present in South America and India
- Yersiniosis
- Typhoid fever
- Rat-bite fever
- Malaria
- Factitious fever

Workup and Diagnosis

- History
  - Documentation of fever
  - Duration of episodes and fever-free intervals
  - Symptoms associated with the fever
  - Symptoms during the fever-free intervals
  - Weight loss
  - Recent documented infections, medications
  - Travel, animal and insect exposure
  - Specific conditions related to episodes (e.g., cold)
- Physical exam
  - Vitals, growth parameters (failure to thrive can be a presentation of UTI and immunodeficiency)
  - Rash (transient pink rash in JRA)
  - Ophthalmologic exam: Uveitis (IBD and Behçet), conjunctivitis (TRAPS)
  - Hepatosplenomegaly, lymphadenopathy
  - Genital ulcers (Behçet)
  - Perianal skin tags (IBD)
  - Mouth ulcers, pharyngitis
  - Arthritis
- CBC with differential
- ESR or CRP
- Urine culture
- Blood culture
- Serology for EBV, CMV, or Parvovirus B19
- Low levels of serum type 1 TNF receptor in TRAPS
- Documentation of fever in the office should exclude the possibility of factitious fever

Treatment

- Repeated viral illnesses
  - Reassurance of the parents
  - Advice on antipyretics
  - Encourage fluid intake
  - Limit of sick exposure if possible
- UTI
  - Antibiotics based on bacteria and sensitivity
  - Prophylactic antibiotics if underlying cause is present
- Bacterial infections: Bacteria-specific antibiotic
- JRA, Behçet, or IBD
  - Prednisone or immunosuppressive medications
- TRAPS
  - Prednisone and etanercept
- Familial cold urticaria and Muckle-Wells syndrome
  - Prednisone may be used
  - If amyloidosis is present, colchicine may be required

13. Fever – Unknown Origin

Fever of unknown origin (FUO) is a term that is often misused to describe febrile illness without an obvious etiology or without other symptoms. The definition in different studies is arbitrary, but basically refers to at least 2 weeks of daily documented fever that is unexplained despite repeated physical examinations and initial laboratory investigation, in an immunocompetent host. In approximately 12% of cases an etiology cannot be found.

Differential Diagnosis

- Infections (40%)
  - –Infectious mononucleosis (EBV, CMV)
  - –Other systemic viral syndromes (e.g., HIV)
  - –UTI (e.g., *E. coli*)
  - –Osteomyelitis (e.g., staphylococcus)
  - –Upper and lower respiratory infections (sinusitis, mastoiditis, pneumonia)
  - –Cat-scratch disease (*Bartonella henselae*)
  - –Tuberculosis, nontuberculous mycobacterial infections
  - –Abscess (abdominal or retroperitoneal)
  - –CNS infections
  - –Endocarditis (subacute)
  - –Salmonellosis
  - –Lyme disease (*Borrelia burgdorferi*)
  - –Leptospirosis
  - –Congenital syphilis
  - –Others: Brucellosis, histoplasmosis, leishmaniasis, yersiniosis, Q fever (*Coxiella burnetii*), Rocky Mountain spotted fever (*Rickettsia rickettsii*)
- Autoimmune diseases (15%)
  - –Rheumatoid arthritis accounts for 3/4 of FUO due to autoimmune diseases
  - –Systemic lupus erythematosus
  - –Rheumatic fever
  - –Vasculitis (e.g., HSP)
  - –Sarcoidosis
- Neoplastic diseases (7%)
  - –Leukemia/lymphoma accounts for 80% of FUO due to malignancies
  - –Neuroblastoma
  - –Hepatoma
  - –Soft tissue sarcoma
- Inflammatory bowel disease (3%)
- Drugs and nutritional supplements (drug fever)
- Factitious fever
- Munchausen by proxy
- Neurologic disorders
  - –Familial dysautonomia
  - –Central thermoregulatory disorder
  - –Head injury
- Hyperthyroidism
- Anhidrotic ectodermal dysplasia
- Diabetes insipidus
- Kikuchi disease

Workup and Diagnosis

- History
  - –Differentiate between FUO and multiple febrile illnesses that occur in short period of time
  - –Daily documentation of fever, onset, duration
  - –Weight loss, diet history, medications, sick contacts
  - –Animal or tick exposure, travel, foreign contacts
  - –Immune status, history of transfusion, surgery
  - –FH of autoimmune or neoplastic diseases
- Physical exam
  - –Vital signs, growth parameters
  - –Skin (rash, desquamation, jaundice)
  - –Ophthalmologic exam (conjunctivitis, uveitis)
  - –Oral lesions
  - –Cardiologic exam (new onset murmur)
  - –Abdominal exam (masses, hepatosplenomegaly)
  - –Testicular exam
  - –Muscle tenderness, bone tenderness, arthritis
  - –Lymphadenopathy
  - –Neurologic exam
- Labs
  - –CBC, ESR, C-reactive protein
  - –Renal and hepatic function tests, albumin and globulin
  - –Urinalysis, blood and urine culture
  - –Viral titers, PPD, cultures for specific organisms, ASO, ANA, bone marrow
- Radiographic imaging with plain films, ultrasound, bone scan, CT scan or MRI of specific organ systems as warranted by the history and physical exam

Treatment

- Specific treatment once diagnosis is made
- Empiric treatment with antibiotics is to be considered only for critically ill patients
- Empiric steroids may be justified only if Still disease is suspected
- Anti-inflammatory agents are sometimes used for a limited period of time and subsequently the patient is observed for recurrence of the fever
- Cessation of offending drugs

14. Hypertension

Hypertension is defined as the average (several measurements over time) systolic or diastolic blood pressure greater than the 95th percentile for age, gender, and height. Severe hypertension occurs when these values are greater than the 99th percentile. Patients with blood pressures between the 90th and 95th percentiles are considered borderline.

Differential Diagnosis

- "White coat" hypertension: Transient, related to anxiety
- Essential hypertension (most common cause in adolescents)
- Obesity
- Drugs: Amphetamines, cocaine, PCP, nicotine, corticosteroids, oral contraceptives, antidepressants, sympathomimetics (including eye and nose drops), decongestants, β-agonists, theophylline, NSAIDs, ephedra, etc.
- Pain/distress
- Trauma: Pain, increased ICP, or spinal cord injury
- Surgery: Transient hypertension secondary to pain or specific procedures such as ductus arteriosus ligation or coarctation repair, renal or urinary tract surgery
- Seizures
- Renal etiologies
  - –Chronic renal parenchymal disease: Most common in preadolescents (chronic renal insufficiency, reflux nephropathy, chronic glomerulonephritis, PCKD)
  - –Acute renal disease: Poststreptococcal glomerulonephritis, nephritis, renal failure
  - –Renal artery stenosis: From fibromuscular dysplasia or by external compression from tumor or hematoma
  - –Congenital ureteropelvic junction obstruction
  - –Renal ischemic events secondary to umbilical catheters (thrombosis/embolus)
- Endocrine disorders: CAH, Cushing syndrome, hypo-/hyperthyroidism, hyperparathyroidism, primary hyperaldosteronism, pheochromocytoma
- Sleep apnea
- Volume overload
- Hemolytic uremic syndrome
- Pregnancy
- Bronchopulmonary dysplasia
- Hypercalcemia
- Williams syndrome (multiple vascular stenosis, autoimmune vasculitis with large vessel involvement)
- Coarctation of the aorta

Workup and Diagnosis

- History
  - –Associated symptoms
  - –Birth history, PMH, review of systems
  - –Medications (including patient's own, those around the house, and alternative medications/herbs)
  - –Social history including substance use, sleep patterns
- Physical exam
  - –Complete physical exam with special attention to eyes, abdomen, and neurologic systems
  - –Complete cardiac exam: Evaluate cardiovascular stability (four-extremity BP, pulse, perfusion, mental status, tachypnea) as well as heart sounds, murmurs, distal pulses
- Labs
  - –CBC, electrolytes, BUN, creatinine, calcium
  - –Urinalysis (blood, protein, calcium, creatinine, creatinine clearance)
  - –Consider urine toxicology screen
  - –ASO titer if poststreptococcal glomerulonephritis is suspected
  - –Thyroid function studies if history is consistent with thyroid dysfunction
- Studies
  - –Consider sleep study to rule out sleep apnea
  - –Consider echo for coarctation of aorta
  - –Consider renal ultrasound, DMSA, renin levels
  - –Captopril scan or renal angiography for renal etiology

Treatment

- Treat the underlying disease when possible
- Stop smoking and illicit drug use
- Avoid the offending drug when possible
- Limit competitive sports and highly static exercises in patients with severe hypertension only until their BP is controlled and there is no evidence of end organ damage
- Salt restriction (4–5 g/day), weight loss, and exercise are part of most regimens
- Essential hypertension can usually be resolved with weight loss, moderate exercise, and dietary modifications
- For other etiologies, many medications are used to control blood pressure
  - –IV: Nicardipine, sodium nitroprusside, labetalol
  - –Oral: Captopril, enalapril, lisinopril, amlodipine, nifedipine extended release, propranolol, clonidine, hydralazine

15. Hypothermia

Hypothermia is defined as a core body temperature below 95°F (35°C). Distinction is made between primary hypothermia, which is due to accidental cold exposure, and secondary, in which a specific disease is the cause. A distinction is also made among mild (89.6–95°F [32–35°C]), moderate (82.4–89.6°F [28–32°C]), and severe (<82.4°F [<28°C]) to reflect the different compensatory mechanisms generated at these low temperatures. Hypothermia often implies a bad prognosis.

Differential Diagnosis

- Cold exposure
  - Infants and younger children are more prone to heat loss due to higher surface-to-weight ratio and poor adaptive behavioral response to cold
  - Immersion and near drowning are the most frequent causes of hypothermia throughout childhood
  - Hypothermia is the leading cause of death during outdoor recreation (winter sports, climbing)
- Drugs
  - Antipyretics, sedatives, anesthetics, phenothiazines, oral hypoglycemics
  - Alcohol ingestion causing vasodilation
- Sepsis or other serious bacterial infection especially in neonates and in the immunocompromised host
- Endocrinologic disorders
  - Hypoglycemia, hypothyroidism, hypopituitarism, hypoadrenalism
- Iatrogenic
  - Surgery (during and immediately after) as a combination of anesthetics and sometimes visceral exposure to the usually cool operating environment
  - Inadequate thermal support during transport and resuscitation
  - Infusion of cold IV fluids and blood products
- Malnutrition/starvation
  - Children die from hypothermia in the tropics despite the high temperature
- Eating disorders
  - 15% of patients with anorexia nervosa have temperature below 95°F (35°C)
- Trauma, burns, and other dermatologic conditions that impair the body's ability to decrease heat loss
- Neurologic and neuromuscular disorders
  - Central dysfunction of thermoregulatory control
  - Immobilizing conditions
  - Intracranial hemorrhage or infarction
  - CNS tumors
  - Congenital absence of the corpus callosum
- Familial dysautonomia
- Menkes syndrome (kinky-hair disease)
- Water intoxication

Workup and Diagnosis

- History
  - Exposure to cold weather or immersion in cold water
  - Severe injury and conditions when victim was found (wet or windy environment); transport/resuscitation
  - Home temperature and presence of heating system
  - Prolonged exposure during physical examination
  - Medications, alcohol ingestion
  - Immobilizing conditions
  - Behaviors consistent with an eating disorder
- Physical exam
  - Low-reading thermometer (most thermometers don't read temperatures below 93.2°F [34°C])
  - Patient may not necessarily "feel" cold
  - Bradycardia, decreased or unobtainable BP
  - Peripheral pulses weak (vasoconstriction)
  - Cyanosis or pallor followed by flushing
  - Shivering followed by muscle rigidity
  - Pupils may be dilated and nonreactive
  - CNS dysfunction with confusion, slurred speech, paradoxical behavior (e.g., undressing)
- Labs
  - Serum glucose (hyper- then hypoglycemia)
  - Electrolytes (shifts occur during rewarming)
  - Arterial blood gas (pH rises, PaO_2 and $PaCO_2$ fall)
  - CBC (hematocrit increases due to hypovolemia)
  - Urine drug screen, blood alcohol level
  - ECG, thyroid function tests
- Radiology: Appropriate imaging for trauma patients

Treatment

- ABCs, CPR if patient is pulseless
- Rewarming
  - Passive external rewarming: Remove cold, wet clothes, dry and insulate patient (ideal for mild hypothermia)
  - Active external rewarming: Hot packs, heating lamps, warmers, warm water baths, electric blankets, and forced-air external rewarming (all controversial, may be responsible for "afterdrop" shifting cold blood from the periphery to the heart)
  - Core rewarming: Heated humidified oxygen, heated IV fluids, heated lavage of cavities (bladder, stomach, peritoneum), extracorporeal blood rewarming
- Aggressive volume resuscitation using isotonic solutions
- Monitor heart rate for high possibility of dysrhythmias
- Glucose infusion for hypoglycemia
- Antibiotics for sepsis or other severe infection

16. Tachycardia/Palpitations

Most tachycardias in children are supraventricular and well tolerated, allowing time for proper evaluation and diagnosis. Cardiovascular collapse is rare but more common in those with a history of congenital heart disease and/or cardiac surgery.

Differential Diagnosis

- Sinus tachycardia
  - –Most common cause of a fast heart rate
  - –Normal response to stress (fever, pain, anxiety, dehydration, exercise, anemia, caffeine, tobacco, albuterol)
  - –<180 beats/min and variable; ECG shows an upright P wave in lead I and AVF
- Supraventricular tachycardia (SVT)
  - –Most common pathologic cause of tachycardia/palpitations in children
  - –Narrow QRS complex (<0.08 seconds)
  - –Almost all hemodynamically stable
  - –Often paroxysmal
  - –Usually AV re-entry or AV node re-entry; both have HR >180 and intermittent sudden onset and resolution
- AV re-entry
  - –Involves an accessory electrical bypass tract connecting the atrium and ventricle (thereby "bypassing" the AV node)
  - –Often associated with Wolff-Parkinson-White (WPW) syndrome (short PR interval, widened QRS interval, "delta" wave)
  - –Most common in <10 years of age
- AV node re-entry
  - –Involves re-entry within the AV node
  - –Most common in >10 yrs of age
- Atrial fibrillation/flutter
  - –Occurs almost exclusively in patients with underlying congenital heart disease
  - –Macro (flutter) or micro (fibrillation) re-entry circuits within the atrium, usually around an old surgical scar
  - –Common in patients status post-Fontan or Mustard-Senning procedures
- Ectopic/multifocal atrial tachycardia
  - –Involves one or more automatic electrical foci in the atrium causing irregular tachycardia with a heart rate <180
  - –The tachycardia has a slow onset and resolution
- Wide-complex tachycardia
  - –Assume ventricular tachycardia until proven otherwise
  - –SVT with bundle branch block (either permanent or rate-related)
  - –Antidromic WPW: Re-entry loop in which the ventricle is depolarized via the bypass tract, creating a wide-complex tachycardia

Workup and Diagnosis

- History
  - –Onset (sudden vs slow acceleration), activity at time of onset, duration, regularity of rhythm, pulse rate, resolution (sudden vs slow; with vagal maneuvers)
  - –Symptoms during tachycardia: Chest pain, pallor, diaphoresis, syncope
  - –History of underlying congenital heart disease
  - –Medication use: Caffeine, tobacco, albuterol
  - –Underlying medical condition: Fever, pain, anxiety, dehydration, anemia, thyrotoxicosis
- Physical exam
  - –Evaluate cardiovascular stability (BP, perfusion, mental status, tachypnea)
  - –All unstable patients with a fast heart rate require electrical cardioversion
  - –Rarely, chronic incessant tachycardias can cause cardiomyopathy with congestive heart failure
- 12-lead ECG
  - –During tachycardia: Narrow vs. wide complex, regular vs. irregular rhythm, P wave axis, QRS wave
  - –Baseline: Evaluate for WPW, prolonged QTc, bundle branch block
  - –During therapy: Record ECG while giving adenosine
- 24-hour Holter monitor for daily symptoms
- 30-day event monitor for intermittent symptoms (recording activated by patient when symptoms occur)
- Exercise testing with ECG monitor for patients with symptoms only during exercise

Treatment

- Sinus tachycardia: Treat underlying cause
- Acute therapy for SVT
  - –Vagal maneuvers increase vagal tone at AV node, lengthening the refractory period and breaking re-entry SVT: Ice to face (<1 year old), blowing hard on thumb (toddler/child), carotid massage (teenager)
  - –Adenosine: Increases refractory period of AV node better than vagal maneuvers by causing temporary AV block that breaks re-entry SVT; short (10 sec) half-life, so must give fast via IV push; side effects include hypotension (transient), chest tightness/pain, sense of "impending doom"
  - –Synchronized cardioversion all unstable tachycardias (especially V-fib and pulseless V-tach)
- Chronic therapy for re-entry SVT
  - –β-blockers, digoxin (not in WPW), calcium channel blockers (not if <1 year old), other antiarrhythmics
  - –Ablation of bypass tract via cardiac catheterization

Section 3

Growth/Development

ADDA GRIMBERG, MD
DOUGLAS A. JACOBSTEIN, MD

17. Failure to Thrive

Failure to thrive (FTT) is a common problem accounting for 1–5% of referrals to pediatric centers. Although no consensus exists, FTT applies to children under 2 years of age whose weight is less than 5% on two occasions or crosses two major growth percentiles. It is more common among children in poverty. The causes can be broken down into three categories: decreased caloric intake, decreased caloric absorption, and increased caloric needs.

Differential Diagnosis

- Psychosocial (non-organic)
  - –Insufficient caloric intake
  - –Most common etiology
  - –Cause accounts for 1/3–1/2 of cases investigated in tertiary settings
- Gastrointestinal disorders
  - –Gastroesophageal reflux
  - –Celiac disease
  - –Milk protein allergy
  - –Pancreatic insufficiency
  - –Inflammatory bowel disease
- Endocrine disorders
  - –Hypothyroidism
  - –Hyperthyroidism
  - –Diabetes mellitus
  - –Diabetes insipidus
  - –Growth hormone deficiency
- Cardiac disorders
  - –Congestive heart failure
  - –Congenital anomalies
- Pulmonary disorders
  - –Brochopulmonary dysplasia
  - –Asthma
  - –Cystic fibrosis
- Infectious
  - –HIV
  - –Parasites
  - –Tuberculosis
- Neurologic
  - –Hypotonia
  - –Cerebral hemorrhage
  - –Diencephalic syndrome
- Metabolic
  - –Galactosemia
  - –Methylmalonic acidemia
  - –Tyrosinemia
- Renal
  - –Renal tubular acidosis
  - –Chronic urinary tract infections
  - –Chronic renal insufficiency
- Syndromes
  - –Down syndrome
  - –Turner syndrome
  - –Russell-Silver dwarfism
  - –Fetal alcohol syndrome
- Anatomic
  - –Cleft lip/palate
  - –Malrotation
  - –Pyloric stenosis
- Lead poisoning

Workup and Diagnosis

- History
  - –Emesis, number and quality of stools, excessive energy, diaphoresis, breathing difficulties, urinary frequency
  - –Diet history: Duration and quantity of feeding, food preferences, juice intake, food allergies
  - –Medical history: Chronic medical problems, surgeries
  - –Observation: Eye contact, absence of smile, lack of interest in environment, parental interaction
  - –Psychosocial history: Caretakers, financial status, employment, family stress, poverty indicators, support systems, parental age, substance abuse
- Birth history
  - –Growth retardation, low birth weight, intrauterine stress, prematurity, parental substance abuse
- Physical exam
  - –Accurate height, weight, and head circumference, multiple points on growth curve
  - –Neuro/developmental age (milestones)
  - –Murmurs, wheezes/crackles, abdominal masses
  - –Exam of hard/soft palate, dysmorphic features
  - –Signs of neglect/abuse including poor hygiene persistent diaper rash, bruising, unexplained scars
- Initial lab screen to include CBC, electrolytes, urinalysis
  - –Consider thyroid function tests, HIV testing, TB skin testing, celiac testing (anti-tissue transglutaminase)
- Radiographs/imaging only if history dictates
- Diet journal, 3-day calorie counts

Treatment

- Hospitalization unnecessary unless severe malnutrition or abuse
- Psychosocial causes require team approach with physician, family, social worker, dieticians
- Goal of refeeding to allow for catch-up growth at 1.25–1.5 times normal caloric intake for age
  - –Monitor for refeeding syndrome with electrolyte imbalances (e.g., phosphorus, potassium, glucose)
- Structured and scheduled feeding crucial in appropriate feeding atmosphere
- Consider nasogastric feedings if weight gain by other methods is insufficient within 4–6 weeks
- Treat organic causes
  - –Diet restriction for food allergy, metabolic disease
  - –Correct electrolyte disturbances
  - –Treat endocrine disease
  - –Remove environmental exposures

18. Obesity

Pediatric obesity is increasing at epidemic proportions. The Centers for Disease Control define "at risk of overweight" as a body mass index (BMI, kg/m^2) of ≥85%ile and <95%ile for age and sex, and "overweight" as ≥95%ile for age and sex. Data from the third National Health and Nutrition Examination Survey (NHANES III) indicates that the prevalence of overweight children (6–11 years) increased from 4% in 1965 to 13% in 1999, and that of overweight adolescents (12–19 years) increased from 5% in 1970 to 14% in 1999.

Differential Diagnosis

- Exogenous obesity (most common)
  - No demonstrable disease as the cause
  - Excessive weight gain from imbalance between caloric intake and energy expenditure
  - Linear growth is robust and frequently accelerated
- Hormonal causes
  - Associated with poor linear growth
  - Hypercortisolism: Cushing syndrome is any type of glucocorticoid excess (endogenous or exogenous); Cushing disease describes pituitary ACTH overproduction
  - Hypothyroidism
  - Growth hormone deficiency
- Insulinoma
- Hypothalamic obesity
  - Tumors (e.g., craniopharyngiomas)
  - Following neurosurgery or irradiation
  - Head trauma
  - Infiltrative/inflammatory
- Genetic syndromes
  - Prader-Willi syndrome
  - Laurence-Moon-Bardet-Biedl syndrome
  - Alström syndrome
  - Cohen syndrome
  - Down syndrome
  - Carpenter syndrome
  - Grebe syndrome
  - Beckwith-Wiedemann syndrome
- Defects in metabolic/eating regulatory pathways is an area of intense investigation; multiple mutations are theoretically possible, but only a few have actually been discovered in humans
  - Congenital leptin deficiency (extremely rare)
  - Leptin resistance (more common than deficiency)
- Drugs
  - Chronic glucocorticoids
  - Neuropsychotropic medications
- Adiposogenital dystrophy syndrome

Workup and Diagnosis

- History: Age and course of onset; linear growth progression; birth and neonatal history (tone, failure to thrive); polydipsia, polyuria, polyphagia; dietary intake, physical activity; cold intolerance, constipation, dry skin, headaches; abdominal pain, onset of puberty if pubertal; developmental delay (genetic syndromes); family history of obesity and genetic disorders
- Physical exam: Vital signs (blood pressure); growth parameters (height, weight, BMI); distribution of fat, moon or coarse facies, pallor, buffalo hump, striae (Cushingoid appearance); acanthosis nigricans (dark velvety areas in skin folds; cutaneous marker of insulin resistance); abdominal masses, micropenis, hypogonadism; depressed deep tendon reflexes; in infants skin "puddling," midline defects
- Diagnostic workup
  - 24-hour urine free cortisol/creatinine ratio (best screen for Cushing syndrome)
  - MRI (hypothalamic/pituitary mass)
  - Adrenal ultrasound (if suspect adrenal mass)
  - Thyroid function tests (T4, TSH)
  - IGF-I and IGFBP-3; possibly provocative growth hormone testing (if suspect GH deficiency)
  - Genetic (FISH) testing for genetic syndromes
  - Serum leptin
- Labs: Urinalysis for glucose, serum glucose, fasting serum insulin, hemoglobin A1c
  - Fasting lipid profile, urine microalbumin

Treatment

- If syndrome or no known disease as etiology
  - Nutritional education and diet manipulation
  - Exercise regimen (energy expenditure must exceed intake)
  - Behavior modification involving family
- Hormonal etiology
  - Hormone replacement for hypothyroidism or growth hormone deficiency
  - Surgical intervention if hypercortisolism caused by tumor
  - Decrease exogeneous glucorticoids if not medically contraindicated
- Leptin treatment in leptin deficiency (therapeutic trials)
- If patient also has type II diabetes mellitus, insulin or oral medications may be required in addition to improved diet and exercise

19. Short Stature

By definition, 3% of normal children are short: A height 2 standard deviations (SD) below the mean for age. Dwarfism is defined as height more than 3 SD below the mean; midget is a dwarf with normal body proportions. Growth failure (worth careful evaluation) defined as: (1) height below 2 SD from the mean for reference population, (2) height less than 2 SD below midparental target, (3) subnormal growth velocity (2 inches or 5 cm per year from age 3 years to puberty), or (4) growth deceleration (falling across major percentiles on growth curve).

Differential Diagnosis

- Familial short stature
- Constitutional delay of growth and puberty
- Hypothyroidism
- Growth hormone deficiency (GHD)
- GH resistance (Laron syndrome)
- Congenital hypopituitarism
  - –Secondary to brain tumors
- Acquired hypopituitarism
  - –After irradiation, surgery, and chemotherapy for neoplasms
  - –Infectious
  - –Infiltrative
  - –Vascular
- Cushing syndrome
- Precocious puberty
  - –Tall initially
  - –Final height compromised
- Pseudohypoparathyroidism
- Rickets
- Genetic syndromes
  - –Turner syndrome
  - –Down syndrome
  - –Noonan syndrome
  - –Prader-Willi syndrome
- Intrauterine growth retardation
  - –Silver-Russell syndrome
- Disorders of bone development
  - –Achondroplasia/hypochondroplasia
  - –Chondrodystrophies
- Psychosocial deprivation
- Malnutrition
- Chronic drug intake
  - –Glucocorticoids
  - –Methylphenidate
- Infectious
  - –HIV
  - –Tuberculosis
- Congenital heart disease
- Gastrointestinal
  - –Celiac disease
  - –Inflammatory bowel disease
  - –Chronic liver disease
- Pulmonary
  - –Cystic fibrosis
- Chronic renal disease
  - –RTA
  - –Renal failure
- Skeletal disorders

Workup and Diagnosis

- History
  - –Neonatal hypoglycemia or jaundice, brain tumor or other malignancy and treatment, central nervous system infection, nutrition status, chronic illness
- Family history
  - –Parents' heights and puberty ages to judge child's growth relative to genetic potential (midparental target height), family history of chronic disease or endocrinopathy
- Physical exam
  - –Anthropometrics (height, weight, sitting height), dysmorphic features, craniofacial midline abnormalities (pituitary disease), dentition maturation (delayed in hypothyroidism), chronic illness, Tanner staging for pubertal assessment, micropenis in boys (growth hormone deficiency)
- Bone age X-ray to evaluate skeletal maturation
- Labs
  - –CBC with differential cell count, LFT, BUN, Cr, electrolytes
  - –ESR, TSH, T4
  - –Growth factors (IGF-I, IGFBP-3)
  - –Celiac antibody panel (anti-tissue transglutaminase)
  - –Karyotype in girls to rule out Turner syndrome
- If IGF-I and/or IGFBP-3 low, provocative growth hormone test to confirm GHD (must fail two tests)
- MRI of the brain with special cuts of the pituitary in any child diagnosed as having GHD

Treatment

- Treat the underlying condition
- Growth hormone therapy
  - –Indicated in GHD and some other forms of short stature (renal failure, Turner syndrome, Prader-Willi syndrome, small-for-gestational age without catch-up growth)
  - –Earlier initiation to optimize final height outcome
  - –Nightly subcutaneous administration of GH at 25–50 μg/kg/day
- Monitor for loss of other pituitary hormones and replace all deficiencies
- Monitoring growth hormone therapy
  - –Close follow-up with pediatric endocrinologist every 3–6 months
  - –Monitor side effects of GH treatment
  - –Monitor serum IGF-I and IGFBP-3 levels
  - –Dose adjustments based on IGF values and growth response

20. Tall Stature

Tall stature and excessive overgrowth syndromes represent physical development in excess of 2 standard deviations (SD) above the mean for the person's age and gender. Referrals for evaluation and treatment are much less common than for short stature. The incidence varies greatly depending on the etiologies.

Differential Diagnosis

- Constitutional tall stature
  - –Most common cause
- Endocrine disorders
  - –Excess GH secretion (pituitary gigantism)
  - –McCune-Albright syndrome
  - –Multiple endocrine neoplasia is associated with excess GH secretion
- Precocious puberty
  - –Tall initially
  - –Final height compromised
- Hyperthyroidism
- Reduced sex steroid activity
  - –Hypogonadism
  - –Klinefelter syndrome
  - –Androgen or estrogen deficiency
  - –Estrogen resistance
  - –Androgen insensitivity syndrome
- Excess insulin
  - –Exogenous obesity
  - –Maternal diabetes mellitus
- Cerebral gigantism (Sotos syndrome)
- Weaver syndrome
- Beckwith-Wiedemann syndrome
- Marfan syndrome
- Homocystinuria
- Fragile X syndrome

Workup and Diagnosis

- History
  - –Signs of tumor: Headache; behavioral, visual problems
  - –Symptoms of impaired secretion of gonadotropins and thyrotropin corticotropin, or hyperprolactinemia
  - –History of pubertal signs
- Family history
  - –Parents' heights and puberty ages to judge child's growth relative to genetic potential (midparental target height); family history of chronic disease or endocrinopathy
- Physical exam
  - –Vital signs, anthropometrics (height, weight, sitting height)
  - –Acromegalic features: Coarse face, broad nose, separate teeth, increased mandible growth, dorsal kyphosis, enlarging hands and feet with thickening fingers and toes, visual field defects
  - –Tanner staging for pubertal assessment
- Bone age X-ray to predict final height
- Labs
  - –IGF-I is most sensitive screen for GH excess
  - –Karyotype in male patients
  - –Thyroid function tests
  - –Gonadotropins and sex hormone levels if puberty abnormal
- Glucose suppression test: Suppress serum GH to <5 ng/dL after 1.75 g/kg oral glucose challenge
  - –Gold standard for verifying GH excess
- MRI evaluation of pituitary mandatory if evidence of GH excess

Treatment

- Constitutional and syndromic tall stature
  - –For predicted adult height >3 SD above the mean, or evidence of significant psychosocial impairment
  - –High-dose sex steroids to induce earlier growth plate closure
  - –Treatment is controversial
- Pituitary adenoma
  - –Transphenoidal surgery is treatment of choice
  - –Postoperative GH and IGF-I define a biochemical cure
  - –Pituitary radiation if case surgery does not normalize GH secretion
  - –Medical therapy: Somatostatin analogs, dopamine agonists, GH antagonists (GH-receptor inhibitor), for suppressing IGF-I and GH

21. Weight Loss

The norm in infants and children is to gain weight, so weight loss in a pediatric patient (unless medically indicated) should demand evaluation. Acute weight loss, defined as loss of 3–5% of body mass in less than 30 days, signals illness and is often the result of the loss of fluid or body mass from catabolism or starvation.

Differential Diagnosis

- Infectious
  - –The most common cause overall and can be divided into acute and chronic
  - –Gastroenteritis most common infection
  - –May be viral, bacterial, fungal, or parasitic
  - –Estimated 21–37 million episodes a year in children under 5
  - –Others include strep, osteomyelitis, EBV, TB
- Psychiatric/psychosocial
  - –Anorexia nervosa
  - –Bulimia
  - –Depression
  - –Rumination
  - –Drugs: Cocaine, amphetamines, laxatives
- Gastrointestinal disorders
  - –Gastroesophageal reflux disease
  - –Inflammatory bowel disease
  - –Hepatitis
  - –Pancreatitis
  - –Pancreatic insufficiency (e.g., CF, Shwachman syndrome)
  - –Celiac disease
  - –Sucrase-isomaltase deficiency
  - –Fat malabsorption: Abetalipoproteinemia
  - –Protein malabsorption: Hartnup disease
  - –Superior mesenteric artery syndrome
- Nutritional
  - –Dieting; inadequate caloric intake
  - –Iron deficiency
  - –Zinc deficiency
  - –Neglect
- Metabolic/endocrine
  - –Diabetes mellitus
  - –Diabetes insipidus
  - –Addison disease
  - –Hyperthyroidism
  - –Hypopituitarism
- Malignancy
- HIV
- Acute/chronic renal failure
- Inflammatory
  - –Systemic lupus erythematosus
  - –Juvenile rheumatoid arthritis
  - –Sarcoidosis
- Neurologic
  - –Increased ICP: Pseudotumor cerebri, mass
- Cardiopulmonary
  - –Cystic fibrosis
  - –Congenital heart disease
  - –Congestive heart failure

Workup and Diagnosis

- History
  - –Bowel function including number and consistency of stools, melena, hematochezia, vomiting, abdominal pain, fever, headache, diaphoresis, sick contacts, travel history, oral intake
  - –Diet history: Food consumption, number of meals
  - –Medications: Prescription and over-the-counter
  - –Social history: Changes in family structure, alcohol, illicit drug use, smoking, changes in grades in school, changes in activities and interests
  - –Developmental history: Milestones, multiple points on growth curve
- Physical exam
  - –Height/weight, pulse, blood pressure, mucous membranes, scleral icteris, adenopathy, neck mass, thyroid, lung sounds, murmurs, abdominal mass/tenderness, hepatosplenomegaly, skin turgor, joint tenderness, neuro exam including funduscopy, gynecologic exam
- Laboratory/radiology are based on H&P
  - –Initial electrolytes, CBC with differential
  - –Consider LFT, amylase/lipase, ESR, iron studies
  - –Throat culture, stool culture, stool for O&P
  - –Stool for blood, urinalysis and culture, fat/reducing substances, thyroid function
  - –HIV test, PPD
  - –Consider chest X-ray
  - –Limited value of CT/MRI unless dictated by H&P

Treatment

- Initial goals are to achieve fluid balance via rehydration and to correct electrolyte disturbances
- Caloric assessment and possible dietary supplementation
- Treat infectious causes if medically indicated
- Psychiatric care
  - –For eating disorders, depression, drug abuse
- Malabsorption
  - –May require special formulas/restriction diets
  - –May require pancreatic enzymes
- Treat endocrine disturbance
- Anti-inflammatory medications for IBD
- Surgical correction of cardiac anomalies

Section 4

Head

KARI A. DRAPER, MD
DAVID J. KAY, MD
MUSTAFA SAHIN, MD, PhD

22. Abnormal Head Shape

The shape of the skull is determined by the intracranial forces, external forces, and the time of closure of the cranial sutures. Birth trauma results in cephalohematoma in 0.2–2.5% of live births, resulting in abnormal head shape and fluid or blood accumulation. Intervention for craniosynostosis may be required to relieve increased intracranial pressure or for cosmetic reasons.

Differential Diagnosis

- Caput succedaneum
- Cephalohematoma
- Plagiocephaly (flattening on one side of the head) usually positional
- Macrocephaly
  - –Neurofibromatosis
  - –Sotos syndrome
  - –Achondroplasia
  - –Robinow syndrome
- Hydrocephalus (excess cerebrospinal fluid)
- External hydrocephalus (benign extradural fluid collection)
- Microcephaly
  - –Autosomal dominant form
  - –Autosomal recessive form
  - –Cornelia de Lange syndrome
  - –Cri-du-chat syndrome
  - –Smith-Lemli-Opitz syndrome
  - –Fetal alcohol syndrome
  - –Congenital infection (e.g., CMV, HSV)
- Linear skull fracture
- Craniostenosis (associated syndromes)
  - –Crouzon syndrome
  - –Apert syndrome
  - –Ataxia-telangiectasia
  - –Hyperthyroidism
  - –Idiopathic hypercalcemia
  - –Mucopolysaccharidosis
  - –Rickets
  - –Sickle cell disease
  - –Thalassemia major
- Scaphocephaly/dolicocephaly (long, narrow head)
- Brachycephaly (broad head)
- Oxycephaly (pointed head)
- Acrocephaly (high, tower-like head)
- Trigonocephaly (triangular head)
- Clover-leaf skull
- Forehead bowing (large lateral ventricles)
- Narrow calvarium (temporal lobe agenesis)
- Small posterior fossa (cerebellar agenesis)
- Occipital bowing (Dandy-Walker malformation)
- Bitemporal widening—subdural hematoma in infancy
- Cranial meningocele

Workup and Diagnosis

- History
  - –Time of onset (birth vs soon after); birth trauma, including prolonged labor, instrumentation; history of intrauterine infection; family history of macrocephaly, microcephaly, genetic disorders, neurocutaneous syndromes, cranial vault abnormalities, associated limb abnormalities (syndactyly)
- Physical exam
  - –Visual inspection of skull, swelling, palpation of sutures for osseous ridge, pulsation, cranial bruits, abnormal transillumination
  - –Skin discoloration in newborns
  - –Signs of increased intracranial pressure
  - –Other findings: Skeletal dysplasia, eye abnormalities, organomegaly, neurocutaneous signs
- Labs
  - –Consider genetic testing and chromosomal analysis, amino acid screen, serologies for intrauterine infection
- Studies
  - –Do emergently with acute change in responsiveness or decreased upgaze ("sunsetting") sign
  - –X-ray of skull will show skull fractures or a band of increased bone density at prematurely closed sutures
  - –CT in children with craniostenosis of multiple sutures or coexisting intracranial abnormalities; also better for evaluating skull dysplasias

Treatment

- Caput succedaneum requires no therapy, and typically resolves within several days
- Cephalohematoma due to birth trauma may require transfusion if there is significant blood accumulation; may require phototherapy for secondary hemolysis and hyperbilirubinemia; needle aspiration is contraindicated because of concerns of infection
- Rapidly increasing head circumference
  - –May be accompanied by increased intracranial pressure, developmental delay, spasticity, and thinning of the cortical mantle
- Plagiocephaly
  - –Fitted shaping helmets are controversial
  - –Effective if used before osseous closure of sutures
- Indications for cranial vault/suture release surgery
  - –Relief of hydrocephalus or increased intracranial pressure
  - –Improvement in the appearance of the head

23. Enlarged Anterior Fontanelle

It is important to know the standards of anterior fontanelle for age. All newborn infants have a palpable anterior fontanelle (usually closes between 7 and 19 months, average 13 months). Some also have a posterior fontanelle that usually closes by 3 months. The mean diameter of the anterior fontanelle at birth is 2 cm.

Differential Diagnosis

- Hypothyroidism
  - –Primary congenital hypothyroidism occurs in 1/4,000 live births, more in females (2:1)
  - –Ectopic thyroid gland is the most common etiology; may also be caused by thyroid dysgenesis, thyroid dyshormonogenesis, hypothalamic-pituitary hypothyroidism
  - –Physical findings include prolonged jaundice, macroglossia, doughy skin, umbilical hernia, weak hoarse cry, hypotonia, poor feeding, sparse hair, dry skin, constipation, abdominal distension, poor growth, developmental delay, slow deep-tendon reflexes, broad flat nose
  - –Acquired hypothyroidism is most commonly due to iodine deficiency or chronic autoimmune thyroiditis
- Increased intracranial pressure
  - –Usually accompanied by increased head circumference
  - –Hydrocephalus
  - –Trauma
  - –Acute CNS infections (meningitis or encephalitis)
- Skeletal dysplasias
  - –Rickets
  - –Achondroplasia
  - –Osteogenesis imperfecta
- Genetic/chromosomal disorders
  - –Down syndrome (trisomy 21): Associated with mental retardation, hypotonia, epicanthal folds, slanted palpebral fissures, small ears, Brushfield spots of iris, clinodactyly, single palmar crease, cardiac defects, brachycephaly, protruding tongue, short neck, large space between first and second toes
  - –Apert syndrome
  - –Trisomy 13
  - –Trisomy 18
  - –Silver-Russell syndrome
  - –Cleidocranial dysostosis
  - –Kenny syndrome
- Fetal hydantoin syndrome
- Intrauterine growth retardation
- Zellweger (cerebrohepatorenal) syndrome
- Hurler syndrome (type I mucopolysaccharidosis)

Workup and Diagnosis

- History
  - –Birth history, including maternal health and medications, gestational age, perinatal fractures
  - –Family history of any genetic or thyroid disease
  - –History of trauma
  - –Symptoms of hypothyroidism
- Physical exam
  - –Growth parameters, including head circumference and growth percentiles
  - –Signs of hypothyroidism
  - –Dysmorphism associated with genetic abnormalities
- Labs
  - –Check state newborn screening test results
  - –Thyroid function tests (TSH, free T4)
  - –Vitamin D, calcium, alkaline phosphatase levels for rickets
  - –Chromosomes as indicated by H&P
  - –Unrinary glycosaminoglycans for Hurler syndrome
  - –Culture of blood and cerebrospinal fluid, including viral culture
  - –Osteogenesis imperfecta: Molecular testing
- Studies
  - –Imaging of the head as indicated by H&P
  - –X-rays of the skeletal system for rickets (rachitic rosary of the ribs, cupping of long bone metaphyses)
  - –Thyroid scan or ultrasound

Treatment

- For hypothyroidism, the treatment is thyroid replacement therapy, typically determined by endocrinologist
- Hydrocephalus is treated, if needed, with neurosurgery and ventriculoperitoneal shunting
- Rickets is prevented with adequate vitamin D intake and moderate sun exposure; treated with calcium, calcitriol and/or vitamin D
- Although no specific treatment exists for the multiple genetic disorders, genetic counseling is important for the family regarding the patient's prognosis and future pregnancies

24. Facial Paralysis

Although Bell palsy is the most frequent etiology, it is a diagnosis of exclusion; one must thoroughly rule out infections, congenital, developmental, and other causes. Serial electrical testing provides objective monitoring of nerve function and may provide some prognostic information regarding future functional status.

Differential Diagnosis

Acquired

- Bell palsy
  - –A diagnosis of exclusion; 40% of cases
- Acute otitis media
  - –From erosion or dehiscence of facial canal
- Chronic otitis media
  - –Nerve compression from granulation tissue
- Herpes zoster oticus
  - –Often infects eighth nerve as well, with hearing loss and vertigo
- Lyme disease
  - –Usually several weeks after inoculation
- Tumors
  - –Temporal bone leukemia, rhabdomyosarcoma of head and neck
- Melkersson-Rosenthal syndrome
  - –Relapsing alternating facial paralysis
  - –Recurrent facial edema
  - –Fissured tongue
- Temporal bone fracture
  - –Although most cases involve longitudinal fractures, transverse may also result in hearing loss and vertigo
- Facial wounds
  - –Early repair if clean wound
  - –Tag nerve for delayed repair if dirty wound
- Iatrogenic
  - –After otologic or parotid surgery

Congenital

- Traumatic (associated with prolonged and difficult labor)
- Inherited disorders
  - –Myotonic dystrophy: Progressive muscle weakness, facial paresis at birth
  - –Albers-Schönberg disease: Osteopetrosis increases bone density, compresses nerve
- Developmental abnormalities
  - –Möbius syndrome: Facial paralysis with 6th cranial nerve palsy
  - –Association with coloboma, heart defect, choanal atresia, genital hypoplasia, ear anomalies (CHARGE)
  - –Goldenhar syndrome, also known as oculoauriculovertebral (OAV) syndrome: First and second branchial arch abnormalities
  - –Asymmetric crying facies: Also called congenital unilateral lower lip palsy (CULLP)

Workup and Diagnosis

- History
  - –Age of onset, rapid vs slow time-course, duration
  - –Prior episodes, trauma, neurologic disorders, ear disease
- Physical exam
  - –Facial movement (e.g., while laughing, crying)
  - –Facial symmetry at rest
  - –Eye closure
  - –Tear production, tongue papillae atrophy
- Audiologic testing
  - –Type of hearing loss predicts site of lesion (SNHL: internal auditory canal or CNS; CHL: middle ear)
- Imaging studies
  - –CT best for detecting pathology within temporal bone
  - –MRI with gadolinium: Inflammation of nerve seen as enhancement on scan; predicts poorer outcome
- Electrical testing
  - –Objective means of monitoring function
  - –Evoked electromyography (EEMG; electrically records muscle compound action potential; below 10% of normal side [i.e., 90% degeneration] predicts poor recovery; test must be done during first few days of paralysis)
  - –Electromyography (EMG): Voluntary action potentials predict excellent prognosis; fibrillation potentials predict poor prognosis; polyphasic voluntary action potentials indicate reinnervation; test most useful weeks after injury

Treatment

- Treat underlying cause, if identified
  - –E.g., tympanomastoidectomy for cholesteatoma, resection or chemoradiation for malignancy
- Psychological counseling when studies indicate expected poor prognosis
- Eye care
  - –Prevent exposure and drying of eye: Artificial tears, lubricating ointment, and moisture chamber at night
  - –Ophthalmologic exam to rule out exposure keratitis
  - –Surgical correction: Tarsorrhaphy, upper lid gold weight or spring placement
- Pharmacologic
  - –Steroids: Recommended, but exact benefit unclear
  - –Acyclovir: Suspected viral etiology of Bell palsy
- Surgery
  - –Facial nerve decompression
  - –Facial reanimation procedures (nerve and/or muscle grafting and/or transpositions)

25. Headache

By age 7, 40% of children will have experienced headaches. By age 15, this figure rises to 75%. Headache can be the presenting symptom of a neurologic emergency such as subarachnoid hemorrhage, or of a chronic and common disease such as migraine. The pattern of onset, duration, and recurrence help to diagnose the type and etiology of headaches.

Differential Diagnosis

- Migraine
  - –Recurring headache with throbbing, pulsating pain; nausea and vomiting; photophobia, phonophobia
  - –Family history of migraine
  - –Improvement with rest/sleep
  - –Without aura (common migraine) 85%
  - –With aura (classic migraine) 15%
  - –Frequently bilateral pain in children
  - –Aura usually develops over 5 minutes and is most commonly visual
  - –Migraine is an episodic disorder
  - –Chronic daily headache is not migraine
- Tension headache
- Pseudotumor cerebri
  - –Elevated ICP with no masses or abnormalities in CSF or labs
- Cluster headache
  - –Unilateral nonthrobbing, periorbital pain
  - –May have ipsilateral conjectival injection, lacrimation, rhinorrhea
- Subarachnoid hemorrhage
  - –Sudden paroxysmal headache
  - –Meningeal signs
  - –An emergency requiring CT and LP
- Increased intracranial pressure
  - –Tumor, abscess, hydrocephalus, hemorrhage
- Sinusitis, otitis
- Dental disease
- Systemic infection
- TMJ disease
- Postconcussive syndrome
- Trigeminal neuralgia
- Mitochondrial disorders
- Venous sinus thrombosis
- Meningitis/encephalitis
- CSF leak, post-lumbar puncture
- Hypertensive crisis
- Trauma
- Arteriovenous malformation
- Stroke
- Toxins and medication
  - –Nitrites, cocaine, interferon, CO
- Fever
- Anemia

Workup and Diagnosis

- History
  - –Duration (recurrent, progressive), frequency
  - –Time of onset and duration
  - –Location and nature of pain, warning (aura)
  - –Factors that alleviate or exacerbate symptoms (e.g., stress)
  - –Nausea, vomiting, photophobia, phonophobia
  - –Family history, response to treatment
- Physical exam
  - –Vital signs (temperature, blood pressure)
  - –Height, weight, head circumference
  - –Funduscopy (to rule out papilledema)
- Neuroimaging (CT, MRI) is required for certain symptoms
  - –Short history of headache (<6 months) or age <5–6 years
  - –Worsening headaches, no response to treatment
  - –Deterioration in cognitive or motor function
  - –Short stature, macrocephaly
  - –Awakening at night or early morning
  - –Repeated morning vomiting
  - –Exacerbation by position change or cough
  - –Focal neurologic symptoms during headache
  - –Cluster headache in prepubertal children and adolescent girls
  - –Systemic symptoms: Fatigue, weight loss
  - –Abnormal neurological exam
- Lumbar puncture with opening pressure
  - –Subarachnoid hemorrhage, pseudotumor, or meningitis

Treatment

- Explanation and reassurance alone may provide relief
- Avoid triggers
  - –Trauma, sunlight, insomnia, stress, diet, dehydration
- Symptomatic treatment:
  - –Acetominophen, NSAIDs, Midrin, Fioricet, Fiorinal
  - –Selective serotonin-1 receptor agonists
  - –Dihydroergotamine (DHE); Migranal nasal spray
  - –Antiemetics
- Prophylaxis
  - –NSAIDs, β-blockers, tricyclic antidepressants, cyproheptadine, calcium channel blockers, antiepileptic drugs, biofeedback
- Cluster headaches
  - –Treated with inhalation of oxygen; sumatriptan
- Pseudotumor
  - –Weight reduction, Diamox
  - –Optic nerve sheath decompression or shunting

26. Increased Intracranial Pressure

Normal intracranial pressure (ICP) is 5–20 cm H_2O. Any addition of volume to the contents of the cranium can potentially elevate the ICP. Elevated ICP can lead to brain damage by either mechanical compression/herniation of the brain or by decreasing cerebral perfusion pressure (CPP) and cerebral blood flow.

Differential Diagnosis

- Hydrocephalus
  - –Due to either increased production or decreased absorption (more likely) of CSF
- Communicating hydrocephalus
  - –Post-hemorrhage
  - –Postinfectious
  - –Choroid plexus papilloma
  - –Vein of Galen aneurysm
- Noncommunicating hydrocephalus
  - –Arnold-Chiari malformation
  - –Aqueductal stenosis
  - –Mass lesion
  - –Ependymoma, astrocytomas
  - –Abscess
  - –Intraventricular hemorrhage, subarachnoid hemorrhage
- Hypoxic ischemic encephalopathy
- Head trauma
- Pseudotumor cerebri (benign intracranial hypertension) due to hypervitaminosis A; steroid withdrawal or administration; tetracycline; oral contraceptive pills; or idiopathic
- Systemic infections
  - –Roseola
  - –*Shigella*
  - –Otitis media
- Meningitis/encephalitis
- Neoplasm
- Intracranial hemorrhage: Subdural hematoma, epidural hematoma, intraventricular hemorrhage
- Metabolic causes: DKA, hepatic encephalopathy, uremia, MSUD, urea cycle defects
- Endocrine
  - –Addison disease, hypoparathyroidism, hypothyroidism
- Abscess
- Venous sinus thrombosis
- Congestive heart failure
- Obstructed venous return
- Lead encephalopathy
- Status epilepticus
- Stroke
- Acute hyponatremia
- Reye syndrome

Workup and Diagnosis

- History
  - –History of trauma, seizures, vomiting
  - –Double or blurry vision
  - –Diabetes; cardiac, liver, or renal disease
  - –Birth history
  - –Fever, neck stiffness, headache
  - –Recent use of aspirin, antibiotics, steroids, vitamin A
- Physical exam
  - –Vital signs, temperature, ABCs
  - –Breathing pattern (Cheyne-Stokes, apneustic, ataxic)
  - –Retinal hemorrhages, otorrhea, spinal fluid rhinorrhea
  - –Cardiac exam, hepatosplenomegaly, meningismus
  - –Neuro exam: Response to voice and noxious stimulation, papilledema, pupillary size and light reflex, eye movements (spontaneous, doll's, caloric), corneal and gag reflexes, motor response to pain, decerebrate or decorticate posturing, muscle tone, DTRs, Babinski sign
  - –Signs of herniation: Change in respiratory pattern, unilateral dilatation of pupil, ptosis, decreased heart rate, increased blood pressure
- Labs
  - –Glucose, electrolytes, ABG, LFT, ammonia, BUN, creatinine, type and cross
- CT without contrast should be performed immediately
- LP for meningitis or subarachnoid hemorrhage
  - –Contraindicated if signs of herniation or mass lesion
- C-spine X-rays if there is history of trauma

Treatment

- Highly elevated ICP can be rapidly fatal
  - –First ABCs, look for signs of herniation
  - –Obtain intravenous access
- Keep head of the bed elevated at 15–30°
  - –Intubate and hyperventilate
  - –IV mannitol with or without furosemide
- If comatose, ICP monitoring is indicated
  - –CPP is defined as mean arterial pressure minus ICP
  - –CPP should be kept above 70 mmHg
- Vasogenic edema (e.g., neoplasm or abscess)
  - –Use dexamethasone
- IV fluids
  - –Use isotonic fluids (normal saline)
- Treat fever aggressively
  - –Temperature elevations can increase ICP further
- Seizure prophylaxis should be considered
  - –High-dose pentobarbital lowers refractory ICP
- Pseudotumor
  - –Treat with serial LP, diuretics, or surgery

27. Macrocephaly

Macrocephaly is defined as head circumference 2 standard deviations (SD) larger than the mean for age. This situation may arise from the size of the brain or other contents of the skull, such as CSF, blood, or bone. Accelerated head circumference growth, usually associated with increased intracranial pressure, needs to be investigated expeditiously.

Differential Diagnosis

- Communicating hydrocephalus
  - –Benign
  - –Post-hemorrhage
  - –Postinfectious
  - –Choroid plexus papilloma
  - –Vein of Galen aneurysm
- Noncommunicating hydrocephalus
  - –Arnold-Chiari malformation
  - –Aqueductal stenosis
  - –Mass lesion
    - –Primitive neuroectodermal tumor
    - –Ependymoma
    - –Astrocytoma
  - –Abscess
  - –Hemorrhage
    - –Intraventricular
  - –Subarachnoid
- Increased brain size
  - –Familial
  - –Sotos syndrome
  - –Neurofibromatosis type I (NF1)
  - –Tuberous sclerosis (TS)
  - –Incontinentia pigmenti
  - –Globoid cell leukodystrophy (Krabbe)
  - –Alexander disease
  - –Canavan disease
  - –Maple syrup urine disease
  - –Tay-Sachs disease
  - –Glutaric aciduria type II
  - –Hurler syndrome
- Increased bone
  - –Anemia
  - –Hyperphosphatemia
  - –Rickets
  - –Osteogenesis imperfecta
- Neoplasm

Workup and Diagnosis

- Confirm and plot head circumference (HC)
- History
  - –Signs of neurologic dysfunction
  - –Headache
  - –Developmental delay
  - –Paroxysmal movements
  - –Prenatal/birth history (gestational age, weight, HC)
  - –Family history of macrocephaly
- Physical exam
  - –Measure the parents' HC and plot it on chart
  - –Obtain previous HC measurements
  - –Acceleration of head growth is a more ominous sign than stably growing large head
  - –Tension of the fontanelle while the child is sitting up
  - –Skin exam looking for café au lait spots (in NF), hypomelanotic macules, Shagreen patches (in TS)
  - –Eye exam for a cherry red spot (in Tay-Sachs)
  - –Funduscopic exam may indicate increased intracranial pressure (e.g., papilledema, loss of venous pulse)
- Neuroimaging
  - –CT or even head US in younger child with open fontanelle for hydrocephalus
  - –MRI for evaluating the white matter in diagnosing leukodystrophies such as Krabbe as well as defining brainstem abnormalities such as aqueductal stenosis or Arnold-Chiari malformation

Treatment

- For hydrocephalus, surgical intervention is necessary
  - –Ventriculoperitoneal shunt
  - –Ventriculoatrial shunt
- For post-hemorrhagic hydrocephalus
  - –Commonly seen in premature infants
  - –Serial lumbar punctures to delay shunt placement
  - –Hydrocephalus resolves spontaneously in the majority
- Other causes of syndromic or nonsyndromic macrocephaly
  - –Currently there are no curative treatments
  - –Management involves addressing the neurologic symptoms
  - –Anticipatory guidance to the caregivers

28. Microcephaly

Microcephaly is defined as head circumference 2 standard deviations (SD) below the mean for age. Most questions about microcephaly arise within the first 2 years of life. Using neurologic and developmental assessments as guides, one can classify microcephaly as benign or pathologic.

Differential Diagnosis

- Benign familial
- Hypoxic ishemic encephalopathy
- Intrauterine infection (TORCH)
- Teratogens
  - –Ethanol
  - –Cocaine
  - –Isotretinoin
  - –Phenytoin
- Down syndrome
- Trisomy 13
- Trisomy 18
- Lissencephaly
- Holoprosencephaly
- Anencephaly
- Porencephaly
- Intrauterine stroke
- Malnutrition
  - –Typically preceded by decreased weight and height velocities
- Growth hormone deficiency
- Thyroid hormone deficiency
- Panhypopituitary
- Chromosomal deletions
- Smith-Lemli-Opitz syndrome (SLO)
- Menkes syndrome (kinky hair disease)
- Neuronal ceroid-lipofuscinosis
- Rett syndrome
  - –Normal head circumference at birth
  - –Acquired microcephaly after 6 months
- Incontinentia pigmenti
- Alper disease
- Phenylketonuria (PKU)
- Pelizaeus-Merzbacher
- Cri-du-chat syndrome
- Cornelia de Lange syndrome

Workup and Diagnosis

- Confirm and plot head circumference (HC)
- History
  - –Signs of neurologic dysfunction
  - –Developmental delay, paroxysmal movements
  - –Early hand preference
  - –Prenatal/birth history (gestational age, weight, HC)
  - –Family history of microcephaly
- Physical exam
  - –Measure parents' HC and plot it on the chart
  - –Obtain previous HC measurements
  - –Deceleration of head growth is a more ominous sign than stably growing small head
  - –Plot weight and height; hormonal deficiency and malnutrition affect these parameters as well as HC
  - –Skin, eye (looking for TORCH, chorioretinitis infections), dysmorphic features, fontanelle size, hepatosplenomegaly
  - –Neurological and developmental assessment (differential diagnosis is dependent on normal vs. delayed)
- Labs
  - –TORCH titers, thyroid/GH levels, LFT
  - –Chromosomes, 7-dehydrocholesterol (high in SLO)
  - –Genetic testing for MECP-2, proteolipid protein
  - –Amino acids, copper (low in Menkes)
- Neuroimaging
  - –MRI is essential in diagnosis of structural abnormalities of the microcephalic brain

Treatment

- Hormonal deficiency
  - –Treat with hormonal supplements immediately
- Smith-Lemli-Opitz
  - –Cholesterol supplementation helps with affect
- PKU
  - –Treat by dietary restriction of phenylalanine
- Menkes syndrome
  - –Treat with copper supplementation
- Other causes of syndromic or nonsyndromic microcephaly
  - –Most cannot be treated
  - –Management involves addressing neurologic symptoms
  - –Anticipatory guidance to the caregivers

Eyes

Section 5

LARRY J. ALEXANDER, OD, FAAO
KATHLEEN O. DeANTONIS, MD
ASIM R. PIRACHA, MD

29. Diplopia

Diplopia of sudden onset is more related to neurologic disease than to ocular disease. Other than space-occupying orbital lesions, most diplopia can be related to a neurologic disorder. The first causes that should come to mind are undiagnosed or poorly controlled diabetes and myasthenia gravis. A good general rule is to assume neurologic disease until proven otherwise.

Differential Diagnosis

- Monocular diplopia
  - –Rare, usually associated with the cornea, lens, vitreous, or refractive anomalies such as high uncorrected astigmatism
  - –May occur in lens implant dislocation
  - –Neurologic disorders may present as monocular diplopia with repetitive images
- Binocular, decompensated phoria with concomitant strabismus, nonpathologic
  - –Recent ocular surgery
  - –Ocular myasthenia (may be transient)
- Binocular with proptosis, gaze restriction
  - –Thyroid disease, orbital pseudotumor, cavernous sinus thrombosis or fistula
- Binocular with isolated third nerve
  - –Atherosclerosis, hypertension, diabetes, tumor, aneurysm
- Binocular with isolated sixth nerve
  - –Trauma, atherosclerosis, hypertension, diabetes, tumor, increased intracranial pressure, sinus disease
- Binocular with isolated fourth nerve
  - –Trauma, stroke, thyroid eye disease, atherosclerosis, hypertension, diabetes
- Binocular with multiple muscle weakness in one eye
  - –Cavernous sinus lesion
- Binocular with multiple muscle weakness in both eyes
  - –Progressive supranuclear palsy, CPEO, acute postinfectious disorders
- Adduction weakness or abducting nystagmus
  - –Inner nuclear ophthalmolplegia (INO), brainstem disease, stroke, MS, posterior fossa mass
- Vertical diplopia with no fourth or third palsy
  - –Stroke, multiple sclerosis, posterior fossa mass

Workup and Diagnosis

- History
  - –Temporal history of the symptoms, including past incidences and transience of defect
  - –Establish whether monocular (one eye covered) or binocular (both eyes open)
  - –History of recent trauma or ocular surgery
  - –Status of known systemic diseases, e.g., hypertension, diabetes, thyroid disease
- Physical exam
  - –Obtain visual acuity and confrontation visual fields
  - –Pupillary evaluation
  - –Observe for head tilt or torsion
  - –Observe for proptosis
  - –Extraocular muscle evaluation to isolate affected muscle
  - –Observe for other neurologic signs or symptoms
  - –Perform a dilated fundus evaluation to rule out associated retinal and/or optic nerve disorders
  - –Perform Tensilon test for myasthenia
- Workup for medical issues such as diabetes, hypertension, atherosclerosis, stroke, thyroid disease
- Workup with imaging for MS, orbital and intracranial tumor, aneurysm, orbital pseudotumor, cavernous sinus lesions
- Neurologic or neuro-ophthalmological consultation is in order

Treatment

- If monocular, first consider a refractive cause or an ocular media compromise
- If binocular, critical to find the underlying cause
- Assess control of diabetes and other systemic concerns and remedy
- If diagnosis of myasthenia, manage systemically with Mestinon
- Neurologic or neurosurgical intervention may be necessary depending on cause
- Relatively benign causes resolve on their own in 3 months, but patching or prism in glasses may be necessary
- Prism in glasses or interventive strabismus surgery may be necessary in recalcitrant cases

30. Eye Discharge

The most common cause of eye discharge in pediatric patients is viral conjunctivitis. Many clinicians treat viral conjunctivitis as bacterial conjunctivitis because the similarities in history and physical examination make a definitive diagnosis difficult without a culture, which is expensive and may take 2–3 days. Additionally, small children frequently acquire superinfection and contagion by repeated rubbing of the eyes, justifying antibiotic prophylaxis.

Differential Diagnosis

- Blocked tear duct (nasolacrimal duct stenosis)
  - Occurs in 5–10% of normal newborns
  - Tearing and mucus discharge secreted to lubricate the eye accumulate at the medial canthus because it cannot drain through the fused nasolacrimal duct
  - Frequently the discharge is mistaken for pus; also superinfection and conjunctivitis may occur
- Allergic conjunctivitis
  - Mucoid discharge, injection, and pruritus are the typical symptoms
  - Symptoms may be seasonal or perennial, depending on the allergy (ragweed vs dust)
  - Patients frequently have a history of other atopic disease (e.g., allergic rhinitis, asthma, or eczema)
- Viral conjunctivitis
  - Adenovirus: Frequently associated with fever and pharyngitis, very contagious, and may have preauricular nodes
  - Human herpesvirus: HSV1 may cause conjunctivitis, frequently accompanied by herpetic lesions on the face
- Bacterial conjunctivitis
  - *Staphylococcus aureus*
  - *Haemophilus influenzae* (non-typable): May cause simultaneous otitis, should be treated for penicillin-resistant organisms
  - *Chlamydia trachomatis* and *Neisseria gonorrhoeae* (newborn): Suspect in an infant of a mother with a history of inadequate prenatal care or any sexually transmitted disease; physical signs are usually impressive; *C. trachomatis* may also cause pneumonia; must be treated systemically
- Foreign body
  - Patient usually relates a history consistent with FB
- Corneal abrasion
  - May manifest as an FB sensation
- Glaucoma
  - May be congenital, acquired, or syndrome-associated; in young children it presents with tearing, progressive enlargement of the eye, and corneal changes

Workup and Diagnosis

- History
  - Onset, duration, character, unilateral or bilateral
  - Painful or painless
  - Presence or absence of FB sensation (corneal abrasion or actual foreign body)
  - Presence or absence of pruritus
  - Presence or absence of allergic/atopic symptoms
  - History of contact with person with eye discharge
  - History of trauma to the eye
- Physical exam
  - Inspection of the sclera, conjunctiva, lids, and lashes
  - Erythema, edema, and injection may occur with allergy, infection, FB, or trauma
  - Bacterial infections are associated with systemic symptoms such as fever, are more likely to be unilateral, and have purulent discharge
  - Viral infections are more likely to be bilateral, have more mucoid discharge, and the conjunctiva may have a granular appearance
  - Fluorescein examination for corneal abrasion or FB
  - Herpetic lesions have a spidery appearance
  - Slit-lamp examination to detect changes consistent with uveitis/iritis
- Studies
  - MRI may be indicated for suspected FB; however, it is contraindicated if FB may be metallic

Treatment

- Blocked tear duct: Supportive care with massage and warm compresses; surgical probe or stent may be indicated if stenosis persists beyond 9 months of age
- Allergic conjunctivitis: Intraocular anti-inflammatory agents, antihistamines, or mast cell stabilizers
- Viral conjunctivitis: Supportive care for most routine viral infections; herpetic lesions should be referred to an ophthalmologist and must be treated with systemic acyclovir and intraocular steroids
- Bacterial conjunctivitis: Usual pathogens are susceptible to polysporin/trimethoprim, may also be treated with quinolones; newborn STD pathogens must be treated systemically
- Foreign body: Removal may require referral to an ophthalmologist
- Corneal abrasion: Routine antibiotics and patching are no longer recommended, but may be used in more severe cases

31. Flashes of Light & Floaters

Flashes of light and floaters may be the presentation in a number of ocular and neurologic disorders. The most frequently encountered presentation of flashes of light is associated with migraine disorders. Flashes with floaters usually indicate a vitreoretinal traction disorder that may lead to retinal detachment.

Differential Diagnosis

- Migraine
  - –Migraine variants may cause visual phenomena such as flashes of light
  - –Flashes are usually in the form of jagged lines called fortifications
  - –In most instances, the flashes are followed by some form of headache
- Cerebral disorders
  - –Variations of TIAs may also present as balls or flashes of light
  - –Formed hallucinations often manifest as flashes
- Retinal damage
  - –Retinal breaks may lead to retinal detachment and may manifest as variable flashes of light
  - –Floating objects are almost always seen
  - –Usually described as resembling gnats; represent liberated red blood cells and/or retinal pigment epithelial cells
- Posterior vitreous separation or detachment (PVD)
  - –PVD is most frequently associated with age but may present with trauma
  - –Patients describe a spider web or tailed floater that may have been associated with a lightning-type flash of light off to one side
  - –PVDs may be isolated or associated with a retinal break
- Hypoxic states
  - –Retinal neovascularization liberates red blood cells into the vitreous
  - –Occurs with diabetic retinopathy, prematurity, and sickle cell anemia
- Cells in the vitreous
  - –Secondary to a number of different inflammatory ocular conditions manifesting as uveitis
  - –Cells escaping from intraocular neoplasm or intraocular retinal vascular tumors

Workup and Diagnosis

- History
  - –Onset, duration, description
  - –History of trauma near the head and/or eyes
  - –Associated symptoms such as headache, ocular pain, photophobia
  - –PMH-known systemic diseases (e.g., hypertension, diabetes, thyroid disease)
- Physical exam
  - –Mental status (possibility of hallucinations or TIA)
  - –Visual acuity and confrontation visual fields
  - –Perform pupillary evaluation
  - –Perform extraocular muscle evaluation
- Dilated retinal/funduscopic evaluation
  - –Usually performed by an ophthalmologist
  - –Indicated if redness, pain, and photophobia are present, to rule out uveitis
  - –Indicated stat (with either binocular indirect ophthalmoscopy and/or three-mirror fundus lens evaluation) to rule out a retinal tear
  - –Indicated with history consistent with retinal neovascularization (vitreous hemorrhage may be subtle or poorly visualized at the periphery)
- CT or MRI to rule out intraocular neoplasia

Treatment

- Migraines
  - –Acute treatment: NSAIDs, analgesics, serotonin agonists, ergotamines
  - –Chronic therapy: β-blockers, calcium channel blockers, tricyclic antidepressants
- Posterior vitreous detachment: Education and follow-up visits to ensure that retinal breaks do not develop
- Retinal tear and/or detachment: Education and urgent retinal consultation for laser/cryopexy/retinal reattachment
- Retinal neovascularization: Usually necessitates laser photocoagulation and often vitrectomy to evacuate the vitreous hemorrhage to save vision
- Uveitis
  - –Requires topical, subconjunctival, or intravitreal steroid treatment, as well as a comprehensive workup for cause
  - –May require systemic immunosuppressive treatment

32. Leukocoria

The red light reflex is an important part of the physical exam in all ages, especially infants and young children who are preverbal and cannot report visual problems or changes. Leukocoria is defined as a white pupillary reflex in childhood. The examination is performed by inspecting the pupil with an ophthalmoscope at a distance of about a foot. A normal appearance is a shiny reddish-orange; white, cloudy, or cottony is abnormal. Any abnormality necessitates a rapid and complete evaluation.

Differential Diagnosis

- Retinoblastoma
  - –Malignant tumor of retina (most common pediatric ocular tumor)
  - –Bilateral in 1/3 of cases
  - –Peak age 12–24 months, 90% occur before age 5 years
  - –Presents with leukocoria (most common sign), strabismus, ocular asymmetry
  - –Associated with gene mutation on chromosome 13; may be inherited or spontaneous
- Congenital cataract
  - –May be unilateral or bilateral
  - –Strabismus or nystagmus is common
  - –May be familial (AD, AR, or XL)
  - –Associated with galactosemia, homocystinemia, Fabry, Wilson, and Niemann-Pick diseases
  - –Syndromes with cataracts are Lowe, Alport, Apert, Crouzon, and Marfan
  - –Congenital infections causing cataracts are rubella, rubeola, toxoplasmosis, cytomegalovirus, syphilis, influenza, and varicella
- Toxocariasis (*Toxocara canis*)
  - –A nematode infection of the eye and viscera
  - –The usual sources are household dogs and cats, particularly puppies
  - –Patients are usually aged 1–10 years
- Retinopathy of prematurity (ROP)
  - –Risk factors are gestational age <32 weeks, birth weight <1,500 g, prolonged oxygen requirement
- Coat disease
  - –Retinal vascular abnormality (telangiectasia)
  - –Seen in boys > girls, generally unilateral
- Persistent hyperplastic primary vitreous (PHPV)
  - –Rare developmental ocular abnormality
  - –Usually congenital, unilateral in 90%
  - –Associated with microphthalmos
- Retinal detachment
  - –Occurs with Coat disease, ROP, trauma, toxocariasis, retinoblastoma
- Coloboma
  - –An embryonic malformation of choroidal fissure

Workup and Diagnosis

- History
  - –Any abnormalities noticed by caregivers
  - –Prenatal and birth history (infections, exposure to animals, prematurity)
  - –Family history of retinoblastoma, metabolic disorders, infant deaths, syndromes
  - –History of exposure to dogs, cats
- Physical exam
  - –Comprehensive eye exam: Vision, visual fields, extraocular movements, proptosis, pupillary response, funduscopic exam
  - –Growth parameters
  - –Other anomalies that may be syndrome-associated
- Ophthalmology consultation
  - –Complete dilated retinal examination
  - –Examination under anesthesia
- Labs
  - –Titers for congenital infections
  - –ELISA (*Toxocara*)
  - –Genetic testing for chromosomal abnormalities
- Studies
  - –CT of head, orbits (retinoblastoma)
  - –CXR, abdominal CT for suspected toxocariasis

Treatment

- Ophthalmology consultation for evaluation and management
- Early intervention to prevent amblyopia
- Retinoblastoma
  - –Radiation, photocoagulation, cryotherapy, chemoreduction, chemothermotherapy
  - –Enucleation is recommended when there is no chance of preserving useful vision
- Toxocariasis: Steroids and photocoagulation
- Retinopathy of prematurity: Photocoagulation or cryotherapy
- Coat disease: Photocoagulation or cryotherapy
- PHPV and congenital cataracts: Surgical intervention (as soon as possible to prevent amblyopia)
- ID and genetics consultation as appropriate

33. Nystagmus

Nystagmus is defined as involuntary rhythmic oscillations of the eyes. The finding is usually bilateral, and the abnormal movements occur identically in both eyes. Ophthalmologists distinguish between types of nystagmus by the direction of the eye movements; they may be rotatory, horizontal or vertical, or jerky and are described in the direction of fast phase and slow phase of the eye movements.

Differential Diagnosis

- Nystagmus occurs at the extreme lateral gaze in many normal individuals
  - May also occur when tracking an object or row of objects horizontally
  - Can be induced by rotatory visual stimuli or otic irrigation (vestibular stimuli) in normal individuals
- Hereditary nystagmus
  - Benign condition of horizontal nystagmus
  - May not be accompanied by other neurologic findings, but involuntary head-bobbing may be a feature
  - May be XL or AD
- Visual impairment
  - Poor vision, ocular blindness, and cortical blindness can result in nystagmus
  - May also have "searching" eye movements that are not true nystagmus
  - Both are more likely to occur in patients born blind or blind from an early age
- Spasmus mutans
  - May be isolated or associated with intracranial mass
  - Characterized by nystagmus, involuntary head-bobbing, and torticollis
- Congenital jerking nystagmus
  - Idiopathic; horizontal nystagmus with lateral gaze on one direction
- Intracranial neoplasms
- Arnold-Chiari malformation
- Cerebellar etiologies
  - Acute cerebellar ataxia
  - Encephalitis or abscess involving the cerebellum
- Septo-optic dysplasia
  - Optic nerve hypoplasia, associated with other midline brain defects
  - Endocrine abnormalities are common (diabetes insipidus, hypoglycemia, hypopituitarism, failure to thrive)
- Toxicity
  - Medications include barbiturates, hydantoin, antihistamines, and salicylates
  - Lead toxicity
  - Alcohol intoxication may involve vestibular disturbances including vertigo, nystagmus
- Opsoclonus
  - Not true nystagmus
  - Eye movements that may be mistaken for nystagmus (e.g., opsoclonus-myoclonus disorder)

Workup and Diagnosis

- History
  - Onset, duration, progression
  - Accompanying signs and symptoms, including symptoms of intracranial space-occupying lesion such as headache and vomiting
  - Family history
  - Birth and past medical history
- Physical exam
  - Characterization of the eye movements that elicit nystagmus, the severity, and the type of eye movements
  - Visual acuity in each eye
  - Funduscopic examination for papilledema
  - Extraocular muscle evaluation
  - Pupillary red light reflex: White in retinoblastoma
  - Preferred head position: Patients with congenital jerking nystagmus frequently turn their faces in such a way as to minimize nystagmus
  - Positional test for benign paroxysmal vertigo
  - Head circumference (hydrocephalus)
  - Neurologic examination including cranial nerves and cerebellar signs
- Labs
  - Toxicology screen and medication levels as applicable
- Studies
  - Imaging of the brain may be required to rule out malignancy, mass, midline defects

Treatment

- Normal and hereditary nystagmus do not require treatment, only reassurance
- Visual impairment: Nystagmus is diminished with optimization of visual acuity
- Spasmus mutans does not itself require treatment; evaluation for intracranial mass is essential
- Arnold-Chiari malformation: Surgical correction
- Acute cerebellar ataxia: Ataxia, nystagmus, and vomiting follow a viral illness; may represent an autoimmune response; slow spontaneous recovery is the norm, some patients have neurologic sequelae
- Septo-optic dysplasia: Nystagmus is not treatable; patients require support for associated disease
- Toxicity: Adjustment of medication levels, lead decontamination, avoidance of alcohol

34. Papilledema (Optic Disc Swelling)

True optic disc swelling or edema can be a very ominous sign. Papilledema is defined as disc swelling produced by increased ICP; it may be asymmetric, UL, or BL. Acutely, the vision, color vision, and pupillary responses are normal, but the blind spot is increased on visual field testing. Chronic forms lead to loss of vision and loss of visual fields. Fortunately, most perceived optic disc swelling is a manifestation of a congenital optic disc variation.

Differential Diagnosis

- Pseudotumor cerebri
  - –Other symptoms: Headache, nausea, and vomiting all worse in morning, transient visual obscurations, diplopia
  - –Diagnosis includes increased ICP, normal imaging, normal CSF
  - –More common in obese females
- Optic neuritis
  - –May be associated with postviral syndromes or meningoencephalitis
  - –Loss of vision, pain on eye movement
  - –Vision usually improves within a few weeks, but not full recovery
- Optic neuropathy
  - –Compressive: Associated with NF1 and optic nerve glioma, presents with progressive visual loss, strabismus, nystagmus, proptosis
  - –Infiltrative: From cancers (leukemias, lymphomas), infection, or inflammation (sarcoidosis, TB, toxocariasis, toxoplasmosis, CMV); optic disc swelling, vision loss, and hemorrhages
  - –Toxic/nutritional optic neuropathy: Symmetric neuropathy from nutritional deficiency (thiamine, B12), drugs (tobacco/alcohol, chloramphenicol, rifampin), toxins (lead, methanol); visual field and vision loss; may recover with treatment
  - –Leber optic neuropathy: Mitochondrial DNA transmission, presents late teens to middle 20s; visual field and vision loss, may spontaneously improve
- Increased ICP: Idiopathic intracranial hypertension, intracranial hemorrhage, space-occupying lesion
- Growth hormone supplementation
- Retinal hemorrhage and loss of vision
- Retinal vein occlusion
- Malignant hypertension: Associated with retinal hemorrhage, exudates, and cotton wool spots
- Optic neuropathy, nonarteritic or arteritic
- Demyelinating disease
- Infectious conditions: Toxoplasmosis, Lyme disease, *Bartonella*; hard exudates may be visible funduscopically

Workup and Diagnosis

- History
  - –History of HA, nausea or vomiting, recent viral illness
  - –Family history of visual loss, neurologic disorder
  - –PMH or signs and symptoms consistent with known systemic diseases; e.g., hypertension, diabetes, thyroid disease, growth hormone therapy
  - –Nutritional deficiencies; exposure to toxins such as tobacco or alcohol; recent drug use; exposure to ticks and animals
- Physical exam
  - –Visual acuity, confrontational visual fields, pupillary response, extraocular muscle movements, proptosis
  - –Dilated fundus evaluation
  - –Neurologic exam for signs and symptoms of demyelinating disease, localizing deficit
- Labs
  - –Titers for CMV, Lyme, toxocariasis, toxoplasmosis
- Radiology
  - –CT or MRI of the brain and orbits for suspicion of intracranial mass, mass effect or hemorrhage
- Studies
  - –Lumbar puncture may be indicated to establish presence or absence of, or to relieve, increased intracranial pressure
- Ophthalmologic consultation to rule out congenital variation to avoid unnecessary and expensive differential testing

Treatment

- Condition-dependent: Treatment of underlying systemic disease is often the only treatment
- Pseudotumor cerebri and other causes of intracranial hypertension: Weight loss, Diamox or Lasix, planned recumbency, LP shunt or optic nerve sheath fenestration if loss of visual function
- Space-occupying lesion or hemorrhage: Neurosurgical intervention
- Meningoencephalitis: IV antibiotics
- Infectious optic neuropathy: Treat underlying cause and consider systemic steroids (controversial)
- Optic neuritis: IV (not oral) steroids
- Optic nerve glioma treatment controversial: Observation if slowly progressive, resection if only one nerve involved, radiation if chiasm involved, shunts if increased ICP
- Toxic or nutritional: Stop offending toxin or supply nutritional supplementation

35. Periorbital Edema

Periorbital edema is frequently reported by parents via telephone. Unless the cause is obvious and benign, an immediate evaluation is warranted.

Differential Diagnosis

- Periorbital cellulitis
  - –Also described as preseptal cellulitis (infection is anterior to the orbital septum and thus does not affect the orbit or globe)
  - –Usual pathogens are streptococcal species, *Staphylococcus aureus*, and *Haemophilus influenzae*
- Orbital cellulitis
  - –Also described as postseptal and affects the preseptal structures as well as the extraocular muscles and the optic nerve
  - –Bacterial pathogens are the same as periorbital cellulitis and may reflect direct spread
  - –May be accompanied by orbital abscess and may spread via the sinuses to the brain
- Other infections
  - –Conjunctivitis
  - –Sinusitis
  - –Dental abscess
- Allergic reaction
  - –Conjunctivitis
  - –Urticaria/angioedema
  - –Drug reaction
- Local ocular causes
  - –Insect bites
  - –Contact dermatitis
  - –Trauma
  - –Foreign body
- Systemic disorders with generalized edema
  - –Hypoproteinemia
  - –Renal disease
  - –Congestive heart failure
- Malignancy
  - –Neuroblastomas: Associated with ecchymoses, "raccoon eyes," and proptosis
  - –Leukemia: Associated with fever, fatigue, anemia, bone pain, lymphadenopathy, splenomegaly

Workup and Diagnosis

- History
  - –Onset, duration, progression of symptoms
  - –Presence of pain or pruritus
  - –History of trauma
  - -Systemic symptoms such as fever
- Physical exam
  - –Temperature, vital signs, growth parameters
  - –Proptosis
  - –Ocular range of motion
  - –Full physical exam including heart, lung, and extremities
- Labs
  - –Electrolytes, BUN, creatinine
  - –Serum protein and albumin
  - –CBC and blood culture if infection is suspected
  - –ESR, LDH if malignancy is suspected
- Studies
  - –CT to distinguish periorbital cellulitis from orbital cellulitis
  - –CT or MRI to discover orbital or cranial tumors
  - –CXR if CHF is suspected
  - –Renal ultrasound to evaluate the architecture of the kidneys, Doppler to evaluate renal flow, DMSA to evaluate renal parenchyma if edema is generalized

Treatment

- Periorbital and orbital cellulitis are treated with IV antibiotics
- Orbital or subperiosteal abscess accompanying orbital cellulitis must be drained operatively
- Conjunctivitis, sinusitis, and dental abscess can usually be treated with oral antibiotics
- Mild allergic reactions are treated with antihistamines; more severe reactions may require epinephrine and/or systemic steroids
- Renal disease should be referred to a nephrologist for evaluation (frequently involving biopsy) and treatment
- Congestive heart failure is initially treated with diuretics and inotropic agents; pursuit of etiology and definitive treatment usually involves a cardiologist
- Suspected or discovered malignancies must be immediately referred to an oncologist

36. Proptosis/Exophthalmos

Proptosis is a finding that usually signals significant pathology. Regardless of duration of symptoms, a rapid evaluation is necessary to discover and treat malignancy or conditions that will result in visual loss.

Differential Diagnosis

- Orbital cellulitis is associated with ethmoid sinusitis, presents with rapid onset of fever, EOM restriction, periorbital edema
- Malignancy
  - –Rhabdomyosarcoma: Most common primary pediatric orbital malignancy, average age 5–7, proptosis is presenting sign, may develop acutely
  - –Neuroblastoma: One of most common childhood cancers, most frequent source of orbital metastasis, associated with opsoclonus (rapid multidirectional eye movements), periorbital ecchymoses, 40% bilateral
  - –Acute leukemia: Most common childhood malignancy, may cause proptosis, ecchymosis, and lid edema
- Benign tumors
  - –Capillary hemangioma: Most common benign pediatric orbital tumor, females > males, presents in infancy, slowly progressive, increases in size with crying, associated with skin hemangioma, thrombocytopenic purpura
  - –Lymphangioma: Second most common benign pediatric orbital tumor consists of lymph-filled channels, may hemorrhage after minor trauma or URI (chocolate cyst)
- Neurofibromatosis type 1 (NF1)
  - –Optic gliomas: Slowly progressive, associated with decreased vision, optic disc atrophy, and swelling
  - –Orbital and periorbital plexiform neurofibromas; associated with sphenoid bone defects, may be pulsatile
- Hyperthyroidism
  - –Graves disease is the cause of hyperthyroidism most commonly associated with proptosis/exophthalmos
  - –Proptosis may be unilateral or bilateral, and lid retraction is common
- Trauma
  - –Fracture of orbital bones and hemorrhage into the orbital space may cause proptosis, pain, and EOM impairment
- Orbital dermoid cyst
  - –Rupture of cyst causes an inflammatory reaction
- Craniosynostosis (e.g., Apert, Crouzon)

Workup and Diagnosis

- History
  - –Onset, duration, progression, pain
  - –Other ocular symptoms such as vision loss, diplopia
  - –Systemic symptoms such as fever, fatigue
  - –Associated symptoms such as skin rash, birthmarks (e.g., café au lait spots in NF1), tremors, palpitations
  - –History of trauma
  - –Past medical history of CA, thyroid disease, neurocutaneous disorders
- Physical exam
  - –Temperature, vital signs, growth parameters
  - –Doppler studies to evaluate orbital blood flow
  - –Check vision and visual fields
  - –Evaluate pupil function and EOM movement (pain, diplopia, restriction)
  - –Palpate orbital rim for mass
  - –Funduscopic exam including optic nerve and retinal appearance
  - –Physical examination for skin findings, abdominal mass, hepatomegaly, neurological exam
- Labs
  - –TSH, T3, T4
  - –CBC, ESR, LDH, blood cultures
- Studies
  - –CT or MRI to look for masses
  - –Doppler studies to evaluate orbital blood flow
- Biopsy if diagnosis uncertain

Treatment

- Ophthalmology consultation is always warranted
- Daily vision testing and optic nerve function evaluation
- Lubrication for exposure
- Cellulitis: Inpatient admission, drainage of abscess, IV antibiotics, close observation for visual detrioration
- Systemic steroids for thyroid disease, capillary hemangioma
- Orbital decompression if optic nerve compression
- Surgical removal of tumors if appropriate
- Irradiation (Graves disease, lymphoid tumors, lacrimal gland tumors)

37. Ptosis

Ptosis, or lid droop, is a relatively common condition. The majority of cases are congenital. In some cases, ptosis may occur after ocular surgery. All cases of acquired ptosis deserve a careful evaluation because of the potential neurologic implications. Certainly high on the list of possible causes are myasthenia gravis, third nerve palsy, and Horner syndrome. Physical alteration of the lid due to hordeola, chalazia, lid cellulitis, and tumors may present as ptosis.

Differential Diagnosis

- Must differentiate true ptosis from lid retraction, which occurs primarily from chemical stimulation (phenylephrine) or thyroid disease
- Of all cases of ptosis, 60% are believed to be congenital; may be exacerbated with fatigue and age
- Dermatochalasis (drooping tissue) may simulate ptosis
- Lid conditions such as hordeola, chalazia, and lid cellulitis may present as ptosis
- Previous lid or ocular surgery
- Traumatic ptosis
- Marcus Gunn (also called jaw-winking) syndrome
- Myasthenia gravis
- Third nerve palsy from hypertension, diabetes, aneurysm
- Horner syndrome
  - –Sympathetic lesion causing partial ptosis, miosis, and anhidrosis
  - –Caused by tumors, aneurysms, inflammatory processes, injuries, or chest surgery
- Acquired myogenic ptosis from local or diffuse muscular disease, such as muscular dystrophy, chronic progressive external ophthalmoplegia, or oculopharyngeal dystrophy
- Chromosomal disorders
  - –Turner syndrome, trisomy 18, 4p-, 18p-
- Fetal drug exposure
  - –Alcohol, hydantoin, trimethadione
- Inherited syndromes
  - –Noonan, Smith-Lemli-Opitz, Aarskog
- Migraine
- Botulism
- Poisoning
  - –Lead, arsenicals, carbon monoxide
- Thiamine deficiency
- Carnitine deficiency
- Vitamin E deficiency
- Tangier disease
- Hydrocephalus

Workup and Diagnosis

- History
  - –Evaluate status of known systemic diseases
  - –Evaluate for congenital ptosis by checking previous photographs, and/or asking family/friends
  - –PMH/PSH: Previous lid or ocular surgery, trauma to the head or orbital region
- Physical exam
  - –Visual acuity, visual fields, dilated fundus exam
  - –Evaluation for localized lesions of the lid, including hordeola, chalazia, and lid cellulitis
  - –With lid droop and no anisocoria, consider myasthenia, neurological causes
  - –With lid droop and anisocoria (pupil difference) consider Horner with miosis, third nerve with mydriasis
  - –Evidence of third nerve palsy: Fixed, dilated pupil or impaired extraocular muscle movements
  - –Evaluate for anomaly associated with jaw movement, e.g., Marcus Gunn syndrome
- Labs
  - –CBC/differential for suspected Horner syndrome
- Studies
  - –For suspected Horner syndrome, perform CXR, neuroimaging; for third nerve palsy, neuroimaging for aneurysm, tumor, uncal herniation, cavernous sinus lesion, and orbital disease
- Myasthenia may be systemic or ocular and necessitates a Tensilon test for diagnosis

Treatment

- Congenital ptosis may be repaired through oculoplastic surgery
- Dermatochalasis may be corrected through oculoplastic surgery
- Hordeola may be resolved by hot compresses, oral antibiotics, supplemented by topical antibiotics as needed
- Chalazia may be addressed with hot compresses but usually require excision
- Lid cellulitis must be treated aggressively with oral antibiotics
- Appropriate neurosurgical or systemic intervention
- Oculoplastic surgery for recalcitrant cases
- Treatment of any underlying disease

38. Retinal Hemorrhage

Hemorrhages in the retina represent a broad range of ocular manifestations of systemic disease and/or trauma. The most important diagnosis to discover is nonaccidental trauma. Recognition of the pattern of hemorrhaging, coupled with patient characteristics, history, and physical examination leads to the proper workup and diagnosis. An eye consultation will serve well in streamlining the evaluation and maximizing intervention.

Differential Diagnosis

- It is critical to realize that hemorrhages do not progress but represent altered structure, and as such may affect acuity
- Nonaccidental trauma must be the first etiology considered
- Pigmented lesions of the retina including choroidal nevi, congenital hypertrophy of the retinal pigment epithelium, retinal pigment epithelial hyperplasia
- Diabetic retinopathy is characterized by dot/blot, flame, preretinal, vitreous hemorrhages
- Hypertensive retinopathy is typically accompanied by signs of hypoxia, e.g., cotton wool spots and optic disc swelling
- May be associated with any systemic vascular disease or collagen vascular disease (e.g., systemic lupus erythematosus)
- Vein occlusion
  - –Occlusion of a central vein may involve the entire retina, occlusion of one branch vein involves a section of the retina
- Peripheral retinal hemorrhaging may be associated with vascular insufficiency due to carotid stenosis
- May be associated with optic disc swelling
- Traumatic truncal injury may create intraretinal hemorrhages called Purtscher lesions
- Intracranial hemorrhage may dissect forward to surround optic nerve (Terson phenomenon)
- Blood dyscrasias, anemias, leukemias, sickle cell, ocular sarcoidosis, Behçet disease, Eales disease may cause retinopathy
- If sudden loss of vision is associated, wet macular degeneration, macular hemorrhage of histoplasmosis, preretinal hemorrhage, or vitreous hemorrhage may be the etiology
- Retinal vascular tumors, which may have an associated neurologic aneurysm
- HIV retinopathy presents with hemorrhage as first sign but may progress to involve and destroy vision

Workup and Diagnosis

- History
  - –Evaluate status of known systemic diseases; e.g., hypertension, diabetes
  - –Investigate for undiagnosed systemic disease: Hypertension, diabetes, carotid occlusion, cardiac anomalies, blood disorders, HIV
- Physical exam
  - –Visual acuity: Acuity is compromised if the hemorrhage lies within the foveal area
  - –Pupillary evaluation: Look for Marcus Gunn pupil
  - –Extraocular muscle evaluation for diplopia (may be associated with diabetes)
  - –Confrontation visual fields are indicated in all cases
  - –Perform a dilated fundus evaluation
- Labs
  - –CBC, differential, lipid profile, ANA, sickle cell, ACE, serum calcium
- Studies
  - –Ultrasonography, fluorescein angiography, ocular CT may be performed in conjunction with an ophthalmology consultation
  - –If secondary to a retinal vascular tumor, orbital and brain imaging with and without contrast is indicated with a neurologic consultation

Treatment

- Condition-dependent
  - –Treatment of underlying systemic disease is often the only treatment
- Laser and surgical intervention may be of benefit in diabetic retinopathy, vein occlusions, hypertensive retinopathy, Eales disease, retinal vascular tumors
- Prognosis depends on degree of retinal damage and neurologic involvement
- Report suspect child abuse to state agency

39. Scleral Injection (Red Eye)

Red eye is a "basket" term that encompasses a wide range of ophthalmic conditions. Most conditions are self-limited; however, red eye can be a sign of serious eye disease. Presence of pain helps to distinguish between the more serious eye conditions and nonvision-threatening conditions.

Differential Diagnosis

- Bacterial conjunctivitis: Common; usually BL; acute-onset purulent/mucopurulent discharge; conjunctival hyperemia; caused by *Staphylococcus aureus, Streptococcus pneumoniae, Haemophilus influenzae*
- Allergic conjunctivitis: Common; BL; seasonal/perennial; lid edema, watery, stringy discharge, conjunctival hyperemia
- Viral conjunctivitis: Common; very contagious; usually BL; lid edema, watery discharge, conjunctival hyperemia, preauricular adenopathy, cornea infiltrates and ulcers possible; caused by adenovirus, HSV, enterovirus
- Neonatal conjunctivitis: Conjunctival inflammation in first month; etiologies chemical, *Gonococcus*, HSV-2, *Chlamydia*, bacterial
- Corneal ulcer: Bacterial, viral, autoimmune, parasitic, fungal
- Corneal abrasion: Contact lens use; trauma; recurrent corneal erosions
- Giant papillary conjunctivitis: Common; secondary to foreign body (contact lens)
- Vernal keratoconjunctivitis: Common, recurrent; BL; mucoid discharge; limbal infiltrates and vascularization
- Atopic keratoconjunctivis: Uncommon; lid eczema; mucoid discharge; corneal vascularization
- Blepharitis/meibomitis: Infection, inflammation of eyelid margin lead to conjunctival and corneal irritation
- Mucocutaneous: Stevens-Johnson syndrome; atopic dermatitis; toxic epidermolysis bullosa; keratoconjunctivitis sicca, rosacea
- Scleritis/episcleritis: Red, tender, no significant discharge; with connective tissue disease and vasculitis
- Canaliculitis/dacrocystitis: Infection of nasolacrimal system
- Subconjunctival hemorrhage: Bright red; resolves over 7–14 days; spontaneous or associated with valsalva
- Iritis: Autoimmune disease associations; perilimbal injection; photophobia, ache
- Angle closure glaucoma: Halos, headache, nausea and vomiting, history of hyperopia

Workup and Diagnosis

- History
  - –Onset, duration, type and progression of symptoms
  - –Degree of redness, presence or absence of pain, discharge, pruritus, edema
  - –Amount and type of discharge
  - –Recent URI or contact with someone with red eye: Suspect viral
  - –Past medical history
  - –Systemic symptoms consistent with autoimmune or connective tissue disease
- Physical exam
  - –Blood pressure, temperature, vital signs
  - –General physical examination for signs of connective tissue or autoimmune disease
  - –Conjunctival scrapings for Gram stain and culture.
  - –Fluorescein staining to elucidate corneal abrasion and ulcer
  - –Giemsa stain of conjunctival scraping if suspect *chlamydia*
  - –Check intraocular pressure (angle closure glaucoma)
- Labs
  - –CBC, platelets, PT/PTT, bleeding time for recurrent subconjunctival hemorrhage
  - –CBC, ANA, ANCA, RF, ESR, CXR, BUN/CR, UA, RPR/FTA-ABS for scleritis/episcleritis
- Severe pain, loss of vision, loss of motility, abnormal pupillary responses require comprehensive eye exam

Treatment

- Intense topical antibiotics for corneal ulcers
- Topical antibiotics for bacterial conjunctivitis (sulfa, fluoroquinolones; avoid gentamicin)
- Consider systemic ceftriaxone if suspect *Gonococcus*
- Tears, cool compresses, topical and oral antihistamines for allergic conjunctivitis
- Frequent handwashing for viral conjunctivitis
- Oral doxycycline and treatment of partners for *chlamydia*
- NSAIDs for epi/scleritis
- Oral doxycycline, topical Metrogel, warm compresses for rosacea, chalazia, and blepharitis
- Massage of inner canthus, hot compresses, oral and topical antibiotics for canaliculitis and dacrocystitis
- Check intraocular pressure if suspect angle closure glaucoma (pressure typically over 40 mmHg)
- Frequent lubrication for dry eye

40. Strabismus

Strabismus is the term for malalignment of the eyes. It may be related to amblyopia, a visual impairment caused by lack of visual stimulation of the affected eye in early childhood, when visual development is taking place. Strabismus can cause amblyopia because the patient can fix on an object with only one eye at a time, and amblyopia can lead to strabismus because the patient learns to use only the dominant eye while the nondominant eye "wanders" or is "lazy."

Differential Diagnosis

- Esotropia
  - –Defined as convergent visual axes or "crossed" eyes
  - –Amblyopia and monocular blindness usually manifests as esodeviation in 0–3-year-olds
- Exotropia
  - –Defined as divergent visual gaze
  - –Amblyopia and monocular blindness usually manifest as exodeviation in children older than 4 years
- Pseudostrabismus: In young children with wide-spaced eyes, flat nasal bridge, or prominent epicanthal folds, the patient may appear to be esotropic
- Transient infantile esotropia: In the first 4 months of life, esotropia may transiently occur in normal children
- Congenital esotropia
  - –Pronounced medial deviation of one eye in the first year of life
  - –Occurs in otherwise healthy infants
- Retinoblastoma
  - –Frequent early finding in retinoblastoma
  - –May be due to visual impairment or space-occupying lesion
- CNS etiologies
  - –Associated with hydrocephalus and periventricular leukomalacia, especially in premature infants
  - –Associated with intracranial masses due to CN VI compression
- Möbius syndrome
  - –VI, VII, and XII nerve palsy and variable limb anomalies
- Accommodative strabismus
  - –Result of visual discrepancy and favored use of the better eye
  - –Also occurs during accommodation when there is significant hyperopia
  - –The eye not in use is esotropic
- Idiopathic childhood exotropia
  - –May be alternating, or may be secondary to visual discrepancy and favored use of the better eye
  - –The eye that is not fixed on an object is exotropic
- Congenital CN III palsy
  - –Familial, usually unilateral, +/− ptosis

Workup and Diagnosis

- History
  - –Onset, duration, severity of symptoms
  - –Persistence or transience of symptoms
  - –Monocular, binocular, or alternating
  - –Associated symptoms (i.e., headache for intracranial masses)
  - –Birth and past medical history
  - –Family history of myopia, strabismus, or amblyopia
- Physical exam
  - –Corneal light reflex: The patient fixes on a light held by the examiner at a distance of 2–3 feet; light reflection on the cornea should be symmetric
  - –Visual acuity in each eye
  - –Cover-uncover test: Patient fixes on a near object with one eye while the other is covered; uncover the contralateral eye and note whether it was convergent while covered
  - –Funduscopic examination for papilledema
  - –Pupillary red light reflex: White in retinoblastoma
  - –Preferred head position: Patients with CN VI palsy frequently turn their faces in such a way as to create a coordinated gaze
  - –Head circumference (hydrocephalus)
  - –Neurologic examination including cranial nerves
- Studies
  - –Imaging of the orbits and brain may be required to rule out malignancy or space-occupying lesion

Treatment

- Ophthalmologic consultation
- Transient infantile esotropia
  - –Self-limiting
- Congenital esotropia
  - –Surgical correction before age 2
- Retinoblastoma and other tumors
  - –Oncologic evaluation and treatment
- Hydrocephalus
  - –May or may not correct with treatment of the hydrocephalus; may require surgical intervention
- Möbius syndrome
  - –Difficult to treat
- Accommodative esotropia
  - –Corrective lenses
- Idiopathic exotropia
  - –Surgery or patching

41. Vision Loss

Sudden decrease of vision is usually an ominous sign. Most often the cause of permanent loss is at the retinal or optic nerve level. For the optic nerve to be associated there must be inflammation. For the retina to be the cause, there must be hemorrhaging or edema. Neurologic conditions are often associated with the transient variation of vision disturbances. Sudden decrease or loss of vision is invariably unilateral; if bilateral, it is associated with posterior cortex circulation or hysteria.

Differential Diagnosis

- Vascular causes
  - –Amaurosis fugax: TIA of the retina lasting 5–60 minutes
  - –Stroke causes loss of side vision usually to the left or right, may be interpreted as loss of vision in the right or left eye
  - –Retinal vascular occlusion: Venous shows gradual decline with retinal hemorrhaging; arterial has sudden onset with minimal to no retinal hemorrhaging
- Transient monocular blindness (TMB)
  - –Lasts seconds
  - –Due to positional changes in optic disc edema with increased intracranial hypertension, orthostatic hypotension, thyroid eye disease, and space-occupying lesions
- Migraine variants are transient and may be associated with headache after presentation
- Optic nerve edema or swelling from demyelinating disease, nonarteritic and arteritic optic neuropathy, toxicity (e.g., lead, chloramphenicol)
- Optic atrophy
- Retinal etiologies
  - –Retinal surface wrinkling disorders
  - –Idiopathic central serous retinopathy often associated with stress
  - –Retinal detachment with probable history of floaters before loss of vision
- Angle closure glaucoma
- Postsurgical
  - –Endophthalmitis: Often associated with ocular surgery and red eye
  - –Cystoid macular edema may occur after ocular surgery
- Vitreous hemorrhage
  - –You will not be able to see into the eye
- Infectious causes
  - –Retinitis and/or uveitis due to toxoplasmosis, cytomegalovirus, Lyme, histoplasmosis
- Trauma
- Hysterical blindness
- Cataracts
- Hypoglycemia
- Retinitis pigmentosa

Workup and Diagnosis

- History
  - –Be aware that patients often have vision reduction over time (e.g., from cataracts) and only perceive the loss as sudden
  - –Onset, duration, trauma; transience vs permanence of visual loss or change
  - –Associated signs and symptoms of demyelinizing disease, toxoplasmosis, bartonellosis, Lyme disease
  - –PMH including migraines, hypertension, diabetes, thyroid disease, rheumatic disease, vascular disease, atrial fibrillation, lipid status
- Physical exam
  - –Obtain visual acuity and confrontation visual fields in both eyes
  - –Redness, pain, photophobia
  - –Pupillary evaluation: look for Marcus Gunn pupil, which usually differentiates optic nerve from other causes
  - –Extraocular muscle evaluation
  - –Perform a dilated fundus evaluation
  - –Evaluate for proptosis
- Radiology
  - –CT or MRI of orbits and brain is indicated for associated neurologic signs, history of trauma
- Evaluation for stroke if right- or left-sided
- Ophthalmology consultation for dilated retinal exam, evaluation, and management

Treatment

- Transient symptoms are usually due to migraine, stroke, or increased intracranial pressure; appropriate therapy for these disorders
- Manage any underlying systemic disease
- If angle closure glaucoma, stat consult for immediate medical and surgical intervention
- Retinitis or uveitis: Management of underlying cause; NSAIDs and steroids
- If hemorrhage in the macula from macular degeneration or histoplasmosis, laser therapy or intravitreal steroids may save the vision
- Vitreous hemorrhage may be evacuated after establishing and treating cause
- Macular edema may be treated with topical steroids, Diamox, intravitreal steroids, NSAIDs
- Retinal vascular occlusion: Intraocular surgery or laser therapy may alleviate symptoms

Section 6

Ears

DAVID J. KAY, MD
RONALD J. WILLIAMS, MD, FAAP, FACP

42. Hearing Loss – Acquired

All patients with suspected hearing loss require formal audiologic testing to characterize the nature (conductive, sensorineural, mixed) and extent of the loss. Early treatment is essential, as is early habilitation for those in whom the hearing loss is not reversible.

Differential Diagnosis

<u>Conductive (CHL)</u>

- Cerumen impaction
- External auditory canal foreign body
- Middle ear effusion (MEE)
  - –Frequently follows acute otitis media
- Tympanic membrane (TM) perforation
  - –Usually due to trauma, chronic otitis media
- Cholesteatoma
  - –Acquired cholesteatoma is accompanied by TM retraction or perforation
  - –Congenital cholesteatoma is usually over an intact TM
- Ossicular erosion or fixation due to middle ear disease
- Ossicular chain discontinuity (generally post-traumatic)
- External auditory canal stenosis from chronic otitis externa
- Middle ear tumor
  - –Paraganglioma (glomus tympanicum), facial neuroma, histiocytosis X, etc.

<u>Sensorineural (SNHL)</u>

- Meningitis, especially bacterial
- Viral, especially mumps
- Autoimmune disease
  - –Vasculitis, scleroderma, Kawasaki disease
  - –Idiopathic
- Acoustic trauma (noise-induced)
- Ototoxic medications
  - –Aminoglycosides
  - –Diuretics (especially loop diuretics)
  - –Salicylates
  - –Cytotoxic (chemotherapeutic) agents, e.g., cisplatinum
- Temporal bone fracture
  - –SNHL more likely with transverse than longitudinal fracture
- Perilymphatic fistula (PLF)
  - –Hearing loss may be progressive or fluctuating
- Cerebellopontine angle (CPA) tumor
  - –Vestibular schwannoma (a.k.a. acoustic neuroma, associated with type II neurofibromatosis), meningioma, etc.
  - –SNHL will be unilateral
- Ménière disease
  - –Characterized by hearing loss, vertigo, tinnitus, sensation of aural fullness

Workup and Diagnosis

- History
  - –Ask about risk factors for SNHL
- Physical exam
  - –Check external auditory canal for patency
  - –Check TM for perforation or cholesteatoma
- Audiometric testing
  - –Classifies hearing loss as conductive, sensorineural, or mixed
  - –Quantifies the extent of the hearing loss for the full spectrum of sound frequencies
  - –If too young for ear-specific behavioral testing, obtain otoacoustic emissions and/or auditory brainstem response testing
  - –Tympanometry to objectively assess mobility (can help with diagnosis of MEE, ossicular discontinuity, and otosclerosis)
- CT scan of temporal bones (fine cuts, axial and/or coronal, noncontrast) for CHL if cholesteatoma or trauma suspected
  - –Determines extent of bony erosion or involvement, and whether mastoid cavity is involved
- MRI with gadolinium of internal auditory canals for asymmetric SNHL
  - –Rule out CPA tumors

Treatment

- Cerumen removal
- Tympanostomy tube placement for chronic MEE lasting >3 months if bilateral, >6 months if unilateral
- Tympanoplasty for TM perforation
- Tympanomastoidectomy for cholesteatoma
  - –Effort to keep external auditory canal wall intact, with second look procedure planned for 6 months later
- Ossicular chain reconstruction (OCR, ossiculoplasty) with prosthesis or incus graft for ossicular anomalies
  - –Including after cholesteatoma resection
- Exploratory tympanotomy for suspected PLF
  - –If present, seal off oval and round windows
- Resection of CPA tumor
- Steroids for autoimmune SNHL (systemic or intratympanic)
- Cochlear implants for profound pre- or postlingual deafness
- Habilitation of any post-treatment hearing loss

43. Hearing Loss – Congenital

About one-third to one-half of congenital hearing loss is genetic, of which 15–30% may be syndromic. Universal newborn hearing screening programs allow diagnosis, and thereby habilitation, of deaf children at a much younger age, dramatically increasing the likelihood of their developing meaningful communication skills.

Differential Diagnosis

- Infections
  - –CMV: Most common intrauterine infection causing hearing loss
  - –Bacterial meningitis
  - –Congenital rubella: Cataracts, cardiovascular anomalies, retinitis, mental retardation
  - –Congenital syphilis
  - –Toxoplasmosis
  - –Lyme disease
- Metabolic
  - –Hyperbilirubinemia (kernicterus): Consider phototherapy or exchange transfusion if serum bilirubin >20 mg/dL in newborn
  - –Hypercholesterolemia
- Ototoxic medications
  - –Aminoglycoside, gentamicin often needed for perinatal sepsis; >5 days risks hearing loss
- Temporal bone anomaly
  - –Middle ear anomaly (results in conductive hearing loss)
  - –Perilymphatic fistula
  - –Dilated vestibular aqueduct (+/− Mondini deformity)
  - –Michel cochlear aplasia
  - –Scheibe aplasia: Membranous aplasia; bony labyrinth normal
- Nonsyndromic hereditary congenital deafness (connexin 26 gene mutation is responsible for half of all genetic deafness)
- Syndromic hereditary congenital deafness
  - –Waardenburg: Telecanthus, confluent eyebrow, colored irides, white forlock
  - –Usher: Retinitis pigmentosa (totally blind by second to third decade), ataxia, vestibular dysfunction
  - –Alport: Progressive nephritis and hearing loss
  - –Apert (acrocephalosyndactyly): Craniofacial dysostosis
  - –Crouzon (craniofacial dysostosis): Prognathic mandibile, small maxilla
  - –Jervell and Lange-Neilsen: Heart disease (prolonged QT interval)
  - –Pendred: Euthyroid goiter
  - –Oto-palatal-digital: Cleft palate, stubby clubbed digits
  - –Congential aural atresia

Workup and Diagnosis

- Newborn hearing screening
  - –Otoacoustic emissions and/or auditory brainstem response; behavioral audiometry when older
- Medical history for risk factors
  - –Infections, low birth weight (<1,500 g), prolonged intubation and ventilation
- Family history for hearing loss, consanguinity
- Physical exam, including otoscopy to rule out gross external or middle ear anomalies
- CMV titers
- CT scan to rule out temporal bone abnormalities, and determine whether patient is a cochlear implant candidate
- β_2 gap junction protein (connexin 26) genetic testing
- Urinalysis and renal ultrasound to rule out Alport syndrome
- Electroretinography to rule out Usher syndrome in patients with associated progressive blindness
- Electrocardiography (ECG) to rule out Jervell and Lange-Neilsen syndrome (prolonged QT interval, sudden death risk with athletics)
- Thyroid function tests
- Chromosomal testing

Treatment

- Identify children with hearing loss early
- Treat medically treatable cause, if any
  - –Syphilis (steroids and penicillin), Lyme disease, toxoplasmosis, hypercholesterolemia
- Intravenous gancyclovir for congenital CMV
- Habilitate by age 6 months if possible
  - –Amplification
  - –Bone-anchored hearing aids
  - –Tympanostomy tube placement
  - –Middle ear reconstruction
  - –Perilymphatic fistula closure
  - –Cochlear implant (after age 12 months)
- Periodic follow-up necessary
  - –Ensure auditory habilitation is working
  - –Check for hearing loss progression

44. Otalgia (Ear Pain)

Not all ear pain is otologic; the ears have rich sensory innervation from multiple nerves, and secondary pain is common. Most otologic ear pain has some associated physical findings; if none is present, a complete head and neck examination, including imaging, may be required to search for a source of referred otalgia.

Differential Diagnosis

External ear

- Otitis externa
  - –Pinnae and especially tragus, are exquisitely tender
- Impacted cerumen
  - –Hearing loss and aural fullness
- Foreign body
  - –Items such as beads, toys, and even extruded tympanostomy tubes
- Trauma
  - –Any object inserted into the ear canal may cause trauma, including Q-tips
- Perichondritis
  - –Inflammation or infection of the cartilage of the pinna and canal, sparing the lobule (since there is no cartilage there)
- Myringitis
  - –Tympanic membrane granulation or de-epithelialization

Middle ear/mastoid

- Acute otitis media
  - –Otalgia may precede middle ear effusion
- Otitis media with effusion
  - –May occur in the absence or presence of an active infection
- Eustachian tube dysfunction
  - –Negative intratympanic pressure
- Barotrauma
  - –Pretreatment with topical nasal decongestants may be effective prophylaxis
- Mastoiditis
  - –Associated with postauricular pain and normal tympanic membrane/middle ear

Non-otologic (secondary)

- Cranial nerve referred pain
  - –III: Dental infection, temporal-mandibular joint (TMJ) syndrome
  - –VII: Herpes zoster oticus (Ramsay Hunt syndrome)
  - –IX: Tonsillitis, pharyngitis
  - –X: Laryngitis, GERD, thyroiditis
- Cervical nerve referred pain
  - –Neck infections, lymph nodes, cysts
  - –Cervical spine disorders
- Paranasal sinusitis
- Migraines
- Neuralgias

Workup and Diagnosis

- History
  - –Onset, duration, and specific quality of pain
  - –Ability to localize (may distinguish otologic from nonotologic)
  - –Associated otologic symptoms: Otorrhea, hearing loss, imbalance, prior ear surgery, antecedent events
  - –Pain associated with mastication, swallowing, voice change, purulent rhinorrhea
- Otologic exam
  - –Inspection and palpation of pinna, tragus, and pre-auricular area, and mastoid bone
  - –Direct otoscopy for signs of external- or middle-ear infection or inflammation
  - –Obstructing cerumen or foreign bodies must be removed to evaluate deeper structures
- Complete head and neck exam
  - –Nose and nasal cavities, oral cavity, and pharynx (particularly teeth and tonsils), TMJ
  - –Examination of nasopharynx and larynx may require fiberoptic endoscopy
- Tympanometry, if middle ear status (fluid, retraction, perforation) is not evident from otoscopy
- CT or MRI
  - –Useful to delineate extent of cholesteatoma, mastoiditis, petrous apicitis, tumor
  - –May be necessary to evaluate either otologic disease or an ill child with nonotologic source (rule out abscess or tumor)

Treatment

- Establish appropriate specific diagnosis as promptly as possible
- If infectious process, initiate antimicrobial therapy
  - –Topical (intraotic) antibiotic drops for otitis externa or otitis media with either a perforation or patent tympanostomy tube
  - –Systemic (oral) for otitis media, nonviral pharyngitis, sinusitis
  - –Parenteral antibiotics for abscess, mastoiditis
- If odontogenic, dental referral
- Adequate follow-up to ensure resolution of otalgia

45. Otorrhea (Ear Discharge)

Otorrhea often arises from the external ear; in the setting of a nonintact tympanic membrane, the middle and even inner ears may be sources as well. Suctioning the otorrhea out of the canal to visualize the tympanic membrane is both therapeutic and diagnostically valuable.

Differential Diagnosis

- Cerumen
  - –Often brownish color
  - –Rarely associated with otalgia or pruritis
- Otitis externa
  - –Bacterial (frequently *Pseudomonas* and *Staphylococcus aureus*) vs fungal (especially after prolonged treatment with antibiotic drops)
  - –Concern: Necrotizing (malignant) otitis externa (i.e., temporal bone osteomyelitis) in immunosuppressed patients, including brittle diabetics
- Acute otitis media with tympanic membrane (TM) perforation
  - –Acute perforation may already have closed by the time the patient is examined
- Chronic perforation drainage
  - –From water contamination (swimming, bathing) if patient is not maintaining dry ear precautions (ear plugs, occlusive head bands, shower caps, etc.)
- Tympanostomy tube drainage
  - –If bloody, suspect granulation tissue surrounding the tube
  - –Increased incidence when not maintaining dry ear precautions is debated (as small tube lumen diameter has considerable surface tension)
- Chronic suppurative otitis media
  - –Chronic middle ear and/or mastoid infection with perforated TM
- Cholesteatoma
  - –"Skin cyst" (keratinizing stratified squamous epithelium) in the middle ear/mastoid
  - –Benign, but often very aggressively locally erosive (mechanical and enzymatic)
  - –Surgical, not medical, condition
- Perichondritis
  - –Spares the lobule (as there is no cartilage there)
- Myringitis
  - –TM granulation or de-epithelialization
- Foreign body
- CSF leak
  - –Watery drainage
  - –Traumatic or congenital
  - –With or without perilymphatic fistula
- Primary dermatologic condition
  - –Eczema, psoriasis

Workup and Diagnosis

- History
  - –Quality of otorrhea: Malodorous and purulent (infectious) vs bloody (traumatic, granulation tissue) vs clear and watery (CSF)
  - –Associated symptoms: Pain and tenderness in acute otitis externa, aural pruritus in chronic or fungal otitis externa
  - –Past medical/surgical history: Prior tympanostomy tubes, middle ear surgery (cholesteatoma), trauma or neurosurgery (CSF leak); dermatologic disease
- Physical exam
  - –Must suction and debride the ear canal of debris to examine tympanic membrane
  - –If canal is too narrow from swelling to see the tympanic membrane, place hydrocellulose wick to draw ototopical medication to affected areas; re-examine in several days
  - –Visualize after suctioning (through otoscope) if source is external or middle ear
- Labs
  - –Gram stain and culture specimen of otorrhea if diagnosis is in question, if patient is initially systemically symptomatic (febrile or other complications), or if patient fails initial treatment
- Imaging studies
  - –CT scan of temporal bone (noncontrast, 1-mm slice thickness) if cholesteatoma or trauma is suspected

Treatment

- Suction and debride the external auditory canal
- Maintain dry ear precautions
  - –No water at all allowed within ear canals
- Ototopical antibiotics
  - –Unless TM is intact, use nonototoxic (e.g., fluoroquinolone) drops
  - –Antifungal solution for candidal infections
- Steroid drops
  - –Often a combination product with antibiotic drops
  - –Essential if granulation tissue is present
- Reacidification of canal
  - –Acetic acid drops
  - –Treats both fungal and bacterial infections
  - –Painful if TM is not intact
- Oral antibiotic
  - –For refractory cases of middle ear etiology
- Prolonged IV antibiotics for severe refractory cases

46. Tinnitus

Tinnitus is a ringing in the ears that is usually constant in pitch and volume and continues for a significant period of time. It can have a wide variety of causes, which requires a very detailed history and head/neck exam.

Differential Diagnosis

- Impacted cerumen
- Eustachian tube dysfunction
  - "Ocean roar" that may wax and wane with respiration
- Acute otitis media
  - Red TM with poor movement, +/− fluid
- Chronic otitis media
  - Persistent otitis with poor TM movement
- Noise-induced hearing loss
  - High pitch
- Trauma
  - Airbag, whiplash, barotrauma, etc.
- Temporal-mandibular joint disorder
  - Nonpulsatile tinnitus
- Migraine
- Ototoxicity
  - High pitch
  - Many drugs, including salicylates and aminoglycosides
- Otosclerosis
- Pseudotumor cerebri
- Infections (meningitis, Lyme disease, rubella)
- Acquired AVM, arterial bruit, venous hum (positional change of tinnitus)
- Tumor
  - Glomus tympanicum or jugulare (pulsatile tinnitus with hearing loss)
  - Acoustic neuroma
- Thyroid disease
- Autoimmune inner ear disease
- Idiopathic
  - Low pitch
- Fetal insults
  - Infections, toxins, etc.
- Sickle cell disease, anemia
- Osteogenesis imperfecta
- Symptomatic Chiari malformation
- Late-onset congenital hearing loss
- Less common causes are
  - Hypertension
  - Myoclonus of palatal muscles
  - Multiple sclerosis
  - Small vessel disease
  - Presbycusis (high pitch)

Workup and Diagnosis

- History
  - Pitch of noise, duration, noise exposure, etc.
  - Complete history including problems during pregnancy
  - Birth history
  - PMH, medication use
- Physical exam
  - Complete head/neck exam looking for abnormalities
  - Neurologic/systemic exam if indicated by history
- Labs
  - CBC if infectious origin suspected
  - Consider TFTs (occult thyroid disease)
- Studies
  - Tympanometry: OM, eustachian tube dysfunction
  - Full audiology evaluation if suspect sensorineural etiology
- Radiology
  - Head CT if suspect glomus tumor (delineates base of skull involvement)
  - MRI (with enhancement): Chiari malformation, MS, pseudotumor cerebri, acoustic neuroma
  - Angiography: Constant pulsatile tinnitus if no specific vascular or musculoskeletal source
  - MRA if CT and MRI negative and suspect vascular etiology

Treatment

- Treat underlying cause; treat underlying depression and insomnia; benzodiazepines may be helpful in depression
- Refer to ENT or neurotologist for vascular etiology
- Stop ototoxic medications
- Tinnitus retraining therapy can reduce tinnitus by habituation training
- Masking devices: Low-level sound to decrease or eliminate tinnitus
- Biofeedback/stress reduction
- Surgery: Correct conductive defect with outer or middle ear disease, remove tumor
- Hearing aids: Presbycusis; cochlear implants: Severe hearing loss, not benefiting from hearing aids
- Botulinum toxin injection: Myoclonus of palatal muscles
- Many medications treat tinnitus, yet none has proven very effective in double-blind placebo controlled trials without significant side effects

Section 7

Nose

KATHLEEN O. DeANTONIS, MD
DAVID J. KAY, MD

47. Chronic Rhinitis

Chronic rhinitis is a common complaint in preschoolers, especially those who attend group child care. A relatively simple differential allows for elucidation of the diagnosis, usually with merely a careful history and physical exam. Even if the primary process is noninfectious, superinfection may occur with chronic disruption of the integrity of the nasal mucosa. Presence of nasal polyps in childhood should prompt an evaluation for cystic fibrosis (CF).

Differential Diagnosis

- Allergic rhinitis
  - Rhinorrhea is typically watery and profuse
  - May have associated sneezing, itchy eyes and nose (allergic salute)
- Infectious conditions
  - Chronic sinusitis: Typically has mucopurulent discharge; headache and fever may or may not be present
  - Succession of URIs: Can get associated bacterial overgrowth, typically group A β-hemolytic *Streptococcus* in young children; may have low-grade fever, lymphadenopathy, and weight loss
  - Congenital syphilis
- Nonallergic rhinitis
  - Typically due to irritants such as smoke or pungent odors
- Vasomotor rhinitis
  - A hyperactive cholinergic response
  - Postnasal drip is commonly associated
- Foreign body
  - Always consider when there is unilateral nasal discharge
  - Halitosis or generalized body odor (bromhidrosis) may be present
- Nasal polyps
  - 10% of children with CF develop polyps
  - Other causes include Kartagener syndrome (immotile cilia), recurrent sinusitis, aspirin intolerance
  - Woake syndrome includes polyps, broad nasal base, frontal sinus aplasia, bronchiectasis
- Adenoid hypertrophy
  - Associated with mouth breathing, noisy respirations
  - Severe cases can result in obstructive sleep apnea
- Juvenile nasopharygeal angiofibroma
  - Typically in adolescent males
  - Associated with recurrent epistaxis
- Hormonal rhinitis (rare)
  - Pregnancy and hypothyroidism

Workup and Diagnosis

- History
  - Onset, duration, and severity of symptoms
  - Character of nasal discharge: Purulent vs clear
  - Unilateral or bilateral
  - History of associated atopic conditions such as environmental allergies, asthma, eczema
  - Family history of atopic conditions
- Physical exam
  - Complete HEENT examination
  - Degree and type of nasal discharge
  - Characteristics of nasal turbinates such as enlargement, color (redness indicates infection, pale or blue color indicates allergy)
  - Allergic features such as allergic "shiners," Dennie lines, high-arched palate
- Labs
  - Nasal smear
  - PMNs indicate an infectious process, whereas eosinophils are consistent with an allergic response
- Radiology
  - Lateral head/neck films reveal adenoidal size and configuration, may show polyps

Treatment

- Antibiotics such as amoxicillin plus clavulanic acid for sinusitis
- Systemic nonsedating antihistamines (e.g., Claritin, Zyrtec, Allegra) for allergic rhinitis, especially if there are other manifestations of atopy
- Intranasal antihistamines may be useful for isolated allergic rhinitis
- Intranasal steroids are used for allergic rhinitis, vasomotor rhinitis, and chronic sinusitis
- Polypectomy may be sufficient therapy for nasal polyps

48. Epistaxis (Nosebleed)

Most bleeding arises from the rich network of blood vessels of Kisselbach plexus in Little area of the anterior nasal septum. Most epistaxis resolves spontaneously or after a few minutes of pressure (nasal pinching). For the vast majority of cases, no medical attention is sought.

Differential Diagnosis

- Trauma
  - –Dry air, especially in winter months
  - –Digital trauma (nose-picking)
  - –Nasogastric or nasotracheal tube
  - –Blunt trauma, with or without fracture
  - –Foreign body: Usually accompanied by unilateral foul-smelling rhinorrhea
  - –Air pollution (indoor or outdoor)
  - –Barotrauma: Diving or airplane descent in patient with upper respiratory infection
  - –Chemical or caustic burn
- Inflammation
  - –Upper respiratory infection (viral or bacterial)
  - –Rhinitis (allergic, nonallergic with eosinophilia, atrophic, chronic): Results in increased mucosal vascularity and increased trauma from sneezing, rubbing, and nose blowing
  - –Vestibulitis
- Anatomic
  - –Nasal septal deviation
  - –Postoperative, following sinus surgery, adenoidectomy, septoplasty, etc.
- Platelet dysfunction
  - –NSAID use, especially aspirin
  - –Idiopathic thrombocytopenic purpura
  - –Leukemia
- Coagulopathy
  - –Von Willebrand disease
  - –Hemophilia
  - –Liver disease
  - –Anticoagulants (coumadin, heparin)
- Benign masses
  - –Nasopharyngeal angiofibroma: Presents only in adolescent males
  - –Pyogenic granuloma
  - –Papilloma
- Malignant neoplasms
  - –Rhabdomyosarcoma
  - –Lymphoma
- Vascular abnormalities
  - –Hereditary hemorrhagic telangiectasia (Osler-Weber-Rendu disease): Autosomal dominant, 90% with recurrent epistaxis
  - –Hemangioma
  - –Internal carotid pseudoaneurysm (suspect with massive bleed after head trauma)

Workup and Diagnosis

- History
  - –Frequency, duration, precipitating factors, maneuvers required to make it stop
  - –Medications, including over-the-counter and herbals
  - –Family history of nosebleeds, easy bleeding, or bruising
  - –Environmental history, including types of heating and cooling systems, allergies, etc.
- Physical exam
  - –Assess general condition, with vital signs, to estimate acute degree of blood loss
  - –Suction, or have child blow out all blood clots and fresh blood
  - –Decongest (topical oxymetazoline) nose; may anesthetize with topical lidocaine or ponticaine as well
  - –Anterior rhinoscopy (using otoscope is often easier and more accessible than headlight and nasal speculum)
- Labs
  - –Hemoglobin and hematocrit
  - –Platelet levels, coagulation studies (PT, aPTT)
  - –For refractory cases, closure time (an *in vitro* bleeding time) and von Willebrand profile
- Hematology consultation
- Studies (for exceptional cases only)
  - –CT scan with contrast
  - –MRI/MRA
  - –Angiography

Treatment

- Humidification
  - –Nasal saline sprays
  - –Aquaphor or antibiotic ointment to anterior septum
  - –Vaporizer at night
- Pinch cartilaginous nose for >5–10 minutes
- Remove (physician suctioning or patient blowing out) all blood clots
- Vasoconstrictive (decongestive) sprays (oxymetazoline)
- Nasal packing
  - –Petroleum gauze (many meters may be needed)
  - –Premade packs: Absorbable (cellulose, gelatin), nonabsorbable, inflatable balloons
  - –Posterior packing requires ICU observation
- Cauterization
  - –Chemical: Silver nitrate
  - –Electrical: Monopolar, bipolar
- Angiography with embolization
- Surgical ligation or clipping of feeding arteries

49. Nasal Obstruction & Rhinorrhea

Nasal obstruction and rhinorrhea in children, unlike in adults, generally cannot be distinguished from each other. In children it is often difficult, if not impossible, to distinguish rhinitis from sinusitis, hence the phrase "rhinosinusitis." Because newborns are obligate nasal breathers, neonatal nasal obstruction may be life-threatening.

Differential Diagnosis

- Physiologic
  - –Nasal cycle
  - –Nasopulmonary reflex
  - –Puberty
  - –Menstruation and pregnancy
- Congenital
  - –Choanal atresia or stenosis
  - –Cleft palate
  - –Craniofacial syndromes such as Treacher Collins, Crouzon
- Cyst
  - –Dermoid, meningocele, or encephalocele
  - –Thornwaldt
- Infectious
  - –Bacterial rhinosinusitis with *Haemophilus influenzae, Streptococcus pneumoniae, Moraxella catarrhalis*, staph
  - –Viral rhinosinusitis with rhinovirus, adenovirus, coxsackie
- Viral prodrome
  - –Measles, mumps, mono, polio
- Fungal (if immunocompromised)
  - –Aspergillosis, mucormycosis
- Inflammatory
  - –Allergic rhinitis
  - –Nasal polyps
  - –Adenoid hypertrophy
  - –Nasopharyngeal GERD
- Granulomatous
  - –Sarcoidosis
  - –Wegener syndrome
  - –SLE
  - –Churg-Strauss syndrome
- Traumatic
  - –Foreign body
  - –Septal hematoma
  - –Septal abscess
- Neoplastic
  - –Chordoma
  - –Craniopharyngioma
  - –Juvenile angiofibroma
  - –Olfactory neuroblastoma
- Cystic fibrosis
- Thyroid disease (hypo- or hyper-)
- Ciliary dyskinesia
  - –Kartagener, immotile cilia syndrome, etc.
- Chronic rhinitis

Workup and Diagnosis

- History
  - –Onset, duration, severity, exacerbating and relieving factors, work of breathing
  - –Family history
  - –Environmental history: Pets, smoke exposure
- Physical exam
  - –Passage of suction catheter to rule out atresia/stenosis
  - –Direct rhinoscopy with otoscope, or with nasal speculum and headlight or head mirror
  - –Fiberoptic rhinoscopy: Flexible well tolerated, rigid (better optics) only for older children
  - –Examine nose before and after decongestion
- Allergy testing
  - –*In vitro* (RAST) better tolerated in young children than *in vivo* (intradermal, prick skin testing)
  - –Nasal cytology
- Studies
  - –Lateral neck X-ray: Useful for adenoid hypertrophy or nasopharyngeal cysts
  - –Sinus X-ray: Limited utility, essentially replaced by CT
  - –CT scan: Contrast only required if tumor suspected; if sinus surgery anticipated, need coronal views
  - –MRI: Excellent for tumors, necessary for congenital cysts (differentiate meningocele from encephalocele); much too sensitive for sinusitis
  - –Angiography: Useful for juvenile nasopharyngeal angiofibromas and other tumors requiring preoperative embolization

Treatment

- Antibiotics for bacterial rhinosinusitis
  - –Endoscopically guided middle meatus cultures correlate well with maxillary sinus contents; routine nasal cultures do not
- Surgical correction of congenital anomalies
  - –Must establish airway (e.g., intubation) if respiratory distress
- Nasal steroids for rhinitis
- Allergic rhinitis may need nonsedating antihistamine or even immunotherapy
- Medications for rhinosinusitis (URI symptoms for >10 days) should include antibiotics (covering β-lactamase organisms), nasal steroids, and topical decongestants (no rebound effect if used with steroids)
- Adenoidectomy for obstructive adenoid hypertrophy or for chronic or recurrent rhinosinusitis refractory to antibiotic therapy
- Endoscopic resection of nasal polyps

Section 8

Oral Cavity

DAVID H. CHI, MD
KATHLEEN O. DeANTONIS, MD
DAVID J. KAY, MD

50. Cleft Lip/Palate

Cleft lip and palate may occur individually or together, and may be unilateral or bilateral. These defects may occur as isolated defects or as part of a larger syndrome. Occurrence of cleft lip or palate should prompt a physical survey for other congenital anomalies, particularly those found in associated syndromes and other midline defects.

Differential Diagnosis

- Cleft lip with or without cleft palate
  - –Incidence 1/500–1/2,500
  - –Highest incidence among Native Americans
  - –Defects are unilateral in 80%
  - –More common in boys
  - –Pathogenesis is multifactorial
- Isolated cleft palate
  - –Incidence 1/2,000
  - –More common in girls
- Pierre-Robin sequence
  - –Micrognathia, glossoptosis (posterior displacement of the tongue to pharynx), and cleft palate
  - –Incidence 1/2,000–1/30,000
  - –Mortality 2.2–26%
- Syndrome-associated cleft lip with or without cleft palate
  - –Accounts for 30% of cases
  - –Over 300 syndromes include this phenotype
  - –Stickler syndrome (25%): Pierre-Robin sequence with severe progressive myopia and arthritis in young adulthood
  - –Velocardiofacial syndrome (15%): Slender hands and fingers, cardiac defects (TOF, VSD, right aortic arch), prominent nose; deletion of 22q11.21
  - –DiGeorge syndrome: Thymic hypoplasia, hypoparathyroidism, cardiac defects (truncus arteriosus, interrupted aortic arch) same spectrum at velocardial facial with same deletion of 22q
  - –Trisomy 13: Microcephaly, cutis aplasia, polydactyly cardiac defects
  - –Trisomy 18: Low-set ears, clenched hands, rocker bottom feet, cardiac defects
  - –van der Woude syndrome: Cleft palate associated with lip pits
- Cause associated with maternal exposure to corticosteroids, phenytoin, valproic acid, thalidomide, alcohol, cigarettes, dioxin, or retinoic acid; and maternal diabetes mellitus, hormone imbalance, and vitamin deficiency
- Fetal alcohol syndrome
- Treacher Collins syndrome

Workup and Diagnosis

- History
  - –Prenatal and birth history
  - –History of prenatal drug/medication use
  - –Family history of cleft lip or palate, or other birth defects
  - –Ethnic background
- Physical exam
  - –Location and extent of the defect
  - –Presence or absence of submucosal cleft palate (must be palpated, because it may not be visible beneath the oral mucosa)
  - –Dental examination
  - –Cardiac examination
- Studies
  - –Syndromic cleft lip with or without cleft palate is detected at fetal ultrasound in 38% of cases
  - –Nonsyndromic clefting is difficult to see on fetal ultrasound
  - –Screening Echo for cardiac anomalies and
  - –Chest X-ray for presence of thymus
- Screenings
  - –Neonatal and periodic hearing screening
  - –Calcium level and immunoglobulins for DiGeorge
- Dental and speech evaluations

Treatment

- Neonatal support is largely nutritional
  - –Patients with velopharyngeal insufficiency are at risk for aspiration
  - –Breastfeeding may or may not be possible depending on the location and size of the defect
  - –Specialized bottles and nipples may be required to accomplish adequate feeding
- Surgical correction (usually in 2–4 stages) with surgical priorities being prevention of regurgitation and aspiration, enabling of speech production, and cosmetic result
  - –In patients with delayed surgical correction, a prosthesis may be necessary to compensate for velopharyngeal insufficiency and to enhance speech development
  - –Speech therapy
  - –Monitoring for otitis media
  - –Referral to a geneticist for genetic testing and consideration of risk with subsequent pregnancies

51. Drooling

Acute and chronic drooling (sialorrhea) must be differentiated. Sudden severe drooling in a septic-appearing child may indicate severe pharyngeal edema and airway compromise. Chronic drooling may be physiologic in a young child, secondary to nasal obstruction causing persistent mouth opening, or from poor neuromotor control of swallow.

Differential Diagnosis

- Physiologic
  - –Commonly seen in children less than 4 years old
- Infectious
  - –Viral and bacterial rhinosinusitis: Nasal congestion and obstruction lead to chronic mouth opening and contribute to drooling
  - –Adenotonsillar hypertrophy may cause drooling via nasal obstruction leading to persistent mouth opening to breathe
  - –Severe pharyngotonsillitis/tonsillitis causes an obstruction of swallowing
  - –Retropharyngeal or peritonsillar abscess similarly causes a physical obstruction of the swallowing mechanism
  - –Epiglottitis: Severe, life-threatening illness caused by *Haemophilus influenzae* type B, which causes rapid enlargement of the epiglottis; classic symptoms include drooling, a "perched" posture, respiratory distress
- Inflammatory
  - –Allergic rhinitis
  - –Nasal polyposis
- Congenital lesions
  - –Craniofacial syndromes
  - –Midline nasal masses, e.g., encephalocele and glioma, may obstruct nasal breathing and require mouth breathing and therefore reduced swallowing
- Neurologic
  - –Cerebral palsy: Significant persistent drooling may occur secondary to impaired neuromotor control
  - –Cricopharyngeal achalasia and esophageal dysmotility are conditions of neuromotor dysgenesis in the smooth muscle
- Trauma
  - –Caustic ingestion causes an increase in saliva production
  - –Laryngeal trauma may damage the structures necessary for swallowing
- Dental
  - –Teething may cause an increase in drooling in an infant or a young child
  - –Dental caries may cause drooling because of pain and local irritation
- Foreign body

Workup and Diagnosis

- History
  - –Severity (number of bibs or tissues saturated), onset, duration
  - –Ability to eat and drink
  - –Recent URI, sinusitis
  - –Mouth breathing, snoring
  - –Severe neuromotor delay, recurrent or chronic aspiration
  - –Prior conservative therapy
  - –Immunization history for HiB
- Physical exam
  - –Fever, general appearance
  - –Head control (a child keeping head in continuous flexion may persist with drooling)
  - –Stridor, nasal obstruction, tonsillar size
  - –Tongue control, excoriations around the mouth
- Studies
  - –Lateral skull X-ray when adenoid hypertrophy is suspected
  - –Flexible fiberoptic nasopharyngolaryngoscopy permits visualization of nasal cavity, adenoids, larynx
  - –CT neck with contrast if abscess is suspected
  - –Modified barium swallow if swallowing difficulty or chronic aspiration is suspected
  - –Further testing for chronic sialorrhea is seldom necessary

Treatment

- Acute drooling with airway obstructive symptoms may require urgent or emergent airway management
  - –Anesthesia and ENT evaluation to secure airway
- No treatment
  - –Age less than 2 years
  - –Mild intermittent drooling
  - –Medical contraindications
- Medical treatment
  - –Anticholinergics: Scopolamine, glycopyrrolate
  - –Botulinum injections in the salivary gland
  - –Speech pathology: Oral motor training to improve oromotor function
- Biofeedback: Condition child to increase frequency of swallow based on noise stimulus
- Surgery
  - –Submandibular gland excision, submandibular duct relocation, parotid gland excision, tympanic neurectomy

52. Dysphagia

Dysphagia is defined as difficulty swallowing. It may occur during any phase of the swallowing mechanism. Prompt diagnosis is important, because delays may lead to pulmonary infection (secondary to aspiration) and failure to thrive.

Differential Diagnosis

- A problem with any phase of swallowing may cause dysphagia

Oral preparatory phase

- Decreased salivation
- Nasal obstruction: Inability to breathe through nose may cause problems with swallowing in neonates and young infants

Oral phase

- Cleft palate and velopharyngeal insufficiency: Inability to separate the nose/nasopharynx from the mouth may lead to nasal regurgitation during swallowing
  - –Hypertrophic tonsils: Mechanical obstruction to swallowing
  - –Neuromuscular problems: Prematurity, cerebral palsy, Duchenne muscular dystrophy, Guillain-Barré syndrome, Riley-Day syndrome all lead to poor coordination of swallow

Pharyngeal phase

- Congenital defects such as vallecular cysts or laryngeal cleft
  - –Inflammatory response; e.g., GERD
  - –Infectious processes
  - –Viral and bacterial pharyngitis
  - –Mass effect from deep neck space abscess
- Tumors: lymphangiomas, hemangiomas, respiratory papillomas, ranulas
  - –Trauma caused by foreign body or caustic ingestion

Esophageal phase

- Congenital lesions such as vascular lesions, webs, or rings
- Inflammatory/infectious
  - –Esophagitis (may be from GERD, allergy, *Candida*, or HSV)
  - –Chagas disease
- Esophageal dysmotility
  - –Cricopharyngeal or lower esophageal sphincter achalasia
  - –Esophageal spasm
- Systemic
  - –Diabetes mellitus, thyroid disease
  - –Scleroderma, polymyositis, dermatomyositis
- Psychological: Globus hystericus

Workup and Diagnosis

- History
  - –Fever, duration, onset, severity, frequency, odynophagia, drooling; vomiting of solids, liquids, or secretions
  - –Voice changes, aspiration, weight loss or failure to thrive, foreign body ingestion, trauma, caustic ingestion
  - –Liquids are least affected by obstructive lesions and first affected by neurologic disorders
  - –Prenatal history: Polyhydramnios, esophageal anomalies
- Physical exam
  - –Craniofacial anomalies/defects in facial anatomy
  - –Nasal exam: Mass or obstruction (6 Fr catheter should pass through in healthy newborn)
  - –Mouth: Pooled secretions, mass, tonsil size, palatal motion
  - –Neck: Neck mass, thyromegaly
- Workup
  - –Modified barium swallow evaluates all phases of swallowing and esophageal function
  - –Flexible fiberoptic exam assesses dynamic problems
  - –Rigid endoscopy: Allows for controlled airway, better optics, and removal of foreign body
  - –Functional endoscopic evaluation of swallow (FEES): Evaluates pharyngeal phase, limited in children because of poor patient cooperation

Treatment

- Important to assess for adequate nutritional intake and safety of swallow without aspiration
- Underlying inflammatory disorders are addressed
- The modified barium swallow study may provide guidance and the speech pathologist may provide recommendations regarding position during feeds, consistency, size limitations, temperature of food, appropriate bottles or utensils, bolus size
- Total oral feeding may not be possible for all children; options include naso- or orogastric feeding or gastrotomy tube feeding
- Surgery
  - –Dysphagia associated with tonsillar hypertrophy may require tonsillectomy
  - –Pharyngeal and esophageal tumors may require resection

53. Halitosis

Halitosis is a relatively infrequent pediatric chief complaint; however, it frequently emerges as part of the HPI. Acute causes are usually upper respiratory infections (such as stomatitis, tonsillitis, or sinusitis), whereas chronic halitosis is more likely to be due to dental issues. However, chronic sinusitis may cause halitosis either from the presence of bacterial colonies or from secondary mouth breathing.

Differential Diagnosis

- Upper respiratory
  - –Stomatitis: Painful ulcerated lesions on oral mucosa and gingiva; coxsackie virus is commonly called hand-foot-and-mouth disease; herpangina refers to herpetic lesions on the soft palate and posterior pharynx; trench mouth refers to necrotizing gingivostomatitis with pseudomembrane caused by spirochetes or fusiform bacteria
  - –Sinusitis: Acute or chronic; pathogens are *Streptococcus pneumoniae*, β-hemolytic strep, *Haemophilus influenzae*, and *Moraxella catarrhalis*; maxillary sinuses are most frequently involved
  - –Pharyngitis/tonsillitis/tonsillar abscess: Group A strep
- Pulmonary disorders
  - –Pulmonary abscess
  - –Bronchiectasis
- Gastric disorders
  - –GERD
  - –Bezoar
- Dental etiologies
  - –Poor oral hygiene: Bacterial accumulation on the teeth or tongue; gingival inflammation; food concretions within tonsillar crypts
  - –Dental abscess: May be sequela of baby-bottle tooth decay, untreated dental caries, dental fracture, or poor hygiene
  - –Orthodontic devices
- Chronic mouth breathing
  - –Seen in children with nasal polyps, adenoid hypertrophy, allergic rhinitis, and chronic sinusitis
  - –Rarely due to a nasopharyngeal tumor such as a hemangioma or fibromas
  - –Resultant dryness causes alteration of the oral mucosa and resultant bad breath; taste and smell may be affected
- Nasal foreign body
  - –Seen most often in the toddler/preschool age group
  - –History of foreign body placement is not always forthcoming
  - –Usually accompanied by unilateral nasal discharge

Workup and Diagnosis

- History
  - –Onset, duration, severity of symptoms
  - –Accompanying signs and symptoms, especially fever, nasal congestion, nasal discharge, sore throat, cough, tachypnea
  - –History of recurrent pneumonia
  - –History of GI upset, digestive problems
  - –Dental history and frequency of dental care
- Physical exam
  - –Examination of the oral cavity for dental hygiene, dental caries, gingival swelling, orthodontic devices that are poorly fitting or poorly maintained
  - –HEENT examination including nasal cavity, oral lesions, tonsillar hypertrophy, asymmetry, exudate, or concretions
  - –General medical evaluation including respiratory and GI systems
- Labs
  - –Throat culture if streptococcal pharyngitis is suspected
- Radiology
  - –X-ray or CT of sinuses for mucosal thickening or air-fluid levels
  - –Lateral X-ray for adenoid hypertrophy
  - –Chest X-ray if pulmonary lesion is suspected
- Studies
  - –Endoscopy may be required for suspicion of GERD or bezoar

Treatment

- Scrupulous oral hygiene
- Stomatitis is usually treated supportively with acetaminophen and oral hydration (Popsicles)
  - –Viscous lidocaine should be used sparingly, if ever
  - –Herpetic lesions may be treated with oral acyclovir
  - –Trench mouth is treated with penicillin
- Streptococcal pharyngitis is treated with penicillin
- Sinusitis requires longer duration of antibiotic therapy
- Bronchiectasis and pulmonary abscess are treated with systemic antibiotics and nonsurgical or surgical drainage
- Adenoidectomy and treatment of concurrent allergies and sinusitis rectifies most mouth breathing
- GERD is treated with H2 blockers and promotility agents
- Endoscopy may be therapeutic and diagnostic for bezoar
- Removal of nasal foreign body is usually sufficient treatment

54. Hoarseness

Hoarseness is a common complaint in the pediatric population. Voice disorders occur in children with 6–9% incidence. History and presentation determine need for diagnostic and therapeutic intervention. Evaluation of stridor and airway obstruction takes precedence over that of voice disturbances.

Differential Diagnosis

- Congenital
  - –Glottic webs
  - –Laryngeal clefts
  - –Laryngocele
  - –Tracheoesophageal fistula
  - –Hemangiomas
- Inflammatory/infectious
  - –Viral URI
  - –Diphtheria
  - –Laryngotracheobronchitis
  - –Gastroesophageal reflux disease: Posterior laryngitis, vocal cord edema
  - –Fungal laryngitis: Consider in an immunocompromised patient
- Tumors
  - –Respiratory papillomas
  - –Squamous cell carcinoma
  - –Hemangioma
  - –Lymphangioma
- Trauma
  - –Traumatic birth
  - –Postintubation: May result in cord edema, granulomas, vocal cord webbing, cricoarytenoid joint dislocation, or ankylosis
  - –Laryngeal fracture
  - –Iatrogenic: Neck or cardiopulmonary surgery may cause injury to the recurrent laryngeal nerve, leading to vocal cord paralysis
  - –Vocal abuse: Vocal cord nodules or polyps
- Endocrine
  - –Hypothryoidism
- Neurogenic
  - –Idiopathic vocal cord paralysis
  - –Arnold-Chiari or Dandy-Walker malformations may lead to brainstem compression of the vagal nerve roots, leading to vocal cord paralysis
  - –Peripheral nerve: Recurrent laryngeal nerve injury or invasion by tumor, myasthenia gravis
  - –Spasmodic dysphonia: Dystonia of the laryngeal muscles
- Systemic disease
  - –Rheumatoid arthritis: Fixation of the cricoarytenoid joint
  - –Relapsing polychondritis
- Functional

Workup and Diagnosis

- History
  - –Onset, severity, progression, quality of cry, recent URI, fluctuations, time preference, stridor, dysphagia, regurgitation, aspiration, exercise tolerance, sick contacts
  - –Immunization history
  - –Trauma history
  - –PMH: Traumatic birth, neck or chest surgery, prolonged or repeated intubations
- Physical exam
  - –Head and neck lymphangioma or hemangioma (possible similar airway lesion)
  - –Neck masses, tracheal shift
  - –Cardiac exam, abnormal muscle tone
- Workup
  - –Flexible fiberoptic nasopharyngoscope: Office exam of the larynx and vocal cord mobility; cannot see subglottis; requires patient cooperation
- Direct laryngoscopy: affords better exam of larynx but requires general anesthesia; subtle structural changes are visible, palpation of cricoarytenoid joint to differentiate paralysis vs fixation is possible
  - –Chest X-ray: Mediastinal lesion, cyst
  - –CT or MRI: Indicated with congenital cyst, tumors, or trauma
  - –MRI of head when intracranial pathology suspected

Treatment

- Medical
  - –Reflux changes: Behavioral and diet modification, anti-reflux treatment, prokinetics, Nissen fundoplication for severe cases
  - –Vocal cord nodules: Limit vocal abuse, voice therapy, antireflux treatment
  - –Supportive or antibiotic treatment for infectious causes
- Voice therapy
  - –Abuse reduction; vocal hygiene; tension reduction; resonance and pitch training
- Hoarseness with airway distress may require immediate intubation or tracheostomy
- Tumors or congenital lesions are treated with surgical resection.
- Brainstem causes may require neurosurgical decompression
- Botox (botulinum toxin) for spasmodic dysphonia

55. Macroglossia

Macroglossia is an abnormal enlargement of the tongue, and is a very significant finding, especially in the neonate. In the neonate, suspect Beckwith-Wiedemann syndrome and monitor for hypoglycemia. In a young infant, suspect hypothyroidism, especially if feeding difficulties or other associated features are present. Macroglossia in older infants and young children is frequently the result of a metabolic storage disorder.

Differential Diagnosis

- Beckwith-Wiedemann syndrome
  - –Sporadic mutation of chromosome 11, affecting insulin production and neighboring genes
  - –Characteristics include severe hypoglycemia, macroglossia, macrosomia, abdominal wall defects, and renal anomalies
- Down syndrome
  - –Macroglossia is actually pseudomacroglossia secondary to hypoplastic oral cavity
- Hypothyroidism
  - –Congenital hypothyroidism may not be recognizable in the immediate neonatal period because of the presence of maternal thyroid hormone
  - –Within days to weeks, symptoms develop
  - –Typical symptoms include sluggishness, hypotonia, persistent hyperbilirubinemia, umbilical hernia, constipation, large tongue, and large fontanelle
  - –Macroglossia may be a significant contributor to feeding difficulties or respiratory compromise
- Storage disorders
  - –Hurler syndrome: Mucopolysaccharidosis type 1; characterized by macroglossia, coarse facial features, hepatosplenomegaly, and growth retardation
  - –Pompe disease: Type 2 glycogenosis; macroglossia, hypotonia, muscle weakness, cardiomyopathy
  - –Gangliosidosis: Lysosomal enzyme deficiency resulting in accumulation of gangliosides in lysosomes in brain and visceral cells; characterized by mental retardation, growth retardation, hypotonia, macroglossia, hepatosplenomegaly
- Benign tumors
  - –Hemangioma
  - –Lymphangioma
  - –Neurofibroma
  - –Rhabdomyoma
- Idiopathic

Workup and Diagnosis

- History
  - –Birth history, including home birth without newborn screening procedures, neonatal hypoglycemia, persistent hyperbilirubinemia
  - –Infant characteristics such as feeding, elimination, activity, and sleeping habits
- Physical exam
  - –Growth parameters
  - –Developmental progress
  - –Presence of physical findings associated with syndromes and disorders
- Labs
  - –Newborn screen results may include thyroid function and metabolic disorders but may also warrant repeat even if normal
  - –Blood glucose
  - –Thyroid function studies
  - –Serum CK and LDH are elevated in Pompe
- Radiology
  - –CT may delineate the soft tissue structures of the tongue, oral cavity, and neck
- Studies
  - –Chromosomal analysis for Beckwith-Wiedemann syndrome, Down (trisomy 21)
  - –Analyze urine mucopolysaccharides (glycosaminoglycans), genetic testing for Hurler
  - –Muscle biopsy: Pompe-Fibroblast culture for lysosomal enzyme activity, gangliosidosis

Treatment

- Tongue reduction surgery may be necessary to protect the airway and allow normal mastication
- Tongue reduction may also help optimize dental and oral cavity development
- Beckwith-Wiedemann: Intractable neonatal hypoglycemia requires immediate recognition and ICU management
- Down syndrome: Macroglossia may or may not require treatment; patients should be followed at a comprehensive Down syndrome care center; genetics referral should also be offered
- Hypothyroidism: Thyroxine replacement with careful tracking to keep levels therapeutic as patient grows
- No definitive treatments are available for storage disorders; care is mostly symptom-oriented and palliative

56. Salivary Gland Enlargement

Salivary gland enlargement in pediatric patients is usually associated with an inflammatory or infectious process. Benign tumors are more common than malignancies, but the probability for malignancy in a solid mass is higher in children than adults. Facial nerve weakness is highly suggestive of malignancy.

Differential Diagnosis

- Congenital
  - First branchial cleft cyst
  - Retention cyst
  - Ectopic rests of salivary tissue
- Infectious/inflammatory
  - Mumps (before immunization) was the most common salivary gland inflammatory disease
  - HIV
  - Coxsackie A
  - Echovirus
  - Viral sialoadenitis
  - Acute bacterial sialoadenitis: Typically *Staphylococcus aureus* or *Streptococcus viridans*
  - Sialolithiasis
- Vascular lesions
  - Hemangiomas: Most common salivary gland mass in children
  - Lymphangioma
- Benign tumors
  - Pleomorphic adenomas: Most common solid benign tumor
  - Warthin tumors
  - Oncocytoma
  - Adenomas
- Malignant tumors
  - Mucoepidermoid carcinoma: Most common
  - Acinic cell carcinoma
  - Adenoid cystic carcinoma
  - Undifferentiated carcinoma
  - Lymphoma
  - Rhabdomyosarcoma
  - Squamous cell carcinoma
- Trauma (may often be associated with facial nerve injury)
- Systemic diseases
  - Diffuse bilateral salivary gland enlargement: often associated with diabetes mellitus, cystic fibrosis, thyroid disease, malnutrition, obesity, autoimmune disorders (Sjögren)
  - Granulomatous disease: tuberculosis, atypical *Mycobacterium*, sarcoidosis, cat-scratch disease
- Drugs such as methimazole, thiourea, phenothiazine, thiocyanate

Workup and Diagnosis

- History
  - Duration, onset, pain, change in size with meals, prior history of recent weight loss or gain, joint tenderness
  - Past medical history of systemic disease: CF, diabetes, autoimmune disorders
  - Exposure: Immunization, radiation, cat-scratch disease
- Physical exam
  - Size, character: Firm, soft, cystic, tenderness, warmth, redness, bilaterality, oral cavity exam, pus from Stenson or Wharton duct, palpable stone, neck mass, facial nerve function (paresis or paralysis is highly suggestive of malignancy)
- Culture of drainage may guide antibiotic therapy
- Plain film X-rays: Limited utility but may identify salivary duct stone; 80–90% of submandibular stones are radio-opaque
- Ultrasound: May differentiate between cystic and solid lesions, ductal dilations, and intra- and extraparenchymal lesions
- CT or MRI: Provides better resolution of salivary gland lesions and surrounding tissues; MRI gives superior details for salivary gland neoplasms
- Fine-needle aspiration: 90% sensitivity and 95–100% specificity for identifying malignancy with experienced pathologist
- Sialography: Limited in children, contraindicated in acute infections

Treatment

- Supportive treatment for viral adenitis
- Bacterial sialoadenitis requires antibiotic therapy with warm compresses and sialogogues to help promote salivary flow; IV antibiotic therapy may be required in severe cases
- Sialolithiasis is treated with surgical excision of the stone or the gland
- Hemangiomas are simply observed unless rapid growth, functional impairment, infection, bleeding, or severe cosmetic deformity is present
- Tumors are treated surgically
  - Parotid neoplasms that are lateral are treated with superficial parotidectomy; submandibular neoplasms require total submandibular gland excision
  - If malignancy is suspected, neck dissection is performed when palpable lymphadenopathy is present and considered for high-grade lesions
  - Possible radiation therapy based on final pathology

57. Snoring

Snoring in children, in and of itself, does not warrant absolute treatment but may indicate the presence of obstructive sleep apnea (OSA). The most common cause of obstruction is adenoid and tonsillar hypertrophy. Adenotonsillectomy eliminates obstruction in 85–95% of otherwise normal children with OSA.

Differential Diagnosis

- Congenital/anatomic
  - –Midface hypoplasia
  - –Retrognathia
  - –Macroglossia
  - –Base of tongue collapse
  - –Nasal septal deviation
  - –Severe laryngomalacia
  - –Craniofacial syndromes
    - –Pierre Robin sequence
    - –Treacher Collins
    - –Goldenhar
    - –Nager
    - –Apert
    - –Klippel-Feil
  - –Choanal atresia
- Infectious/inflammatory
  - –Adenotonsillar hypertrophy
  - –Viral and bacterial rhinosinusitis
  - –Allergies
  - –Nasal polyposis
  - –Gastroesophageal reflux disease
- Tumors
  - –Encephalocele
  - –Dermoids
  - –Gliomas
  - –Juvenile nasopharyngeal angiofibroma
  - –Chordoma
  - –Craniopharyngioma
  - –Thyroid tumors
- Neurologic
  - –Cerebral palsy: Hypotonia may lead to collapsing pharyngeal soft tissue
  - –Myopathies
  - –Anoxic encephalopathy
- Systemic
  - –Mucopolysaccharide storage disease
  - –Cystic fibrosis
- Iatrogenic
  - –Prior cleft palate repair
  - –Nasopharyngeal stenosis
  - –Pharyngeal flap
- Obesity (either as an isolated problem or a contributor to one of the above pathologies)

Workup and Diagnosis

- History
  - –Loud snoring, mouth breathing, apneic episodes, gasping or snorting, daytime fatigue or restlessness, nocturnal enuresis, failure to thrive, dysphagia
  - –Medical history: Cardiovascular anomalies, craniofacial syndromes, prior surgery in the mouth
- Physical exam
  - –Midfacial hypoplasia, retrognathia or micrognathia
  - –Tonsillar hypertrophy, nasal mass, adenoid facies
  - –Obesity
  - –Hyponasal speech
- Studies
  - –Lateral skull film evaluates adenoid size
  - –Flexible fiberoptic nasopharyngoscopy evaluates nasal cavity, adenoid size, base of tongue, larynx
  - –CT of face: Consider for craniofacial anomalies
  - –Audio- and videotape of sleep from home
  - –Polysomnogram is the gold standard to evaluate for sleep apnea and associated sleep disorders; not necessary in all cases; consider in those with complex medical problems, age <2, or severe history out of proportion to normal exam
  - –ECG and chest X-ray if cardiopulmonary disease suspected

Treatment

- Snoring requires treatment only when associated with obstructive sleep apnea
- Medical options
  - –Weight loss, if obese
  - –Treatment of nasal obstruction
  - –30 days of amoxicillin plus clavulanate may be considered in those with mild symptoms to reduce adenotonsillar size
  - –CPAP or BiPAP if surgery is contraindicated
- Adenotonsillectomy: First-line surgical treatment
- Uvulopalatopharyngoplasty: Not commonly performed in children
- Midface or mandibular advancement if craniofacial anomalies contributing to OSA
- Tracheotomy: Definitive procedure, because obstruction is bypassed; performed only in extreme cases

58. Sore Throat

Most sore throats and coughs are due to infection. Children may have 5–8 upper respiratory infections per year. The primary differential is between viral and bacterial etiologies, especially group A β-hemolytic streptococcus.

Differential Diagnosis

- Infectious
  - –Viral
    - –Adenovirus
    - –Rhinovirus
    - –Parainfluenza
    - –Influenza
    - –Coronavirus
    - –Others: EBV RSV, CMV, HSV
  - –Bacterial
    - –*Streptococcus*
    - –*Haemophilus*
    - –*Moraxella*
    - –*Staphylococcus*
    - –*Corynebacterium*
    - –Anaerobes
  - –Fungal
    - –*Candida*
- Inflammatory
  - –Allergy
  - –Gastroesophageal reflux disease
  - –Sinusitis resulting in postnasal drainage
- Tumors
  - –Leukemia
  - –Rhabdosarcomas
  - –Squamous cell carcinoma secondary to oral ulcerations
- Trauma
  - –Foreign body ingestion
  - –Caustic ingestion
  - –Soft tissue injury from accidental and nonaccidental trauma
- Systemic/rheumatologic disorders
  - –Kawasaki disease: Mucocutaneous lymph node syndrome may have sore throat at presentation (other oral findings include strawberry tongue, fissured lips, mucosal erythema, fever, and lymphadenopathy)
  - –Behçet syndrome
  - –Reiter syndrome
- Others
  - –Cigarette smoke
  - –Environmental pollutants
  - –Pharyngeal drying: Mouth and pharynx can be dry from mouth breathing, more common in the winter months

Workup and Diagnosis

- History
  - –Duration, onset, severity, frequency, odynophagia, dysphagia, daycare, sick contacts, fever, malaise, headache
  - –Foreign body and caustic ingestion
  - –Days of school or work missed
  - –Immunization history
  - –Medical history: Systemic disease, connective tissue disorder
- Physical exam
  - –Nasal exam: Evidence of rhinosinusitis
  - –Mouth: Ulcerations, masses, tonsil size, erythema, exudates
  - –Neck: Lymphadenopathy
  - –Skin: Rash
  - –Chest: Wheezes, asymmetry
- Studies
  - –For pharyngitis: A major goal is to differentiate streptococcal pharyngitis from viral etiologies
  - –Throat culture: 92% sensitive; 100% specific; requires 24–48 hours
  - –Rapid strep test: 72–85% sensitive; 88–100% specific
  - –CBC with differential for suspected mononucleosis
  - –Chest X-ray (inspiratory and expiratory) for suspected foreign body
  - –CT neck: When complication of infection is suspected such as abscess

Treatment

- Viral causes
  - –Supportive care including hydration, acetaminophen or ibuprofen, bedrest, salt water rinses
  - –Steroids may be considered to minimize upper airway obstruction
- Antibiotics for bacterial etiologies
  - –For group A β-hemolytic strep: Shortens duration of symptoms and prevents rheumatic fever
- Consider inpatient admission when there is concern about adequate airway or oral intake
- Airway management: Intubation or tracheotomy
- When gastroesophageal reflux is suspected, treatment may include dietary changes, antireflux therapy
- Adenotonsillectomy for recurrent tonsillitis is considered depending on frequency of recurrence, i.e., 6–7 infections/year, or 4–5 infections/year for 2 years, or 3 infections/year for 3 years

59. Stomatitis

Oral ulcers may represent a local infection, an immune reaction, or a general medical condition. The most common cause is idiopathic aphthous ulcers, followed by oral infections. Occasionally a general medical condition may be discovered in the evaluation of stomatitis, and HIV should be remembered as a potential etiology because stomatitis or rampant herpetic infections may be among the earliest clinical manifestations.

Differential Diagnosis

- Aphthous ulcers (idiopathic)
  - –May be due to alteration of T-cell immune function
  - –Triggers include dietary substances, stress, and illness
  - –Nutritional deficiencies (iron, B vitamins) may play a role
  - –May run in families, thus making it more difficult to distinguish from herpetic lesions that have been shared among family members
  - –May be small or large, may be singular or grouped
- Infectious stomatitis
  - –Coxsackievirus: Also known as hand-foot-and-mouth disease; all locations of lesions may not be present; usually seen in the summer and fall
  - –Herpetic gingivostomatitis: Common in toddlers; may last a week or longer; generally accompanied by fever, lymphadenopathy; painful lesions may cause reduction in oral intake and resultant dehydration
  - –Herpangina: Caused by an enterovirus rather than human herpesvirus; lesions are present primarily on the soft palate, anterior tonsillar pillars, and posterior pharynx
  - –Trench mouth: also known as Vincent angina; caused by fusiform bacteria or spirochetes; causes necrotizing gingivostomatitis with pseudomembrane formation; found in developing nations and malnourished patients
- Hematologic disorders
  - –Associated with leukemia
  - –Associated with neutropenia secondary to chemotherapy for malignancy
  - –Associated with cyclic neutropenia
- Behçet disease
- Stevens-Johnson syndrome
- Inflammatory bowel disease: May be found in Crohn disease or ulcerative colitis
- HIV
  - –Alterations in T-cell immunity can lead to aphthous ulcers
  - –HIV patients are more susceptible to herpetic infections

Workup and Diagnosis

- History
  - –Onset, frequency, duration of symptoms
  - –Established or suspected triggers
  - –Concomitant symptom: Fever, lymphadenopathy, rash, diarrhea, weight loss
- Physical exam
  - –Size of lesions
  - –Distribution of lesions
  - –Morphologic characteristics
  - –Presence of other findings on physical exam: Fever, rash, abdominal tenderness
- Labs
  - –Tzanck smear (shows multinucleated giant cells) or a positive herpes simplex culture can confirm herpetic gingivostomatitis
  - –Trench mouth may be confirmed by simple culture for fusiform bacteria or darkfield examination for spirochetes

Treatment

- Symptomatic care
  - –Rinsing with a 1:1 solution of dipheniraminc with antacid provides temporary relief
  - –Acetaminophen may be used liberally
- Occlusive topical solutions may aid in healing
- Topical anesthetics such as benzocaine or viscous lidocaine should be used sparingly if at all in children
  - –Damage to the mucous membranes may result
  - –Accidental swallowing can lead to aspiration secondary to the impairment of the gag reflex
- For severe or recurrent aphthous ulcers, systemic steroids or colchicine are sometimes used
- Herpetic lesions are treated with oral acyclovir
- Trench mouth is treated with penicillin

Section 9

Neck

KATHLEEN O. DeANTONIS, MD
DAVID J. KAY, MD
MUSTAFA SAHIN, MD, PhD
NICOLE J. ULLRICH, MD, PhD

60. Neck Masses

Suspect a neoplasm when cervical lymphadenopathy does not improve with 6–8 weeks of appropriate therapy. The location of a mass (anterior neck, lateral neck, cheek) directs its differential diagnosis within three categories: inflammatory, congenital, or neoplastic. Cellulitis may rapidly progress to a dangerous abscess if left untreated.

Differential Diagnosis

- Lymphadenopathy
  - –Inflammatory is most common pediatric neck mass
  - –Viral or bacterial adenitis, mononucleosis, cat-scratch disease, tuberculosis, atypical mycobacterium
  - –Granulomatous (sarcoid, etc.)
  - –Lymphoma is most common neck malignancy
  - –Kawasaki disease
  - –Metastatic malignancy
- Deep neck abscess or cellulitis
  - –Bacterial, atypical mycobacteria, cat-scratch disease, etc.
- Hemangioma
  - –Most common benign neck neoplasm
  - –Rapid growth, then spontaneous involution
- Vascular malformation
  - –Lymphatic malformation (lymphangioma, cystic hygroma)
  - –Venous malformation
  - –Arteriovenous malformation
- Branchial cleft cyst
  - –First (types I and II), second (most common), third
- Preauricular cyst
  - –Anterior to tragus
- Thyroglossal duct cyst
  - –Most common congenital midline mass
  - –Elevates with swallowing
- Thyroid mass
- Ectopic thyroid
- Parathyroid mass
- Dermoid cyst
- Plunging ranula
- Teratoma
- Lipoma
- Thymic cyst
- Ectopic thymus
- Sternocleidomastoid (SCM) muscle tumor of infancy (congenital torticollis)
  - –Fibrous tumors, unknown etiology
- Laryngocele
  - –Abnormal dilatation of ventricle and saccule
- Salivary gland neoplasm
  - –Parotid, submandibular
- Paraganglioma
  - –Carotid body tumor, glomus jugulare, glomus vagale

Workup and Diagnosis

- History
  - –Recent trauma or infection
  - –Exposure to cats or tuberculosis
  - –Weight loss
- Physical exam
  - –Levels of the neck: I = submandibular, II = upper third of SCM, III = middle third of SCM, IV = lower third of SCM, V = posterior to SCM, VI = anterior neck
  - –Infectious signs: Pain, redness, swelling
  - –Systemic findings: Fever, hepatosplenomegaly
- Labs
  - –CBC with differential: Atypical lymphocytes suggest EBV
  - –PPD
  - –EBV titers, monospot test
  - –HIV test, if suspected by history
- Fine needle aspiration (FNA) biopsy
  - –Can differentiate abscess from cellulitis
  - –Cytology may diagnose pathology of soft tissue tumor
- X-rays
  - –Lateral neck useful screen for retropharyngeal abscess
- CT scan with contrast (abscess shows low-density center with rim enhancement) or MRI
- Ultrasonography
  - –For midline neck masses, may be used to confirm presence of a normal thyroid
  - –Also differentiates abscess from cellulitis

Treatment

- Oral antibiotics for infected neck masses
  - –IV antibiotics if poor response
- Abscess requires incision and drainage (I&D)
  - –Send contents for Gram stain and culture
- Cat-scratch disease and atypical mycobacteria self-limiting, but take months to resolve
- Congenital cysts and masses: Excision
  - –If infected, delay excision until infection clears
- Hemangiomas treated only if obstruct breathing or feeding, or cause thrombocytopenia or cardiac failure
  - –Excision, laser ablation, steroids, interferon
- Lymphatic malfomations are benign; surgical debulking with sacrifice of normal tissues; may recur
- SCM tumor of infancy (congenital torticollis) usually resolves with physical therapy only
- Cold abscess (no fever or pain) requires I&D
- If airway obstructed, intubate
  - –Severe obstruction may require tracheostomy

61. Nuchal Rigidity

Nuchal rigidity is characterized by involuntary muscle spasms that limit passive neck flexion. Although it has myriad causes, meningeal irritation may occur secondary to infection, so patients must be evaluated emergently for meningitis/focal infection. Cervical muscle spasms and dystonia are common etiologies that can be treated with local therapies and pharmacologic agents that act at the neuromuscular junction.

Differential Diagnosis

- Stress
  - Causing muscles to tighten and stiffen
- Injury/whiplash secondary to trauma
- Cervical adenitis
- Meningitis
  - Presence of nuchal rigidity has 30% sensitivity, 95% specificity
- Encephalitis
- Subarachnoid hemorrhage
- Retropharyngeal abscess
  - Associated with fever, sore throat (84%)
- Epiglottitis
- Focal dystonia
- Torticollis, congenital or acquired
- Tetanus
  - Associated with trismus, risus sardonicus, opisthotonus, muscle spasms
- Dental abscess
- Pharynx/larynx spasms
- Chemical meningitis
  - After spinal anesthesia or lumbar puncture
- Parameningeal infection
  - Lesion on MRI/CT
- Posterior fossa tumor
- Thyroiditis
- Rheumatoid arthritis
- Cervical arthritis
- Pneumonia
- Cervical spine osteomyelitis
- Poliomyelitis
- Trichinosis
- Chagas disease
- Infantile Gaucher disease
- Maple syrup urine disease
- Kernicterus
- Toxins
  - Phenothiazines
  - Strychnine
  - Lead poisoning
  - Methanol poisoning
  - Hypervitaminosis A

Workup and Diagnosis

- History
  - Duration
  - Age of onset
  - Presence and location of pain
  - Trauma
  - Vomiting, headache, fever
  - History of blood clots, aneurysm
  - Decreased sensation or movement in other areas
  - Recent infection or recent dental work
  - Visual changes
  - Seizures
- Physical exam
  - Vital signs, blood pressure, pulse, temperature
  - Head circumference in infants to evaluate for progressive increase in intracranial pressure
  - Head and neck should be palpated
  - Sinus tenderness, thyromegaly, and focal lymph nodes
  - Kernig sign: Flex hip and knee, then extend knee, assess for resistance to knee straightening
  - Brudzinski sign: Flex neck/chin to chest, observe if hip and knees flex
  - Careful mental status examination
- Evaluation
  - Lumbar puncture to identify bacterial or viral meningitis, particularly in the febrile patient
  - MRI scan if focal neurologic abnormality, seizure, mental status changes

Treatment

- Meningitis/encephalitis
  - Broad-spectrum antibiotics
  - Neurologic checks
  - Dexamethasone may improve neurologic outcome and lower incidence of postmeningitic deafness
- Subarachnoid hemorrhage
  - Immediate neurosurgical evaluation
  - Consider MRA/conventional angiography
  - Surgical clipping and excision
  - Pharmacologic management of cerebral vasospasm
  - Nimodipine is often used to prevent delayed ischemia
- Torticollis: Treat with valium, botulinum toxin type A
- Adenitis/dental abscess: Antibiotic treatment
- Injury: Soft collar, NSAIDs
- Cervical muscle spasms
  - Heat, massage, soft cervical collar, analgesics

62. Torticollis

Torticollis is the term used to describe an abnormal fixed head position, characterized by rotation of the neck to one side and lateral flexion of the neck to the contralateral side.

Differential Diagnosis

- Congenital muscular torticollis
  - –Most likely secondary to birth trauma
  - –SCM muscle is stretched during delivery, a hematoma results, and the SCM muscle spasms in response
  - –SCM muscle may become fibrotic
- Brachial nerve plexus injury
  - –Also associated with birth trauma
- Benign paroxymal torticollis
  - –Occurs in infants and young children
  - –Abrupt onset with pallor and vomiting
  - –May be a migraine variant
- Muscular spasm
  - –May occur after prolonged exposure to a cold stimulus such as wind
- Dystonic reaction
  - –May be drug reaction to antipsychotics, metoclopramide, prochlorperazine, trimethobenzamide
  - –May be part of a dysmotility syndrome such as myasthenia gravis or Huntington chorea
- HEENT infection
  - –May occur with cervical adenitis, otitis, or mastoiditis
  - –Local pressure on the neighboring SCM muscle causes irritation and spasm of the muscle
- Atlantoaxial subluxation
  - –Associated with Down syndrome, achondroplasia
  - –May be secondary to fracture, infection, or malignancy of the cervical spine
- Post-upper respiratory infection
  - –May occur in young children
  - –Retropharyngeal edema displaces the atlantoaxial junction
- Ocular torticollis
  - –A compensatory mechanism enacted by patients with trochlear nerve palsy or superior oblique muscle weakness
  - –Head positioning results in better alignment of the affected eye with the unaffected eye, and minimizes diplopia
- GERD, hiatal hernia
  - –May manifest as neck torsion (known as Sandifer syndrome)
- Klippel-Feil syndrome

Workup and Diagnosis

- History
  - –Onset, duration, associated symptoms such as pain or stiffness
  - –Birth history, including birth trauma, deformity at birth, other congenital malformations, syndromic features
  - –Past medical history, including trauma and recent illness
  - –Family history of syndromes, movement disorders migraines
- Physical exam
  - –SCM muscle examination for length, tension, masses, and range of motion
  - –Cranial nerve testing, especially EOMs
- Studies
  - –AP and lateral plain films to evaluate bone structure and look for fracture
  - –Open-mouth views to evaluate the odontoid
  - –Flexion and extension views (passive range of motion) to evaluate cervical stability
  - –CT or MRI to evaluate deep soft tissue structures of the neck
- Labs
  - –CBC with differential, ESR and blood culture if cervical osteomyelitis is suspected

Treatment

- Physical therapy including massage and stretching of the contracted muscle
- For infants, selective positioning and placement of visual stimuli to promote stretching of the affected muscle
- Surgical release of the SCM muscle
- Surgical stabilization of the alantoaxial joint
- Discontinuation of causative medications
- Ophthalmic consultation for EOM impairment

Section 10

Chest

DAVID H. CHI, MD
SHANNON FOURTNER, MD
ADDA GRIMBERG, MD
C. BECKET MAHNKE, MD
TIMOTHY D. MURPHY, MD

63. Abnormal Heart Sounds

Abnormal heart sounds are common in pediatric patients and usually benign. Approximately 50% of children will have an innocent murmur at some time, compared to a 1% incidence of congenital heart disease (nearly all of which present by 1 year of age).

Differential Diagnosis

- Abnormal S_2
  - –Most important auscultatory finding; normally, S_2 is single on inspiration and narrowly split on expiration, indicating normal pulmonary arterial pressures; difficult to learn, especially in babies with fast heart rates or a screaming child
  - –Single and/or loud S_2: Increased pulmonary artery pressure (large L to R shunt, pulmonary hypertension), also seen in patients with only single outlet from heart (i.e., pulmonary atresia)
  - –Wide fixed-split S_2: ASD, right bundle branch block, post-cardiac surgery
- Systolic murmur
  - –Up to 50% of children at some point in life
  - –Mid-systolic/ejection type: S_1 and S_2 separate from the murmur (lub-shhh-dub), due to flow across semilunar valve, harsh indicates semilunar valve stenosis, whereas low-pitched, vibratory, musical indicates innocent murmur
  - –Holosystolic/regurgitant murmur: Begins with S_1 (which is not clearly heard); always pathologic (mitral valve regurgitation, VSD, subaortic stenosis)
- Diastolic sounds
  - –Always abnormal
  - –Early and medium/high pitch murmur indicates semilunar valve insufficiency, low frequency rumbling indicates mitral/tricuspid stenosis
  - –S_3/S_4/opening snap: Soft S_3 can be normal in healthy children; any sound clearly heard is probably an abnormality of the mitral/tricuspid valve (opening snap) or ventricular filling (S_3/S_4)
- Continuous murmur
  - –Murmur in systole that continues into diastole (may not fill entire diastole)
  - –Venous hum: Low pitched, continuous murmur at both upper sternal borders; disappears when supine; innocent
  - –Patent ductus arteriosus: Harsh, machinery-like murmur at left upper sternal border (LUSB)
- Systolic ejection click
  - –High-pitched sound
  - –Early: Bicuspid aortic valve, loudest at apex/LLSB, often confused with split S_1
  - –Mid/late: Mitral valve prolapse

Workup and Diagnosis

- Majority of murmurs heard after the first year of life are systolic and innocent
- Major innocent murmurs of childhood: All must have a normal S_2 and no symptoms
  - –Still (vibratory) murmur: Vibratory, musical, twangy midsystolic murmur loudest at the LLSB, louder when supine, heard in toddlers
  - –Venous hum: Continuous low rumbling sound at upper sternal borders, disappears when supine
  - –Peripheral pulmonary stenosis (PPS): Midsystolic murmur at LUSB, radiates to back and both axillae, normal up to 1 year of age (refer for evaluation if present afterwards)
  - –Innocent pulmonary flow murmur: Midsystolic murmur, LUSB, loudest when supine, adolescent age range
- Physical exam: Assess growth pattern, heart rate, organomegaly, and femoral pulses
- Four-limb blood pressures very helpful in evaluating possible aortic coarctation (higher BP in arms, lower in legs)
- Chest X-ray: Rarely useful in the routine evaluation of murmurs in children (unless pathology likely)
- 12-lead electrocardiogram useful for assessment of atrial or ventricular enlargement/hypertrophy
- Pulse-oximetry is very useful in the newborn to rule out mildly cyanotic lesions
- Echocardiography

Treatment

- Innocent murmurs
  - –Parental reassurance that this is a normal, common finding in children representing normal blood flowing through a normal heart, usually disappearing with age (as the patient grows, the stethoscope is farther from the heart, so the sound isn't heard)
  - –The murmur may get louder during times of increased cardiac output (i.e., illness, fever, dehydration, activity, or other stress)
  - –No bacterial endocarditis prophylaxis required
- Abnormal findings requiring referral
  - –Abnormal S_2 (single or widely split)
  - –Holosystolic/regurgitant murmur
  - –Any diastolic sounds
  - –Systolic ejection clicks: "Harsh" murmurs
  - –Any murmur with cardiac symptoms
- Further treatment is dependent on underlying anatomy and physiology

64. Apnea

Apnea is defined as the cessation of breathing; how long a pause is physiologically significant depends on age. History will often be more helpful than physical exam. Central apnea refers to a lack of respiratory effort accompanied by a lack of air flow; obstructive apnea refers to a lack of air flow in the face of a respiratory effort. "Central apnea" may be due to muscle weakness and failure despite CNS activation.

Differential Diagnosis

- Much apnea is physiologic and normal
  - –Post-sigh apnea is normal
  - –Newborns, especially premature babies, may have irregular breathing as their respiratory control center matures
  - –Periodic breathing at high altitude
- Prolonged apnea is respiratory arrest, and inadequate ventilation is respiratory failure, and both require immediate intervention
- Apnea may be divided into central, obstructive, and mixed apnea; etiologies vary by age
- Central apnea in infants
  - –Apnea of prematurity
  - –Congenital central hypoventilation syndrome (CCHS, or Ondine curse)
  - –CNS depression (sepsis, shock, drug effect, RSV, seizure or postictal state)
  - –Respiratory muscle failure (e.g., myotonia, infantile botulism)
- Obstructive apnea in infants
  - –Upper airway obstruction (severe laryngomalacia, choanal atresia, macroglossia, micrognathia, subglottic stenosis or web, laryngospasm)
  - –Lower airway: Rarely causes obstructive apnea (tracheal stenosis, rings, slings)
- Central apnea in children
  - –CNS (drug-induced CNS depression, CCHS, abnormal CNS brainstem anatomy and function, sepsis/septic shock)
  - –Respiratory muscle failure (muscular dystrophy, myotonia, myasthenia gravis)
- Obstructive apnea in children
  - –Upper airway obstruction, obstructive sleep apnea syndrome (OSAS), tonsillar and adenoidal hypertrophy, macroglossia, micrognathia, subglottic stenosis, laryngospasm
- Mixed apnea
  - –CNS depression and decreased upper airway tone
  - –Gastroesophageal reflux leading to increased parasympathetic activity and/or laryngospasm
  - –Respiratory muscle failure and adenoidal hypertrophy
- Apparent life-threatening events (ALTE)
- Trauma may cause apnea at any age

Workup and Diagnosis

- Acute or prolonged apnea must be treated immediately with life-support protocols
- History may determine if apnea is central or obstructive
  - –Snoring, stridor, gasps are consistent with obstructive apnea
  - –Pauses are consistent with central apnea
  - –Ingestion of raw honey can cause infantile botulism
  - –Apnea/ALTE may occur in a familial pattern, but such a history should provoke a search for intentional injury
- Apnea is most often associated with sleep and/or change in stage of sleep, so obtaining data during sleep may be needed to diagnose the cause of the apnea
- CCHS may be associated with hypoventilation while awake, but is primarily a sleep-related disorder
- Neuromuscular disease may be accompanied by structural disease (e.g., arthrogryposis, scoliosis)
- Obstructive disease may have an obvious etiology (e.g., micrognathia), but consider central or CNS disease
- Radiographic studies not as helpful as physiologic studies; fluoroscopy may diagnose malacia
- A pneumogram examines heart rate, respiratory rate, chest wall movement, and oxygen saturation, but may miss obstructive disease
- Preferred test is polysomnography, which adds measures of sleep stage and body movement, EEG, pH, and CO_2
- Covert videotaping in hospital may be needed for suspected abuse

Treatment

- Central apnea therapy depends on cause; an infant may need no more than monitoring or supplemental O_2.
- Severe central apnea, especially with respiratory muscle failure, may need to be treated with artificial respiration (via nasal/face mask or tracheotomy tube)
- CCHS may be treated long term with diaphragmatic pacing
- Other causes of central apnea require targeted therapy (i.e., antibiotics for sepsis, O_2 for severe hypoxia)
- Severe obstruction is bypassed with tracheostomy, or overcome with positive pressure ventilation
- Weight loss is an important adjunct in treating severe OSAS
- Respiratory stimulants (e.g., caffeine) may help some babies with apnea of prematurity
- Vigorously treat causative factors (e.g., GERD)
- Apnea monitors are of little proven value in the management or treatment of apnea, yet frequently used

65. Chest Pain

Chest pain is a frequent complaint in pediatrics, especially in the adolescent age group. Although rarely cardiac in etiology, this often represents the patient's/family's greatest fear. A careful history and physical exam, with attention to the needs of the patient/family and appropriate reassurance, are often all that are required.

Differential Diagnosis

- Musculoskeletal
  - –Sharp, stabbing pain that is usually very well localized, often worsened by deep breath or cough
  - –Costochondritis: Tender parasternal pain at insertion of ribs into cartilage en route to sternum; increases with palpation or mild chest compression (possibly postviral)
  - –Injury to chest wall
- Pulmonary
  - –Very common cause, usually associated with respiratory symptoms: Shortness of breath, cough, exercise intolerance
  - –Asthma (most common), often only EIA; may have personal/family history of atopy (asthma, eczema, seasonal allergies); shortness of breath is usually primary complaint, with feeling of chest tightness/pain as a secondary symptom
  - –Pleuritic chest pain: Sharp, stabbing pain with deep breaths, indicates pleural space inflammation, probably postinfectious (especially viral)
  - –Pneumonia: Chest pain secondary to cough or pleural involvement
  - –Pneumothorax can occur spontaneously, especially in tall, thin athletes
- Gastrointestinal
  - –GERD and PUD: Burning, substernal pain with eating, worse at night
  - –Rarely pancreatitis (with back pain too), cholecystitis, hiatal hernia, hepatitis
- Cardiac: Rare in children
  - –Precordial catch syndrome: Sharp, brief (seconds) chest pain usually associated with rising from lying or sitting; unclear etiology, but of no significance
  - –Pericarditis: Inflammation of the pericardium; often postviral, may represent connective tissue/autoimmune, cancer, bacterial infection (very ill appearing with fever), or post-cardiac surgery; patients often lean forward to decrease the pain
  - –MI (rare): Congenital coronary anomaly, post-Kawasaki, cocaine use, hypertrophic cardiomyopathy
  - –Aortic dissection: Consider if features or history of Marfan syndrome is present

Workup and Diagnosis

- History
  - –Activity at onset, (chest pain with exercise is a red flag!), precipitating/relieving factors, quality of pain (sharp vs dull)
  - –Associated symptoms (shortness of breath, diaphoresis, cough/wheeze, nausea/vomiting), recent illness, response to eating, sleeping, different foods (caffeine, chocolate, spicy, or high-fat foods)
  - –Personal/family history of asthma, allergies, eczema
  - –Recent diagnosis of heart disease or death in a family member often generates fear in the patient or parent, prompting the evaluation of chest pain
  - –Social history: Recent life stressors (school problems, family discord, etc.); drug use, especially cocaine
- Physical exam
  - –Reproducible with palpation likely musculoskeletal
  - –Chest exam: Wheezing, rales, crepitus
  - –Cardiac exam: Usually normal, even with cardiac causes; pericarditis is associated with rub
- Chest X-ray for infiltrates, pneumonia, pneumothorax
- ECG and cardiac enzymes are rarely required but relatively inexpensive and readily available, and can rule out MI and provide reassurance for families
- Cardiac stress test
  - –Continuous ECG monitoring while the patient exercises to evaluate for coronary insufficiency
  - –Used for patients with exercise-induced chest pain and/or coronary abnormalities

Treatment

- Most patients/families with chest pain simply want reassurance that symptoms are not cardiac in origin
- A careful history and physical exam are most important; however, a normal CXR and ECG provide therapeutic reassurance to the patient/family
- Further cardiology consultation is rarely required but should be considered with patients experiencing chest pain with exercise, a history of Kawasaki disease, Marfan syndrome (this is an emergency), and for those patients with persistent chest pain
- Costochondritis: Treated with NSAIDs until resolved
- Pericarditis: Treated with aspirin or NSAIDs; requires cardiology follow-up until resolved, rarely requires pericardiocentesis
- Appropriate therapy of identified pulmonary, gastrointestinal, or musculoskeletal problems

66. Cough – Acute

A cough occurs by increased intrathoracic pressure against a closed glottis (Valsalva maneuver), followed by the abrupt opening of the glottis and a sudden expulsion of air. Increased intrathoracic pressure leads to dynamic compression of the airways. The effect of air flow at high pressure through a compressed trachea (only 1/6 of original area) is a greatly increased velocity; in adults airflow may reach 400–500 miles per hour. The result is a generally effective method of removing debris and secretions from the airway.

Differential Diagnosis

- Upper airway disease
  - URI or common cold accounts for much pediatric coughing (influenza, parainfluenza, rhinovirus)
  - Chronic sinusitis, tonsillitis, laryngitis, and croup are other common infections
  - Allergic disease
  - Vocal cord dysfunction (VCD)
- Lower airway disease
  - Asthma is inflammatory triad of edema, mucus, and bronchospasm, characterized by reversibility with asthma drugs (the most common triggers for asthma are viral disease, irritants such as ETS, allergic disease, and gastroesophageal reflux)
  - Infectious diseases: Bronchiolitis, caused by RSV in babies, causes cough from inflammatory changes and debris; bronchitis is more common in older children and may be secondary to smoking or ETS exposure; other viral lower airway diseases include adenovirus, influenza, and parainfluenza
  - Foreign body aspiration
  - Chronic diseases (e.g., cystic fibrosis and bronchiectasis) and structural abnormalities (e.g., PCD, TEF, or cleft, rings, and slings) may present with intermittent rather than chronic cough
- Parenchymal and pleural disease
  - Infectious diseases account almost exclusively for all parenchymal and pleural causes of cough (i.e., pneumonia and empyema)
  - Usual infectious agents include bacterial disease (e.g., streptococcal, staphylococcal) and atypical pneumonias (e.g., *Mycoplasma pneumoniae*), TB
  - Irritation of a branch of cranial nerve ten in the external auditory canal can trigger cough

Workup and Diagnosis

- History
  - What started it? History (e.g., infection or FB aspiration) may suggest a mechanism
  - What makes it worse? Activity leading to cough may suggest asthma or structural disease; seasonal onset suggests allergic disease; night cough suggests GER
  - Is the cough productive? Infection is the primary cause of sputum production; also consider asthma, bronchiectasis, smoking, or CF
- Physical exam
  - Loud, "brassy," vibrato, honking quality suggests tracheomalacia
  - High-pitched stridor suggests a fixed tracheal obstruction (ring, sling, FB, subglottic stenosis)
  - Violent paroxysms with an inspiratory whoop suggests pertussis syndrome
  - A productive, "wet" cough suggests bronchitis or pneumonia
  - A wheezy, "tight" cough suggests asthma
- Studies
  - CXR may demonstrate an atypical pneumonia
  - Pulmonary function tests to diagnose asthma or large airway obstruction
  - Bronchoscopy and lavage to diagnose malacia, infection, FB, VCD
  - V/Q scan may diagnose a pulmonary embolus (rare)
- Exercise testing may provoke symptoms of exercise-induced asthma or VCD

Treatment

- Treatment is often empiric and based on history
- Cough suppression is usually avoided, but may assist with sleep; other OTC therapies of little value
- An empiric "diagnostic trial" of medication may treat asthma, GER, or bacterial infections
- Treatment of "habit component" may help with psychogenic cough or other chronic conditions (e.g., postinfectious bronchitis)
- Speech therapy is very helpful for VCD or habit cough (i.e., using cold water "hard swallow," benzocaine throat lozenges, breathing exercises)
- Serious psychiatric disease may be associated with VCD but referral to mental health specialists is rarely needed

67. Cough – Chronic

In adults, "chronic" is often defined as more than 3 months of coughing in 2 years, but chronic cough is not as well defined in children. In general, for children, cough of more than 3–4 weeks' duration will be brought to the attention of caregivers as "chronic," as is a cough with every URI (more properly defined as recurrent).

Differential Diagnosis

- Lower airway disease
  - –Asthma
    - –Inflammatory triad of edema, mucus, and bronchospasm, characterized by reversibility with asthma drugs
  - –The most common triggers for asthma are viral disease, irritants (e.g., ETS), allergic disease, and GER
  - –Airway infections: Bronchiolitis, caused by RSV in babies, may cause chronic cough from persistent inflammatory change and debris; bronchitis is more common in older children and may be secondary to smoking or ETS exposure
  - –Foreign body: Associated with endobronchial infection and damage
  - –Cystic fibrosis: The most common life-threatening inherited illness of whites, is associated with production of chronically infected sputum
  - –Bronchiectasis: Chronic infection and damage to the airway; may be secondary to another disease (e.g., TB or CF)
  - –Structural abnormalities: PCD, TEF, or cleft, rings, slings
- Upper airway disease
  - –Infectious diseases: Chronic sinusitis, tonsillitis, laryngitis, including that secondary to GER (although acute disorders, the inflammation from URI may be associated with a chronic cough if frequent enough)
- Parenchymal and pleural disease
  - –Infectious disease accounts almost exclusively for all parenchymal and pleural causes of cough (e.g., pneumonia and empyema)
- CNS causes
  - –CNS causes of cough include "habit cough" (or psychogenic cough), Tourette disease associated "cough tic" or throat clearing, VCD
  - –Irritation of a branch of cranial nerve ten in the external auditory canal can trigger chronic cough

Workup and Diagnosis

- History
  - –Cough lasting longer than 2–6 weeks suggests either a predisposing factor (e.g., bronchomalacia) or an ongoing trigger (e.g., asthma)
  - –An acute lung or airway injury (i.e., infection or FB) suggests a mechanism for chronic cough
  - –An insidious onset is more consistent with a chronic underlying condition (i.e., CF, TB, GER)
  - –Seasonal change suggests allergic disease
  - –Night cough suggests GER
  - –A positive response to asthma therapy suggests asthma
  - –Antibiotic responsiveness suggests chronic infection (i.e., CF, bronchiectasis, sinusitis)
  - –Distractability suggests habit cough, as may a lack of coughing while asleep
  - –Is the cough productive? Culture sputum and consider asthma, bronchiectasis, smoking, or CF
- Physical exam: Loud, "brassy," vibrato, honking quality suggests tracheomalacia; high-pitched stridor suggests a fixed tracheal obstruction (ring, sling, FB, subglottic stenosis); violent paroxysms with an inspiratory whoop suggest pertussis syndrome
- Studies: Chest films often not diagnostic; PFT to diagnose asthma or large airway obstruction; bronchoscopy and lavage to diagnose malacia, infection, FB, VCD
- Exercise testing may provoke symptoms of EIA or VCD

Treatment

- Treatment is often empiric and based on history
- An empiric "diagnostic trial" of medication may treat asthma, GER, or bacterial infections. Treatment of "habit component" may help with other chronic conditions (e.g., postinfectious bronchitis)
- Speech therapy is helpful for VCD or habit cough (i.e., using cold water "hard swallow," benzocaine throat lozenges, breathing exercises)
- Serious psychiatric disease may be associated with VCD, but referral to mental health specialist is rarely needed
- Other treatments first require accurate diagnosis (e.g., TB, CF, FB)
- Cough suppression may be of use at night to achieve sleep, but is generally avoided

68. Crackles/Rales

Breath sounds are made by air flow through airways. Crackles, also known as rales, are discontinuous breath sounds, more prominent during inspiration, and often accompanied by tachypnea and increased work of breathing. Rales are usually polyphonic, representing many sites of origin. "Fine," or high-pitched, rales may originate from smaller airways; low-pitched rales (sometimes mistakenly called rhonchi) originate from larger airways. Rales are not made by the sound of alveoli "popping open," but originate from the first through ninth generation of airways. All sources of rales can cause wheezes as well.

Differential Diagnosis

- Think anatomically and physiologically
- Upper airway
  - –Not generally a source of rales; louder discontinuous sounds from the upper airway may obscure fine rales from the lower airways
- Lower airway
  - –Predominantly inspiratory and polyphonic
- Extraluminal compression of airways
  - –Parenchymal: Pulmonary edema and heart failure, pneumonia, bronchogenic cyst
  - –Vascular: Ring, sling
  - –Lymphatics: Enlarged lymph nodes (e.g.,TB, sarcoidosis, malignancy)
  - –Structural: CLE, CCAM, scoliosis or chest wall deformity with airway "kinking"
- Transluminal change in airway
  - –Asthma with inflammation, edema, hyperemia, mucus gland hypertrophy and proliferation, smooth muscle bronchospasm
  - –Bronchus-associated lymphoid tissue
  - –Bronchiolitis obliterans
  - –Tracheobronchomalacia
  - –Bronchial atresia
  - –Bronchiectasis/bronchitis
  - –CF
  - –Ciliary disease (primary ciliary dyskinesia or dysfunction secondary to ETS or hyperoxia)
  - –Miscellaneous (e.g., hemangioma, polyps, TEF)
  - –Immunologic disorders (e.g., IgA deficiency)
- Intraluminal change in airway
  - –Mucus (increased production or decreased clearance)
  - –Pus (infected sputum), debris
  - –Blood (rare)
  - –FB
  - –Aspirated food or stomach contents secondary to gastroesophageal reflux (GER)

Workup and Diagnosis

- History may suggest a specific diagnosis (e.g., pneumonia)
  - –Age of onset: Rales at birth suggest congenital or genetic abnormality, or neonatal infection
  - –What helps?A history of a positive response to diuretics suggests lung water, whereas a response to β-agonists or steroids suggests asthma; worsening with β-agonists suggests bronchomalacia
  - –What makes it worse? Relation to diet or fluid intake may suggest congestive heart failure
  - –Time course: History may establish allergic trigger by season, locale, or association with allergic exposure
- Other symptoms
  - –Hemoptysis or weight loss (CF, TB, bronchiectasis, malignancy)
  - –Chronic cough (CF, bronchiectasis, recurrent infection or immunodeficiency)
  - –Weakness or hypotonia (neuromotor disease, Down syndrome, aspiration of feeds)
  - –Choking on feeds (upper airway disease, TEF, chronic aspiration, VCD)
  - –Fevers suggest infectious etiology (or rarely, autoimmune disease or malignancy)

Treatment

- Congestive heart failure is treated with diuretics, cardiac inotropes, or afterload reducers
- Asthma is treated with layered therapy for acute symptom control ("rescue" medicine) and prevention of disease ("controller" medicine)
  - –Rescue medicines are inhaled β-agonists (immediate) or steroids (rapid)
  - –Controller medicines include ICS, leukotriene modifiers, anti-inflammatory agents, and long-acting bronchodilators
- Bronchomalacia is treated with atrovent and/or ICS
- Treatment of underlying triggers is key to control of chronic disease (e.g., GER, allergic disease, aspiration)
- Treatment of atypical causes of rales requires persistence in search for diagnosis, and is then disease-specific

69. Cyanosis

Cyanosis is due to arterial hypoxemia and may not easily be seen during physical exam. Examine soft tissue with high blood flow, such as the gums or tongue, for cyanosis. Cyanosis elsewhere (e.g., fingertips or lips) may be due to reduced blood flow. If possible, use pulse oximetry to measure oxyhemoglobin saturation.

Differential Diagnosis

- Recall the pathway for oxygen, from the air to the tissue; etiology is often multifactorial
- Reduced O_2 availability: High altitude (>6,000 feet), e.g., air travel, ski resort, mountain travel
- Reduced O_2 transport to alveoli: Respiratory failure/arrest, air flow obstruction (usually compensate for large obstruction unless complete); restrictive chest wall disease (e.g., kyphosis, weakness, or obesity)
- Abnormal gas exchange or V/Q mismatch: Most common physiologic pulmonary cause of hypoxia
- Abnormal ventilation
  - –Alveolar diseases: Pneumonia, pulmonary edema, diffuse alveolar damage, alveolar proteinosis
  - –Conducting airway diseases: Asthma, bronchiolitis
  - –Combined pathology: ARDS, bronchopulmonary dysplasia, HMD
- Abnormal perfusion
  - –Pulmonary hypertension, pulmonary embolus, abnormal anatomy (e.g., pulmonary sequestration)
- Shunt
  - –Intrapulmonary shunt (or "total" V/Q mismatch), e.g., AV malformations
  - –Extrapulmonary shunt, e.g., TOF, TAPVR, TGA
- Abnormal transport to tissue
  - –Abnormal hemoglobin: β-thalassemia, sickle cell disease, CO poisoning
  - –Decreased hemoglobin: Anemia, blood loss
  - –Decreased blood flow: Dysrhythmia, bradycardia, cardiac arrest, hypotension
- Abnormal O_2 delivery at tissue
  - –Abnormal hemoglobin affinity for O_2
  - –End-organ failure (e.g., mitochondrial disease, cyanide poisoning)
- Chronic cyanosis starting at birth suggests either congenital lesion or neonatal injury (e.g., meconium aspiration, group B streptococcus sepsis, HMD)

Workup and Diagnosis

- History
  - –Birth history
  - –Past medical history including respiratory, cardiac and hematologic disorders, acute or chronic onset, and accompanying features
- Physical exam
  - –Patency of the airway, adequate air movement, distribution of air flow, symmetry of breath sounds, crackles, dullness to percussion, chest wall movement
  - –Auscultate heart, feel all pulses, obtain BP, seek signs of chronicity (e.g., clubbing of nail beds)
  - –Examine well-perfused soft tissue (e.g., gums) to assess for cyanosis, not fingertips
- Oximetry is useful but may not help during shock or hemoglobinopathies; may not be accurate with dark skin
- If O_2 does not help, consider shunt (cardiac disease is more common than intrapulmonary shunt)
- Arterial blood gases
  - –Disparate PaO_2 and SaO_2 suggests possibility of abnormal hemoglobin affinity for O_2
- Chest film and CT for parenchymal disease
- MRI/MRAfor vascular anatomy
- V/Q scan
- ECG, Echo, or catheterization for cardiac disease
- PFT for obstructive or restrictive disease
- Sleep studies, EEG for CNS causes
- Muscle biopsy for tissue or mitochondrial diseases

Treatment

- Immediately treat cyanosis with O_2, monitor the patient, then determine cause
- Treat underlying causes
  - –High altitude: Descend
  - –Central or obstructive causes of respiratory failure: Treat with mechanical ventilation and search for cause
  - –V/Q mismatch: Treat cause(s)
  - –Shunt: Treatment may be surgical
  - –Hemoglobinopathies: May need transfusion, exchange transfusion, or electrophoresis
  - –Decreased hemoglobin: May need whole blood or packed red blood cells
  - –Decreased delivery: May need blood pressure support, cardiac stimulants, manual chest compression, or cardiac massage
  - –Abnormal tissue delivery: Target specific disease

70. Dyspnea

Dyspnea is defined as "shortness of breath," so it is important to determine the effect of activity on breathing. Worsening when supine does not reliably differentiate left-sided cardiac disease from pulmonary causes of dyspnea in children. Attention to the respiratory pattern and exam (e.g., Cheyne-Stokes breathing, or wheezing) should help determine the source of the dyspnea. Dyspnea may not be apparent if the patient is paralyzed or profoundly weak.

Differential Diagnosis

- Dyspnea is driven by an aberration in the mechanics of breathing; consider the pathway taken by oxygen to the tissues, and the mechanics of getting it there
- Hypoxia
  - –Low O_2 delivery to tissues increases effort to deliver it, including increased respiratory effort
  - –Any cause of hypoxia will lead to dyspnea (decreased availability, V/Q mismatch due to pneumonia or other lung disease)
- Obstructive disease causes increased effort to move air
  - –Upper airway: Nasal congestion, choanal atresia, FB, tonsils, adenoids, macroglossia, decreased tone, retropharyngeal abscess, laryngomalacia, VCD/paralysis, laryngeal web or polyp, subglottic stenosis
  - –Lower airway: Asthma, BALT, bronchiolitis obliterans, tracheobronchomalacia, bronchial atresia, bronchiectasis, bronchitis, CF, PCD, hemangioma, polyps, TEF
- Restrictive disease
  - –Small or stiff lungs, chest wall disease (e.g., obesity, kyphoscoliosis, chest deformity), respiratory muscle weakness (Duchenne muscular dystrophy, paralysis)
- Parenchymal disease
  - –Pneumonia, congenital lesions
- Vascular disease
  - –Pulmonary hypertension, sequestered lung
- Cardiac disease
  - –Congenital cyanotic heart disease (e.g., TOF, TAPVR, TGA)
  - –Pericarditis
  - –Myocarditis
- Compression of the lung
  - –Pneumothorax
  - –Tumors (e.g., cyst, teratoma)
  - –Elevated diaphragm
  - –Effusions (e.g., empyema, hemothorax)
- Pulmonary embolism (rare)

Workup and Diagnosis

- History
  - –Determine first the urgency of the problem; some patients who appear to be less dyspneic because of fatigue or weakness are at greater risk of respiratory failure
  - –Is there dyspnea at rest? Increased O_2 consumption with activity increases symptoms; dyspnea at rest suggests a more severe problem, a fixed degree of hypoxia, or diminished compensatory mechanisms (e.g., profound weakness)
  - –Does oxygen help? If not, it may represent a fixed mechanical problem (e.g., severe obstruction or chest wall disease), shunt, or other severe V/Q mismatch
- Physical exam
  - –Inspection and palpation are important; abnormal mechanics or hyperinflation may suggest etiology
  - –Loud monophonic sounds (stridor, wheeze) suggest large airway obstruction; polyphonic wheezes suggest small airway disease
- Oximetry is very useful but may not be accurate
- Labs
  - –ABGs (low PaO_2 and SaO_2 or high $PaCO_2$ suggests interventions)
- Studies
  - –Chest film and CT for parenchymal disease
  - –MRI/MRA for vascular anatomy; V/Q scan
- ECG, Echo, or catheterization for cardiac disease
- Pulmonary function test for obstructive or restrictive disease

Treatment

- Dyspnea is a sign of respiratory distress, but it is not treated with sedation (increases risk of respiratory failure or arrest)
- Oxygen
  - –First line in the treatment of hypoxia
  - –Use caution if it is accompanied by hypercapnea (as in chronically cyanotic patients or with COPD), because the respiratory effort may be driven by the hypoxia, and there will be a decrease in respiratory drive leading to increases in $PaCO_2$ (rare in children unless there is CCHD)
- Airway lesions may require intervention to provide relief; target underlying illnesses (e.g., treat pneumonia with antibiotics) but persist in efforts to improve mechanics (e.g., chest physiotherapy to clear secretions)
- Surgical stabilization of abnormal chest wall or of anatomic abnormality
- Asthma therapy may provide relief even when asthma is not the "primary" problem (e.g., muscular dystrophy)

71. Gynecomastia

Gynecomastia is benign breast tissue enlargement in males, affecting up to two-thirds of boys in adolescence. The majority of cases are secondary to normal developmental changes involving a transient imbalance of the estrogen/testosterone ratio. Peak for pubertal cases occurs at Tanner stage II–III, and most spontaneously regress.

Differential Diagnosis

- Pubertal
  - Prevalence 40–69% in adolescent males
  - Onset by 10–12 years old
  - Peaks at 13–14 years, Tanner III staging
  - Resolution in 1–2 years in 75%
  - Obese patients more affected
- Several drugs can cause gynecomastia
  - Antiandrogens: Flutamide, finasteride, ketoconazole, spironolactone
  - GI agents: Cimetidine, ranitidine
  - Calcium channel blockers: Verapamil, nifedipine
  - Illicit drugs: Marijuana, heroin, methadone, amphetamines
  - Hormones: Androgens, anabolic steroids, estrogens
  - Psychiatric: Phenothiazines, diazepam, tricyclic antidepressants
- Androgen insufficiency
  - Klinefelter syndrome (47, XXY)
  - Seminiferous tubule dysgenesis
  - Testicular failure
  - Androgen-insensitivity syndrome, androgen receptor defects
  - Biosynthetic defects in testosterone production
  - Isolated LH deficiency
- Excess estrogen
  - Feminizing adrenocortical tumors (rare)
- Testicular neoplasms
  - Germ cell tumors: Associated with hCG production; hCG leads to Leydig cell dysfunction and increased aromatase
  - Leydig cell tumors secrete estradiol
  - Sertoli cell tumors: Associated with excessive aromatase activity
- Pseudogynecomastia
  - Fat deposition without glandular development
  - Seen in obesity
- Other breast enlargement (not truc gynecomastia)
  - Neurofibroma
  - Carcinoma of breast
  - Hemangioma
  - Lipoma
- Reifenstein syndrome
- Kallmann syndrome
- Liver cirrhosis

Workup and Diagnosis

- History
  - Breast characteristics
  - Duration
  - Progressive or regressing
  - Unilateral/bilateral
  - Associated erythema, tenderness, and/or discharge
  - Medication exposure
  - Change in appearance of testicles
  - Pubertal onset
  - Erectile function
  - Liver or kidney problems
- Physical exam
  - Abdominal exam for mass
  - Testicular exam for mass
  - Genital exam for Tanner staging
  - Chest exam for size and texture of tissue
- Labs
  - Investigation indicated for severe, prolonged, or sudden onset for the adolescent, for prepubertal boys, for pubertal boys with minimal viralization and/or small testes, and for child with CNS complaints
  - Karyotype
  - Serum gonadotropin (LH)
  - Serum testosterone
  - Serum estradiol
  - Serum hCG

Treatment

- Pubertal
  - No treatment if pubertal development and physical exam are normal
  - Re-evaluation in 6 months
- Cessation of drugs when implicated
- Testosterone replacement if indicated for hypogonadism
- Weight loss for pseudogynecomastia
- Surgery (reduction mammoplasty) if severe and psychologically distressing
- Persistent pubertal gynecomastia
  - Therapy is investigational; no large trials completed yet
  - Antiestrogens (clomiphene and tamoxifen)
  - Aromastase inhibitors (testolactone)

72. Heart Failure

Heart failure exists when adequate cardiac output cannot be maintained either at rest or with activity. It can be either acute, chronic, or an acute decompensation of the chronic state, and represents a wide range of anatomic and pathophysiologic conditions. The three main categories are increased afterload, left-to-right shunt lesions, and intrinsic myocardial disease.

Differential Diagnosis

Increased afterload

- Most common in the neonate due to left-sided obstructive lesions, which present acutely
- Aortic coarctation is most common
  - –Increased pulse/BP in right arm
  - –Decreased pulse/BP in lower extremities
- Critical aortic stenosis
  - –Poor pulses, loud murmur
- Hypoplastic left heart syndrome, aortic arch interruption

Left-to-right shunt lesions

- Normal cardiac muscle funtion but overcirculation of lungs due to a congenital connection between the right and left side of the heart and low PVR
- Usually presents at 1–2 months of age
  - –PVR drops and systemic resistance becomes higher than PV
  - –Blood shunts from left to right (systemic circulation to pulmonary circulation)
  - –Pulmonary overcirculation and poor systemic output (poor peripheral perfusion, low urine output)
- Ventricular septal defect (most common)
- Atrioventricular septal defect (AV canal, endocardial cushion defect), associated with Down syndrome
- Patent ductus arteriosus
- Atrial septal defect (usually asymptomatic)

Intrinsic myocardial disease

- More common cause of heart failure in older children and adolescents
- Myocarditis
  - –Acute inflammation and dysfunction of cardiac muscle, usually postviral
  - –1/3 remain stable, 1/3 return to normal cardiac function, and 1/3 deteriorate
- Cardiomyopathy
  - –Dilated most common, but also hypertrophic and restrictive
  - –Multiple genetic and metabolic causes, often positive family history, some represent old, "burned-out" myocarditis
- Myocardial infarction (rare)
  - –Kawasaki disease
  - –Congenital coronary abnormalities (anomalous left coronary artery)

Workup and Diagnosis

- Neonate
  - –Consider left-sided obstructive lesions in any neonate with poor or differential pulses/perfusion
  - –Often have respiratory distress, hepatomegaly, and metabolic acidosis
  - –Critically ill requiring supplemental O_2 and ventilatory support; transfer to tertiary care ICU
- Infants/children
  - –History: Activity tolerance, poor feeding, diaphoresis, respiratory symptoms (wheezing or frequent infections due to pulmonary overcirculation), weight gain (poor due to increased metabolic demands or excess due to activity intolerance and edema), dyspnea on exertion for older patients
  - –Physical exam: Vital signs (tachypnea, tachycardia), perfusion/pulses, edema (especially of face/eyes for infants), increased work of breathing/retractions, hepatomegaly, increased jugular venous distension
- Chest X-ray often reveals nonspecific cardiomegaly and pulmonary venous congestion
- ECG: Evaluate for ventricular hypertrophy (left-to-right shunt lesions, hypertrophic cardiomyopathy); low QRS voltage (myocarditis, dilated cardiomyopathy)
- Echocardiography and/or cardiac catheterization to further define anatomy and function
- Serum electrolytes, BUN/creatinine, and LFTs (including total protein and albumin) to further define current metabolic state before therapy

Treatment

- Increased afterload due to left-sided obstructive lesion
  - –Use prostaglandins to open ductus arteriosus to relieve the obstruction, and/or use the right ventricle for systemic circulatory support
  - –Inotropic support (dopamine/dobutamine) if very ill
  - –Surgical intervention depending on specific anatomy
- Left-to-right shunt lesions
  - –Diuretics to decrease lung fluid and improve respiratory mechanics
  - –Inotropic support with dopamine/dobutamine for critically ill, digoxin for chronic use
  - –Systemic afterload reduction with ACE inhibitors if systemic BP adequate
- Myocardial disease
  - –Diuretics and inotropes for afterload reduction
  - –β-blockers and ACE inhibitors
  - –Mechanical circulatory support and cardiac transplantation for advanced heart failure

73. Hemoptysis

Hemoptysis is defined as coughing or spitting up blood. Blood can originate from any anatomic site that communicates with the mouth (the "aerodigestive" tract): the mouth, sinuses, nasopharynx, oropharynx, esophagus, stomach, airways, or lung parenchyma. History often differentiates source, as may exam, but hemoptysis—no matter how small—always warrants attention.

Differential Diagnosis

- Think anatomically and physiologically of why we bleed and the source of the blood
- Upper airway
  - –Nose bleed
  - –Chronic sinus disease
  - –Postoperative bleeding
  - –Dental disease
  - –Trauma (including CNS)
- Digestive tract
  - –Esophageal varices
  - –Gastric bleeding (unlikely to come from intestine; that is, distal to antrum)
  - –Oral ulcers/trauma
- Lower airways
  - –Tracheobronchial tree bronchiectasis (e.g., with CF)
  - –Bronchial erosion (e.g., from tracheotomy tube)
  - –Wegener granulomatosis
- Parenchyma
  - –Pulmonary hemorrhage
  - –Pulmonary tuberculosis
  - –Lung abscess
  - –Hemorrhagic fevers (rare in U.S.)
  - –Paragonimiasis (a trematode infection)
  - –Lung contusion from trauma
  - –Primary pulmonary hemosiderosis
  - –Swyer-James syndrome
- Cardiovascular causes
  - –Pulmonary embolism
  - –Multiple pulmonary telangiectasia (e.g., Osler-Weber-Rendu)
  - –Ruptured arteriovenous fistula
  - –Mitral stenosis
- Bleeding disorders (may present from any source)
  - –Hemophilia, leukemia, and other blood dyscrasias
  - –Increased consumption of coagulation factors (e.g., disseminated vascular coagulation)
- The most common source of blood originating in the lower airways is from small bronchial lesions secondary to inflammation from infection

Workup and Diagnosis

- History
  - –Recent surgery such as sinus surgery, tonsillectomy, transbronchial biopsy
  - –Recent trauma
  - –Recent respiratory disease (e.g., choking episode suggests FB, fever and productive cough suggest infection)
  - –Chronic illness suggests bronchiectasis, CF, chronic infection (e.g., TB)
  - –Chest pain associated with cough suggests tracheal disease (i.e., tracheitis)
  - –Association with gagging or emesis suggests Mallory-Weiss tear
  - –Association with liver or spleen disease suggests varices or decreased platelets
- Physical exam
  - –Careful ENT evaluation for an upper airway source of bleeding
  - –Bleeding in other sites suggests bleeding disorder (e.g., joints, skin)
  - –Examine whole patient for signs of systemic disease
- Labs
  - –Blood work may help: PT/PTT and CBC for anemia and/or thrombocytopenia
- Flexible nasopharyngoscopy or bronchoscopy to evaluate airways
- Chest X-ray to evaluate pulmonary hemorrhage
- MRI may diagnose ectopic blood vessel in chest

Treatment

- The patient may need blood, packed red cells, or blood products emergently
- Diagnosis-specific therapy (e.g., FB removal)
- Therapy for bronchiectasis is aimed at treatment of underlying endobronchial infection
- Cauterization of bleeding vessels is more useful in the upper airway
- Digestive tract: Antacids, reduce portal hypertension, surgically repair source of bleeding
- It is a life-threatening surgical emergency if a large blood vessel bleeds into the trachea from tracheotomy tube-related erosions
- Consider gel-foam or metal coil injection into the bronchial circulation for chronic bleeding caused by bronchiectasis

74. Stridor

Priority of stridor evaluation is based on history and clinical presentation. A child with new stridor and respiratory distress requires immediate intervention. The most common cause of chronic stridor in infants is laryngomalacia. Synchronous airway lesions need to be considered and evaluated by an otolaryngologist.

Differential Diagnosis

Nasal cavity and nasopharynx
- Congenital
  - Piriform aperture stenosis
  - Choanal atresia
  - Lacrimal duct cyst
  - Craniofacial anomaly
  - Nasopharyngeal mass (teratoma)
- Inflammatory/infectious
  - Rhinosinusitis
  - Adenoid hypertrophy

Oral cavity, oropharynx, and hypopharynx
- Congenital
  - Macroglossia
  - Glossoptosis
  - Vallecular cyst
- Inflammatory/infectious
  - Tonsillar hypertrophy
- Tumors
  - Lingual thyroid
  - Dermoid
  - Lymphovascular malformation
- Foreign body

Laryngeal
- Congenital
  - Laryngomalacia (#1 cause in infants); usual onset is in the first 2 weeks of life, typically positional; most resolve spontaneously by age 1
  - Saccular cyst
  - Webs
  - Clefts
  - Vocal cord paralysis
- Inflammatory/infectious
  - Epiglottitis
  - Laryngotracheitis (croup)
  - Gastroesophageal reflux
- Tumors
  - Papillomas
  - Hemangiomas
- Trauma
  - Subglottic stenosis
  - Foreign bodies
  - Laryngeal fracture
  - Caustic ingestion

Tracheobronchial
- Congenital
  - Tracheomalacia
  - Vascular rings
  - Tracheoesophageal fistula
- Inflammatory

Workup and Diagnosis

- History
  - Duration, onset, severity, character, progression
  - Failure to thrive, feeding problems, cyanosis, apnea
  - Reflux history: Frequent spit-ups, vomiting, heartburn, chest pain, hoarseness
  - Birth, neonatal, and past medical history: Complicated labor, respiratory distress at delivery
  - Prior intubations, neurologic problems, prior episodes of croup, prior neck surgery, foreign body ingestion
  - Immunization history
- Physical exam
  - Fever, respiratory rate, heart rate, level of consciousness, cyanosis
  - Auscultation: Chest, nose, mouth, neck (phase of stridor: inspiratory, expiratory, biphasic)
  - Nose: Nasal obstruction
  - Mouth: Tonsillar hypertrophy
  - Neck: Retractions, compressive mass, thyroid
- Studies
  - Flexible nasolaryngoscopy: Check for choanal patency, adenoid size, laryngomalacia, vocal cord mobility
  - Direct laryngoscopy and bronchoscopy (DLB): Controversial whether all children with stridor need DLB
  - MRI: Vascular compression or external mediastinal mass
  - Modified barium swallow or esophagram in children with history of swallowing difficulties

Treatment

- Treatment is frequently based on diagnosis from endoscopy
- Immediate evaluation when respiratory distress is present
  - Observation, intubation, tracheostomy, FB removal
- Acute stridor
  - Viral laryngotracheobronchitis: Steroids, racemic epinephrine, and supplemental O_2
  - Bacterial tracheitis: Culture-directed antibiotic therapy, consider intubation
- Chronic stridor of newborn
  - History, physical, and endoscopy (fiberoptic or direct) confirmation of laryngomalacia
  - Consider treatment for reflux
  - Repeat endoscopy and possible supraglottoplasty if persistent stridor and failure to thrive

75. Tachypnea

Tachypnea is defined as rapid breathing. The younger the child, the faster the average respiratory rate, and the wider the acceptable range of normal. The average newborn may breathe anywhere between 30 and 80 respirations per minute, a 2-year-old at 20–40, and older children at rates close to adult averages (16–28). Minute ventilation (V_e) is measured in liters per minute; a rapid respiratory rate with a smaller tidal volume (V_t) may lead to little change in V_e.

Airway obstruction in infants may lead to tachypnea instead of expiratory prolongation. Rather than forcing air out (increasing V_t), the baby may breathe rapidly at a high lung volume, keeping airways open (airway caliber is greater at higher lung volumes).

Differential Diagnosis

- Consider tachypnea using a compartmental, anatomic model; recall that causes are usually multifactoral and that the CNS ultimately drives RR
- CNS
  - Increased "respiratory drive" usually affects rate, not just V_t
  - Physiologic variables that drive up RR are those found in respiratory failure (hypoxia, hypercapnea, acidosis); thus, hypoxia for any reason (e.g., high altitude or pneumonia) increases RR
  - Other "CNS" factors that may increase respiratory rate include dehydration, fever, and anxiety
- Obstruction
  - Airway obstruction may lead to an increased work of breathing, expiratory prolongation, increased V_t, or dyspnea, but may cause tachypnea as well
  - Upper airway: Laryngomalacia, choanal atresia, macroglossia, micrognathia, subglottic stenosis, web, or laryngospasm
  - Lower airway: Tracheal stenosis, rings, slings, asthma, or FB
- Parenchymal disease
  - Decreased lung volume (e.g., atelectasis, pneumonectomy), poor compliance (e.g., pulmonary edema, pneumonia, pulmonary fibrosis)
- Chest wall disorders
  - High or low chest wall compliance (e.g., kyphoscoliosis or flail chest)
- Pulmonary vascular disease is often due to hypoxia and other mechanisms
  - Pulmonary edema (altered compliance and hypoxia)
  - Pulmonary hypertension (hypoxia), V/Q mismatch (e.g., pneumonia), shunt such as CCHD
- Lymphatic system
  - Lymphangiectasia (altered compliance)
  - BALT (airway obstruction and hypoxia)
  - Chylothorax (altered chest wall mechanics and hypoxia)
- Other inflammatory mediators (e.g., cytokines or eicosanoids) may affect respiratory rate through uncertain mechanisms

Workup and Diagnosis

- Remember, tachypnea may be normal
- History is directed at logical associations with tachypnea
- Setting of onset: History of acute onset and associated with a viral illness might suggest temperature or mild acidosis as relevant factors, whereas a sudden onset associated with a sudden-onset cough in a toddler may suggest FB
- What makes it better (O_2 or antipyretics)?
- Related signs and symptoms: Look for evidence of CCHD, sepsis (e.g., GBS sepsis), toxic ingestion (e.g., aspirin)
- Physical exam
  - Look for agitation, anxiety, mental status changes, or other signs of CNS dysfunction
  - Auscultate over all of airways to find potential source of obstructive disease
  - Inspect for evidence of chest wall disease or increased work of breathing (e.g., retractions or use of accessory muscles of respiration)
- Radiology is effective in demonstrating parenchymal or pleural disease; less helpful with airways
- Other radiographic tools targeted at suspected cause: CT for empyema, congenital lesions of lung; MRI/MRA for vascular anomalies in chest; and nuclear medicine (V/Q scan); Echo/ECG for CCHD
- Pulmonary function tests: Measure volumes and flows
- Blood work for miscellaneous (ABG, CBG)

Treatment

- Treat underlying etiology
- Prevent impending respiratory failure aggressively with O_2, fluids, intubation, and mechanical ventilation
- Severe metabolic acidosis may need correction with bicarbonate and therapy targeted at the cause (e.g., antibiotics for sepsis)
- Relieve obstruction medically or surgically depending on site and cause; severe upper airway obstruction may require intubation to bypass obstruction; severe lower airway obstruction may need bronchoscopy (e.g., FB, mucus plug) or asthma therapy
- If the demands of respiration are excessive, respiratory muscle failure may ensue, requiring mechanical ventilation; severe lower airway obstruction may even preclude mechanical ventilation
- Tachypnea in well babies is often physiologic and may require no intervention, but one must first exclude pathology

76. Wheezing

Breath sounds are made by air flow through airways. Normally they are fairly quiet and somewhat louder during inspiration as air flows toward the stethoscope. Wheezing is defined as continuous breath sounds that are more prominent during expiration and often accompanied by expiratory prolongation. Wheezes may be monophonic or polyphonic, representing one or many sites of origin for the wheeze. High-pitched wheezes originate from smaller airways; low-pitched wheezes (sometimes called rhonchi) originate from larger airways. All breath sounds (normal and abnormal) are louder in young children because of their relatively thinner chest walls.

Differential Diagnosis

Lower airway (expiratory, polyphonic)

- Extraluminal compression of airways
  - –Parenchymal: Pneumonia, pulmonary edema, bronchogenic cyst
  - –Vascular: Ring, sling, "cardiac wheeze"
  - –Lymphatics: Enlarged lymph nodes (TB, sarcoidosis, malignancy)
  - –Structural: CLE, scoliosis, or chest wall deformity with airway "kinking"
- Transluminal change in airway
  - –Asthma: Inflammation, edema, hyperemia, mucus gland hypertrophy and proliferation, smooth muscle bronchospasm
  - –Bronchiectasis/bronchitis
  - –Cystic fibrosis
  - –Ciliary disease: Primary ciliary dyskinesia, dysfunction due to ETS or hyperoxia
  - –Anatomic: Hemangioma, polyps, TEF, bronchial atresia, BALT, bronchiolitis obliterans, tracheobronchomalacia
  - –Immunologic disorders (e.g., IgA deficiency)
- Intraluminal change in airway
  - –Mucus (increased production or decreased clearance), pus (infected sputum), blood
  - –Foreign body
  - –Aspirated food or stomach contents secondary to gastroesophageal reflux

Upper airway (usually inspiratory and monophonic)

- Nasal (congestion, choanal atresia, FB)
- Oropharyngeal (tonsils, adenoids, macroglossia, foreign body, decreased tone, retropharyngeal abscess)
- Laryngeal (laryngomalacia, vocal cord dysfunction or paralysis, laryngeal web or polyp, subglottic stenosis)

Central nervous system

- Structural disease (e.g., Arnold-Chiari malformation leading to vocal cord paralysis)
- Functional (e.g., vocal cord dysfunction, chronic aspiration)

Workup and Diagnosis

- History
  - –Triggers: Viral disease, irritants, and allergic disease
  - –Improvement with β-agonists or steroids suggests asthma
  - –Worsening with ETS suggests asthma or bronchitis; with exercise, EIA or VCD; with β-agonists, bronchomalacia
  - –Delayed onset with exercise suggests EIA; rapid onset with exercise suggests VCD (teens) or bronchomalacia (babies)
  - –Age of onset: First month, structural problems (e.g., bronchomalacia); first year, RSV bronchiolitis, GER, or aspiration; early childhood, asthma, possible FB aspiration; adolescence, asthma and VCD
  - –Other symptoms: Hemoptysis, chronic cough, weight loss (CF, TB, bronchiectasis, malignancy, recurrent infection, or immunodeficiency); weakness, hypotonia (neuromotor disease, Down syndrome, aspiration); choking on feeds (upper airway disease, TEF, chronic aspiration)
- Exam findings
  - –High pitch indicates smaller airways; low pitch, larger airway(s); inspiratory, extrathoracic airway; expiratory, intrathoracic airways; biphasic, fixed obstruction or two sites; expiratory prolongation, small airways or severe larger airways
- Diagnostic tests: CXR may show hyperinflation, peribronchial cuffing, congenital lesions; CT, tissue density abnormalities, airway lesions; MRI, airway, blood vessel interface; MRA defines vascular anatomy; nuclear med, reflux and V/Q studies; PFT, volume and air flow; bronchoscopy, lavage and visualize
- Blood gas; disease-specific studies (e.g., sweat test)

Treatment

- Asthma is treated with layered therapy for acute symptom control ("rescue" medicine) and prevention of disease ("controller" medicine)
  - –Rescue medicines are inhaled β-agonists (immediate) or steroids (rapid)
  - –Controller medicines include ICS, leukotriene modifiers, anti-inflammatory agents, and long-acting bronchodilators
- Bronchomalacia is treated with atrovent and/or ICS
- Treat/eliminate underlying triggers

Section 11

Abdomen

SARAH FRIEBERT, MD
DOUGLAS A. JACOBSTEIN, MD
CHRISTINA LIN MASTER, MD
BANKOLE OSUNTOKUN, MD
JONATHAN E. TEITELBAUM, MD

77. Abdominal Distension

A prominent "potbelly" contour is normal in infants and young children. Pathologic enlargement of the abdomen is a fairly common problem that can result from reduced tone of the wall musculature or from increased content (gas, liquid, or solid). Acute-onset abdominal distension is a sign that should be taken seriously, especially when accompanied by bilious vomiting.

Differential Diagnosis

- Mechanical intestinal obstruction
  - –Incarcerated inguinal hernia
  - –Malrotation with volvulus
  - –Intestinal atresia (newborns)
  - –Imperforate anus (newborns)
  - –Intussuception
  - –Hirschsprung disease
  - –Meconium ileus (in newborns, due to CF)
  - –Left microcolon syndrome (typically in infants of diabetic mothers)
  - –Fecal impaction (from chronic constipation)
  - –Bezoars: Lactobezoars in premature infants
- Functional intestinal obstruction
  - –Paralytic ileus, postoperative ileus, reflex ileus (from sepsis or acute infection)
  - –Peritonitis/intestinal perforation
  - –Severe hypokalemia
  - –Gastroparesis
  - –Necrotizing enterocolitis (NEC)
  - –Toxic megacolon (IBD)
  - –Dysmotility (pseudo-obstruction syndrome)
- Renal enlargement
  - –Hydronephrosis (most common cause of abdominal distension in the newborn)
  - –Ureteropelvic junction obstruction
  - –Bladder distension
  - –Congenital polycystic kidney
- Ascites
- Hepatomegaly
  - –Budd-Chiari or Beckwith-Wiedemann
  - –Glycogen storage disease
  - –Amyloidosis
  - –Congestive heart failure
- Splenomegaly
- Tumors/cysts
  - –Wilms tumor, neuroblastoma, lymphoma, teratoma, sarcoma, ovarian cyst or tumor, omental cyst, dermoid cyst
- Pancreatic pseudocyst
- Obesity: Protuberant abdomen (common)
- Aerophagia
- Pregnancy
- Hematometrocolpos
- Malnutrition (e.g., kwashiorkor, celiac)
- Abdominal abscess
- Prune-belly syndrome
- Poor posture

Workup and Diagnosis

- Rapid recognition of obstruction is essential
- History: Age of onset, duration, fever, weight loss, vomiting (bilious/nonbilious), abdominal pain, last bowel movement, bloody or currant-jelly stools (intussuception), last menstrual period, respiratory distress, trauma
- Birth history, PMH, PSH, time of passage of meconium (delayed in Hirschsprung)
- Maternal history: Pregnancy (oligo- or polyhydramnious), labor/delivery, gestational diabetes
- Physical exam: Vital signs, general appearance, abdominal exam for presence of ascites (flank bulging, shifting dullness, fluid wave), masses and tympanic percussion, umbilicus sunken in obesity, herniated if tense ascites, perineum exam for inguinal hernia
- Labs: CBC, Serum electrolytes, LFT, UA, stool for occult blood, amylasc, and lipasc
- Studies
  - –Obstructive series for air fluid levels, distended bowel loops, or pneumoperitoneum
  - –Abdominal ultrasound for pancreatic pseudocyst, ascites, and masses
  - –Upper GI series for proximal obstruction
  - –Barium enema for distal obstructions
  - –CT scan of the abdomen for better delineation of masses or anatomical anomalies
  - –Surgical consult if obstruction or perforation suspected

Treatment

- Treatment is focused on underlying cause
- Management of intestinal obstruction
  - –Make the patient NPO
  - –Nasogastric tube placement for decompression
  - –Correction of fluid and electrolyte imbalance
  - –Antibiotic for cases of suspected perforation, NEC, or peritonitis
  - –Laparascopy/laparatomy: Prompt relief of obstructions or repair of perforation is paramount
- Prokinetic for dysmotility or gastroparesis
- Surgical resection and subsequent reanastomosis for Hirschsprung disease (one-step or staged repair)
- Percutaneous, surgical, or endoscopic drainage of pancreatic pseudocyst if persistent
- Fecal disimpaction and treatment of constipation
- Correction of malnutrition
- Contrast or air enema for reduction of intussuception or flushing of meconium ileus
- Surgical resection of tumor

78. Abdominal Masses

Abdominal masses are common presenting signs of malignant solid tumors in children and should be presumed to be such. They require urgent evaluation to rule out compression of internal organs, hemorrhage, and/or malignancy. In newborns, an abdominal mass is most likely renal in origin; if malignant, Wilms tumor and neuroblastoma are most likely. In older children, malignant abdominal masses are usually splenic and/or hepatic infiltration with leukemia or lymphoma.

Differential Diagnosis

- Wilms tumor
  - More common in younger children
- Neuroblastoma
  - More common in younger children
- Leukemia/lymphoma
  - Involvement of retroperitoneal nodes, liver, or spleen
- Hepatic tumors
  - Hepatoblastoma, hepatocellular carcinoma, angiosarcoma, rhabdomyosarcoma of the liver, metastatic disease
- Germ cell tumors
  - Ovarian, teratoma
- Soft tissue sarcoma
  - Rhabdomyosarcoma
- Rare malignancies in children
  - Carcinoid tumors, adrenocortical carcinoma, pancreatoblastoma, malignant rhabdoid tumor
- Cystic masses
  - Ovary, renal, mesenteric
- Benign tumors
  - Adenomas (especially of liver), hamartomas, pheochromocytoma
- Vascular lesions (e.g., hemangioma)
- Renal etiologies
  - Distended, nonemptying bladder, bladder outlet obstruction
  - Congenital mesoblastic nephroma
  - Severe hydronephrosis
- Gynecologic
  - Ovarian torsion, endometriosis, pelvic inflammatory disease
- Gastrointestinal
  - Constipation/stool impaction, intestinal obstruction (e.g., Hirschsprung), GI duplication, incarcerated hernia
- Pancreatic pseudocyst
- Infectious
  - Abscess, hepatitis, virus (EBV, CMV) causing splenomegaly or hepatomegaly
- Structures normally palpable in small children are liver edge, spleen tip (especially with viral illness), aorta, sigmoid colon, and spine

Workup and Diagnosis

- History
  - Mass duration, growth rate, pain; fever, weight loss, bone pain, night sweats
  - Anorexia, vomiting, constipation or diarrhea, early satiety, jaundice; prematurity, umbilical catheterization; opsoclonus, myoclonus (neuroblastoma)
  - Vaginal bleeding/amenorrhea, sexual activity, previous pregnancies/fertility, history of STDs; urinary dysfunction, congenital urinary tract anomalies
  - Signs of catecholamine excess (sleeplessness, jitteriness, flushing, hypertension)
- Family history: Wilms tumor, neurofibromatosis, hepatic tumors, Beckwith-Wiedemann
- Physical exam: Vital signs, toxicity, pallor, puffiness; location, size, tenderness, consistency of mass; hemihypertrophy (with Wilms), lymph nodes; wheezing, rales, SVC syndrome; presence of ascites, visible venous dilation; testicular exam, rectal; pelvic examination in teenagers; petechiae, purpura/ecchymoses, café au lait spots
- Labs: CBC with differential; electrolytes, BUN, Cr, LFT albumin, urinalysis; LDH, uric acid, PT/PTT/INR, ferritin, viral titers (EBV, CMV, hepatitis), tumor markers, stool guaiac
- Studies: KUB/upright film, chest X-ray; CT of chest/abdomen/pelvis; abdominal ultrasound; bone marrow aspirate/biopsy

Treatment

- Depends on specific etiology
- Respiratory and hemodynamic stability of the patient must be secured before any evaluation or treatment
- Prompt involvement of a pediatric surgeon, neurosurgeon, oncologist, urologist/urologic surgeon, gynecologist, or gastroenterologist will help streamline the approach

79. Abdominal Pain

Abdominal pain is a frequent complaint and associated with an enormous number of causes. Many causes of acute abdominal pain require surgical intervention, so a prompt diagnosis is needed. Diagnostic clues would include the location of the pain. Traditionally, the farther away the pain is from the umbilicus, the more likely one is to find an organic cause. Chronic pain without associated vomiting, weight loss, or bloody diarrhea is often functional in origin.

Differential Diagnosis

Epigastric pain
- Peptic ulcer disease/GERD
  - May be due to *Helicobacter pylori* or NSAID use
- Gallbladder disease
  - Most commonly with hemolytic disorders
- Pancreatitis
  - Trauma and idiopathic are common causes

Periumbilical pain
- Functional abdominal pain/IBS
  - Most common cause of nonorganic pain
  - Occurs in children 3–15 years old
- Appendicitis
  - Periumbilical pain moves to RLQ
- Gastroenteritis (virus, bacteria, parasite)
- Carbohydrate intolerance
  - Lactase, fructase, trehelase deficiency
- Abdominal migraine
- Drugs
  - Antibiotics, anticonvulsants, bronchodilators
- Small bowel bacterial overgrowth
- Streptococcal pharyngitis

Suprapubic pain
- Urinary tract infection
  - With dysuria, fever, foul-smelling urine
  - Pyelonephritis may have CVA tenderness
- Constipation
  - Accounts for 3% of visits to pediatrician
  - May have a palpable fecal mass
- Urinary retention
- Hydrometrocolpos
  - Associated with imperforate hymen
  - Cyclic pain with onset of menstrual cycle

Right lower quadrant pain
- Appendicitis
- Ovarian torsion
- Pelvic inflammatory disease
- Ectopic pregnancy
- Mittelschmerz
  - Pain midcycle with ovulation
- Inflammatory bowel disease
  - Classic for terminal ileal Crohn disease
- Iliopsoas abscess
- Inguinal hernia
- Right lower lobe pneumonia

Workup and Diagnosis

- History
  - Type of pain, location, radiation, duration
  - Relieving and worsening factors including foods
  - Awakens from sleep, activity level, emesis, diarrhea
  - Nausea, hematochezia, melena, fever, dysuria, hematuria
  - Sexual activity, anorexia, headache, cough, rashes
  - Stool frequency, joint complaints
- Surgical history: Previous abdominal surgery
- Social history: Stressors, changes in school or family
- Physical exam
  - Height, weight, temperature, pulse
  - General appearance, hydration status
  - Pharyngeal erythema/exudates, abdominal tenderness
  - Psoas sign, obturator sign, palpable masses
  - Rectal exam including hemoccult
  - Rashes, joint swelling, vaginal exam
- Labs: Geared toward history and physical findings
  - Consider CBC with differential, urinalysis, and culture
  - stool for culture and O&P
  - Amylase and lipase, LFTs, *H. pylori* antibody (IgG)
  - Hydrogen breath test for sugar intolerance
  - Pregnancy test, vaginal cultures
  - Throat culture
- Consider KUB or obstruction series
- Abdominal CT scan with contrast versus ultrasound
- Pelvic ultrasound for torsion, ectopic pregnancy, abscess, hydrometrocolpos

Treatment

- If concerned about "surgical abdomen," consult surgery
  - Appendicitis, ovarian torsion, hydrometrocolpos
- Treat infections with antibiotics
- Eliminate offending carbohydrate in intolerance
  - Lactase supplementation for lactose intolerance
- Irritable bowel syndrome or functional pain
  - Identifying stressors may be helpful
  - Antispasmodics have similar action to placebo
  - Tricyclic antidepressants at low doses are helpful particularly if pain is associated with diarrhea
- Counseling may be needed for chronic pain
- Stop offending drugs if possible
- Constipation
  - Disimpaction if significant fecal mass
  - Stool softeners/laxatives, increased dietary fiber
- Drain abscess
- PUD/GERD: Acid blockade therapy
- Pancreatitis: Bowel rest, pain management

80. Ascites

Ascites, the accumulation of serous fluid within the peritoneal cavity, may be caused by a combination of factors, including hypoalbuminemia, portal hypertension, increased aldosterone and antidiuretic hormone secretion, overproduction of lymph, and enhanced renal reabsorption of sodium and water. In children, hepatic, renal, and cardiac diseases are the most common causes. Patients are at an increased risk of spontaneous bacterial peritonitis. The most common infecting organism is *Streptococcus pneumoniae*.

Differential Diagnosis

- Hepatic, resulting in portal hypertension
  - Hepatic cirrhosis: Extrahepatic biliary atresia, α-1-antitrypsin deficiency, galactosemia, tyrosinemia
  - Portal vein thrombosis
  - Cavernous transformation: Catheterization, dehydration, clotting disorder, omphalitis
  - Budd-Chiari syndrome, due to neoplasm, collagen disease, hypercoagulopathy, OCP
  - Arteriovenous fistula
  - Fulminant hepatic failure (drugs, virus)
  - Congenital hepatic fibrosis
  - Lysosomal storage diseases (e.g., Gaucher)
- Bile ascites (bile peritonitis): Spontaneous rupture of the common bile duct
- Renal
  - Nephrotic syndrome
  - Urinary ascites (due to bladder rupture)
  - Obstructive uropathy: Congenital ascites may be seen with bilateral hydronephrosis
- Peritoneal dialysis
- Cardiac
  - Congestive heart failure
  - Chronic constrictive pericarditis
  - Inferior vena cava web
  - Erythroblastosis fetalis
- Peritonitis
  - Tuberculous peritonitis
  - Schistosomiasis (Mansoni)
  - Tularemia
  - Abscess
- Gastrointestinal disorders
  - Infarcted bowel
  - Bowel perforation
  - Pancreatitis, ruptured pancreatic duct
  - Protein-losing gastroenteropathy
- Chylous ascites
  - Collection of lymph within the abdominal cavity; secondary to lymphatic obstruction from trauma, surgery, tumor, tuberculosis, or filariasis
- Gynecologic
  - Ovarian tumors, cyst torsion or rupture
- Malignancy
  - Leukemia, lymphoma, neuroblastoma
- Systemic lupus erythromatosus
- Ventriculoperitoneal shunt
- Hypothyroidism

Workup and Diagnosis

- History and physical exam
  - Clinical hallmark of ascites is abdominal distension
  - Five classic signs of ascites: Flank bulging, flank dullness, shifting dullness, fluid wave, puddle sign
  - Only appreciated when there is considerable fluid
  - Respiratory distress may develop with tense ascites
  - Umbilical herniation can be seen with large ascites
  - Peripheral edema or anasarca may accompany severe hypoalbuminemia
- Urinalysis and urine electrolytes (for proteinuria)
- CBC with diff (lymphopenia in lymphatic obstruction)
- Serum electrolytes (for sodium management)
- True liver function tests
  - Examines the synthetic function of the liver
  - Serum albumin, vitamin K, and coagulation factors
- Abdominal ultrasound detects small volume of ascites
- KUB may show centrally floating intestines
- Paracentesis: Milky fluid indicates chylous ascites, fluid analysis will reveal elevated protein and triglycerides and lymphocytosis (fluid serous in a fasting patient)
  - Bile may indicate perforation of common bile duct
  - High creatinine: Seen with bladder rupture
  - Ascitic fluid analysis for cell count, cytology, protein, LDH, amylase, lipase, creatinine, pH, culture, Gram stain, bile, lipids, and sudan red staining for fat

Treatment

- Treatment is directed at underlying cause
- Bed rest, fluid, sodium restriction is the first line
- Diuretics: Careful use in selected cases
- Chylous ascites
  - High-protein, low-fat diet supplemented with medium-chain triglycerides
  - Parenteral nutrition may be needed to decrease lymph flow and supplement nutrition
  - Laparotomy may be indicated for failed dietary management, to seal leak site
- Surgical intervention: Bile or urine ascites
- Therapeutic paracentesis: May be repeated to relieve respiratory distress or impending umbilical rupture
- Portacaval shunt or a peritoneovenous shunt (LeVeen) for intractable ascites
  - Shunt between peritoneal cavity and superior vena cava
- Transjugular intrahepatic portosystemic shunt (TIPSS) for cirrhosis while awaiting transplantation

81. Bowel Sounds – Decreased

Decreased bowel sounds can be as innocent as a hungry patient anticipating his or her next meal or as ominous as an impending abdominal catastrophe necessitating emergent laparotomy. However, the sensitivity and specificity of the auscultation of bowel sounds are quite low, differ subjectively by clinician, and will vary from one moment to the next. Before declaring an absence of bowel sounds, one should auscultate for a minimum of 5 minutes ("if you didn't hear them, you didn't listen long enough").

Differential Diagnosis

- Benign etiologies
  - –Normal variant: 5–30 bowel sounds per minute is typical; however, several minutes may elapse without any sounds
  - –Failure to auscultate long enough
  - –Hunger
  - –Auscultation immediately after abdominal palpation or percussion; always listen for bowel sounds before palpating abdomen
- Complete bowel obstruction
  - –Partial bowel obstructions often have increased bowel sounds
- Adynamic ileus
  - –Abdominal surgery
  - –Electrolyte abnormalities (hypokalemia, hyponatremia, hypomagnesemia, uremia)
  - –Drugs (e.g., narcotics, α- and β-blockers, anticholinergics, psychotropic agents)
  - –Lower lobe pneumonia
  - –Sepsis
  - –Retroperitoneal hemorrhage
  - –Vertebral compression fracture
- Peritonitis
  - –Acute appendicitis (or ruptured appendix)
  - –Perforated gastric ulcer
  - –Ruptured ectopic pregnancy
  - –Pancreatitis
  - –Pelvic inflammatory disease
  - –Peritonitis
  - –Solid organ injury (e.g., after trauma)
- Intestinal ischemia
- Less common etiologies
  - –Diabetic coma
  - –Hypoparathyroidism
  - –Rib fractures
  - –Myocardial infarction
  - –Spinal injury
  - –Perforated gallbladder
  - –Black widow spider bite

Workup and Diagnosis

- A careful history and astute physical exam are crucial
  - –Characterization of the pain
  - –Patients with peritonitis appear very ill and have abdominal tenderness, rebound, and guarding
  - –Auscultate before palpation
  - –Auscultation of each quadrant is not crucial; bowel sounds radiate throughout the abdomen
- Initial labs should include CBC, electrolytes, BUN/creatinine, calcium, liver function tests, amylase, lipase, and urinalysis
- Imaging studies may include X-rays, CT scan, and ultrasound
  - –Flat and upright X-rays may reveal rupture (free air) or obstruction (dilated proximal loops of bowel with air-fluid levels); thoracic and/or lumbar X-rays may reveal spinal fractures
  - –Abdominal CT scan will give more anatomic detail and may better differentiate ileus from obstruction
  - –Ultrasound is useful for gynecologic concerns
- Differentiate postoperative ileus from obstruction
  - –Some degree of ileus is expected following laparotomy (3–5 days); prolonged ileus should be investigated
  - –Both can cause nausea/vomiting, constipation or obstipation, distension, tenderness, and tympany
  - –A transition point or lack of gas in the rectum may suggest an obstruction

Treatment

- Although treatment decisions should rarely (if ever) be based on bowel sounds, serial assessment may be a useful sign of a patient's clinical evolution
- Ileus is treated conservatively by bowel rest (NPO), IV hydration, and nasogastric decompression (for nausea and vomiting)
  - –Correct electrolyte abnormalities as necessary
  - –Discontinue constipating drugs (especially narcotics)
  - –Prokinetic drugs (e.g., metoclopramide, erythromycin) have mixed results but are often used
  - –Encourage ambulation
  - –Decreased nasogastric output, "normal" bowel sounds, passage of flatus, improved X-rays, or patient hunger may indicate readiness to begin oral intake
- Peritonitis generally requires emergent surgical intervention; treatment is directed at the specific underlying diagnosis

82. Bowel Sounds – Increased

Normal bowel sounds (BS) are intermittent low-to-medium-pitched gurgles interspersed with occasional high-pitched, tinkling metallic sounds heard every 10–30 seconds. In acute intestinal obstruction (mostly small bowel) the BS are markedly increased. High frequency, loud low-pitched gurgles (borborygmi), often rising to a high-pitched crescendo that coincides with colicky abdominal pain is pathognomonic of small bowel obstruction. This represents bouts of peristaltic activity that occurs in an attempt to "overcome" the obstruction.

Differential Diagnosis

- Hypertrophic pyloric stenosis (HPS)
  - –Most common cause in the neonate, between second and eighth week of life
  - –Typically nonbilious vomiting
  - –Most common in first-born males
  - –25% of offspring of affected female will have HPS
  - –Increased among blood groups B and O
- Mechanical intestinal obstruction
  - –Small bowel obstruction is most common
  - –May be congenital or acquired
  - –May be partial or complete
  - –Simple or strangulating (bowel ischemia)
- Congenital small bowel obstruction
  - –Incidence 1/1,500 live births
  - –Malrotation with or without volvulus
  - –Duodenal atresia/stenosis (common in infants with Down syndrome)
  - –Jejunal, ileal atresia/stenosis
  - –Annular pancreas
  - –Intestinal duplication
  - –Intra-abdominal hernia
  - –Meconium ileus (common in CF)
- Acquired small bowel obstruction
  - –Intussuception
  - –Incarcerated inguinal hernia
  - –Postsurgical adhesions
  - –Duodenal hematoma (post traumatic)
  - –Ascariasis: Heavy infestation, with formation of obstructing ball of worms
  - –Crohn disease (stricture)
  - –SMA syndrome
- Colonic obstruction
  - –Bowel sounds usually not very increased
  - –Hirschsprung disease
  - –Small left colon syndrome (seen in infants of diabetic mothers)
  - –Adhesions (post-NEC)
  - –Fibrosing colonopathy (seen in CF)
  - –Chagas disease
- Acute gastroenteritis
- Drugs
  - –Prokinetic agents: Metoclopramide, erythromycin
- Early peritonitis
  - –High-pitched, high frequency
- Intestinal pseudo-obstruction

Workup and Diagnosis

- History
  - –Age of onset, PMH, PSH, history of trauma
  - –Bilious/nonbilious, projectile/nonprojectile vomiting
  - –Diarrhea, last wet diaper, mental state
  - –Colicky abdominal pain
  - –Travel history
  - –Medications
  - –Maternal history: Polyhydramnios, gestational DM
- Physical examination
  - –Vital signs, anthropometry measurements
  - –Signs of dehydration
  - –Abdominal exam: Visible peristalsis waves (with pyloric stenosis), tenderness, masses (epigastric olive mass in HPS)
  - –Inguinal exam for incarcerated hernia
- Labs
  - –Electrolytes (hypochloremic metabolic alkalosis in HPS)
  - –Amylase and lipase to rule out pancreatitis
  - –CBC: Leukocytosis and thrombocytopenia with metabolic acidosis is highly suggestive of bowel infarction
- Studies
  - –Obstructive series
  - –Abdominal ultrasound (for HPS and intussuception)
  - –Upper GI series or CT when obstructive series and ultrasounds fail to pinpoint site of obstruction

Treatment

- Fluid resuscitation and stabilization of the patient in the presence of intestinal obstruction
  - –Make the patient NPO
  - –Nasogastric tube decompression prevents vomiting
  - –Cultures and antibiotics
  - –Children with bowel ischemia often present in sepsis and shock
  - –Neonates with bowel obstruction and children with suspected strangulating obstruction should also receive antibiotics
- Immediate surgical intervention for relief of obstruction to prevent bowel ischemia and gangrene
- Treatment is directed at underlying cause in nonsurgical cases

83. Constipation

Constipation is a common complaint, accounting for 3% of all pediatric office visits. Stool frequency can be variable in infants, who average 4 per day (SD 1.8) at 1 week, 2.2 per day (SD 1.6) at 1 month, and 1.8 per day (SD 1.2) at 1 year. After 4 years of age, 95–99% of healthy children and adults defecate at least three times per week.

Differential Diagnosis

- Functional constipation
  - By far the most common etiology
  - Rome II criteria define chronic functional constipation in infants and young children as at least 2 weeks of scybalous, pebble-like, hard stools for the majority of stools, or firm stools two or fewer times per week
  - Presents with stool-withholding behavior
  - Often due to inadequate fluid/fiber intake
- Drugs: Antacids (with aluminium and calcium), anticholinergics, antidepressants, bismuth, calcium antagonists, cough suppressants, opioid analgesics, phenobarbitol
- Irritable bowel syndrome
- Endocrine disorders
  - Hypercalcemia
  - Hypothyroidism
  - Hyperparathyroidism
  - Pregnancy
  - Reduction of steroid hormones in luteal and follicular phases of menstrual cycle
- Hirschsprung disease
  - 1/5,000 births, male to female ratio 4:1
  - 94% do not pass meconium within 24 hours of birth
  - 61% diagnosed by 12 months of life
- Neurologic disease
  - Myelomeningoce
  - Hypotonia (e.g., Down, myopathies, prune-belly syndrome)
  - Cerebral palsy
- Celiac disease
- Cystic fibrosis
- Inflammatory bowel disease
- Lead toxicity
- Structural abnormalities
  - Anal disorders (imperforate anus, anteriorly displaced anus, perianal fissures, strep infection, anal stenosis)
  - Colonic strictures (primary or secondary)
  - Pelvic masses (sacral teratoma)
- Infectious disease
  - Infantile botulism
  - Chagas disease
- Metabolic disorders
  - Uremia
  - Hypokalemia
  - Amyloid neuropathy
- Ogilvie syndrome

Workup and Diagnosis

- History and physical exam are often diagnostic for functional constipation
- History
  - Age at onset, duration, stool frequency/consistency, pain/bleeding with defecation, abdominal pain, toilet training, fecal soiling, stool-withholding behavior, appetite change, nausea/vomiting, weight loss, attempted treatments, dietary intake of fluid and fiber
  - Medical history: Gestational age, time of meconium passage, existing medical conditions, surgeries, delayed growth and development, sensitivity to cold, coarse hair, medications, association with stress
- Physical exam
  - Vital signs (including growth parameters), abdominal exam for fecal mass, anal inspection (position of anus, soiling, sacral dimple, skin tags, perianal fissures; rectal examination: anal wink, anal tone, presence/consistency of stool, fecal mass, other masses, explosive stool on withdrawal of finger, occult blood), and neurologic examination (tone, strength, cremasteric reflex, DTRs)
- KUB may demonstrate fecal mass in uncooperative patients
- Labs rarely needed, but may include thyroid (TSH, free T_4), electrolytes (including Ca^{++}, Mg^{+++}, Ph^{+++}), lead level, and celiac testing (tissue transglutaminase IgA)
- Rectal biopsy, manometry, or BE for Hirschsprung
- Spinal MRI for sacral anomalies

Treatment

- Functional constipation
  - Parental education and demystification of the process of normal defecation
  - Disimpaction with oral laxatives, senna, magnesium citrate, enemas
  - Maintenance stool softeners for 6–12 months, osmotic agents such as lactulose, polyethylene glycol 3350 (Miralax), mineral oil, milk of magnesia, Mylanta
  - Dietary manipulations: Increase fluid intake and increase dietary fiber (14 g/1,000 cal required)
- Cessation of offending drugs when possible
- Correction of electrolyte disturbance
- Treatment of endocrinologic disease
- Hirschsprung disease is treated by surgical resection of agangliotic segment with subsequent reanastomosis

84. Diarrhea – Acute

Acute diarrhea is an abrupt onset of increased fluid content of stool above about 10 mL/kg/day and increased frequency from 4–5 to more than 20 times daily. It is a major problem worldwide because of excessive loss of fluid and electrolytes in stool. In the U.S., every year diarrhea accounts for 1–2 episodes per child, about 10% of all hospital admissions for children under 5 years of age, and 400 deaths. According to the WHO, about 3 million diarrhea-related deaths occur per year globally.

Differential Diagnosis

- Viral gastroenteritis
  - –Rotavirus, most common (winter)
  - –Norwalk-like virus
  - –Calcivurus
  - –Enteric adenovirus
  - –Astrovirus
- Bacterial gastroenteritis
  - –*Campylobacter jejuni* (associated with Guillain-Barré syndrome)
  - –*Salmonella*
  - –*Shigella:* May cause seizures (up to 30%), HUS
  - –*Escherichia coli* (various types): Enteropathogenic, enterohemorrhagic (O157:H7) verotoxin can cause HUS (6–8% of cases), enterotoxigenic (traveler's diarrhea), enteroinvasive
  - –*Clostridium difficile* (toxin A or B)
  - –*Yersinia enterocolitis* (mimics acute appendicitis)
  - –*Vibrio cholerae*
  - –*Aeromonas hydrophila*
  - –Toxin-mediated food poisoning: *Bacillus cereus, Staphylococcus aureus, Clostridium perfringens*
- Parasitic infestations
  - –*Giardia lamblia*
  - –*Cryptosporidium* (severe in AIDS patients)
  - –*Entamoeba histolytica*
- Food allergies
  - –Cow's milk and soy protein allergy are most common in infancy
- Malbasorption (celiac disease, CF)
- Lactose or fructose intolerance
- Overfeeding (relative lactase deficiency)
- Vitamin deficiency (e.g., niacin)
- Zinc deficiency
- Laxative abuse
- Irritable bowel syndrome
- Constipation with encopresis
- Bacterial overgrowth
- Antibiotics
- Hirschsprung toxic colitis
- Adrenogenital syndrome

Workup and Diagnosis

- History
  - –Duration of diarrhea
  - –Frequency and consistency of stool
  - –Vomiting, weight loss
  - –Diet history
  - –History of sick contact
  - –Fever and blood mixed in stool more common with invasive pathogens: *Salmonella, Shigella, Campylobacter, Yersinia, E. coli* O157:H7, and *E. histolytica*
- Physical exam
  - –Vital signs, look for signs of dehydration
  - –Severe cases may present in hypovolemic shock
- Labs
  - –Urinalysis: Specific gravity and ketones
  - –Serum electrolytes: Acidosis, hyper- or hyponatremia, hypoglycemia
  - –Stool for Rotazyme
  - –Stool culture: *Salmonella, E. coli, Shigella, Campylobacter,* and *Yersinia*
  - –Stool ELISA for *C. difficile* toxin A and B
  - –Stool for ova and parasites
  - –Blood culture indicated in the presence of fever
  - –CBC may reveal high bandemia with shigellosis
  - –Stool for occult blood and WBC is of little value in differentiating viral from bacterial causes

Treatment

- Mainstay of treatment is rehydration to correct fluid and electrolyte deficits
  - –Oral route is best in mildly to moderately dehydrated children who can tolerate PO fluid
  - –IV fluids: Useful in severe to moderate dehydration
  - –Estimate fluid deficit using % of weight loss, and add this to maintenance requirement and ongoing losses
  - – Correct over 24–48 hours
- Antibiotics
  - –Not necessary in most cases, can precipitate HUS
  - –Indicated for *V. cholerae, Shigella, and G. lamblia*
  - –Indicated in selected circumstances: *Salmonella* in very young infant, if febrile, or positive blood culture
  - –Metronidazole for *C. difficile* (if antibiotic elimination doesn't help)
- Refeeding: No benefit to withholding milk, incidence of lactose intolerance overstated
- Probiotics: *Lactobacillus rhamnosus* for rotavirus

85. Diarrhea – Chronic, No Blood or Weight Loss

Chronic diarrhea (nonbloody, without weight loss) is defined as increased total daily stool output (greater than 10 g/kg/day), associated with increased stool water content; diarrhea is classified as chronic when it lasts longer than 2 weeks. Per liter, normal stool of infants and children contains approximately 20–50 mEq of sodium, 50–70 mEq of potassium, 20–50 mEq of chloride. Diarrhea may be osmotic or secretory.

Differential Diagnosis

- Osmotic: Presence of nonabsorbable solute, pH <5, volume <200 mL/day, normal electrolytes, stops with fasting
- Secretory: Mostly due to toxins, pH >6, volume >200 mL/day, no response to fasting, stool Na >70 mEq/L, negative reducing substances
- Toddler's diarrhea: Chronic nonspecific diarrhea, onset 3 months to 3 years of age, average 4–6 stools daily, due to excessive juice intake or low-fat diet
- Excessive intake of nonabsorbable solutes (lactulose, sorbitol, magnesium hydroxide)
- Congenital lactose deficiency: Very rare in infancy, but may occur in extremely premature infants; adult-onset type of hypolactasia may be seen in older children (over age 5), autosomal recessive, 15% white adults, 85% of black adults, 90% of Asian adults
- Secondary lactase deficiency: Follows a viral gastroenteritis, most commonly rotavirus, may persist for months
- Fructose intolerance
- Sucrase-isomaltase deficiency: Autosomal recessive, found in 0.2% of North Americans, symptoms commence on starting sucrose or glucose polymer-containing foods
- Glucose-galactose malabsorption: Rare, autosomal recessive disorder
- Infections
  - –Giardiasis (most common infectious cause of chronic diarrhea in toddlers)
  - –Cryptosporidium
  - –Microsporidium
- Irritable bowel syndrome (IBS)
  - –Abnormality of intestinal motility and pain perception with no organic basis
  - –Abdominal pain associated with intermittent diarrhea or constipation
- Bacterial overgrowth: Enteric bacteria colonizes the upper small intestine
- Trehelase deficiency (trehelose is the sugar found in mushrooms)
- Zinc deficiency
  - –Acrodermatitis enteropathica is typical rash
- Low-fat diet

Workup and Diagnosis

- History
  - –Weight loss
  - –Daycare setting, ill contacts
  - –Diet history: Type and amount of fluids daily (intake of >150 mL/kg/day with normal weight and height suggests toddler's diarrhea)
  - –Frequency of stool and consistency
  - –Associated symptoms: Abdominal pain, bloating, flatulence, rash, fever, or vomiting
  - –Onset of symptoms and relation to ingestion of milk, sucrose, or glucose
  - –Worsening with stress (typical for IBS)
  - –Exposure to lakes, well water (suggestive of parasite)
  - –Travel history
  - –Excessive "sugar free" gum chewing (sorbitol)
- Stool examination
  - –Gross examination (blood, mucus, undigested food)
  - –Color is not helpful
  - –Occult blood test (not detected in IBS)
  - –pH: Stool pH <5 indicates osmotic diarrhea from reducing sugars (sucrose and trehelose are nonreducing)
  - –Stool cultures, O&P, *Clostridium difficile* toxin
- More studies only if all of above failed to reveal cause
- Hydrogen breath test
  - –Detects carbohydrate malabsorption (lactose, sucrose, fructose, glucose) and bacterial overgrowth
- Stool electrolytes if secretory diarrhea is suspected

Treatment

- Treatment is directed at cause
- Chronic nonspecific diarrhea
  - –Restriction of fluid intake to <90 mL/kg/day
  - –Reduction of fruit juices (<8 ounces/day)
  - –Elimination of sorbitol-containing juices
- Carbohydrate malabsorption
  - –Trial elimination or reduction of offending sugar
  - –Lactase (Lactaid) for lactose intolerance
  - –Sucrase (Sucraid) for sucrase-isomaltase deficiency
- Small intestine bacterial overgrowth
  - –Antibiotic therapy with metronidazole alone or in combination with ampicillin or Bactrim
  - –Surgery for partial small bowel obstruction
- Low-fat diet: Increase fat intake to approximately 40% of total daily calorie intake
- Irritable bowel syndrome
  - –Anticholinergic therapy or antidepressants
- Acrodermatitis enteropathica: Zinc supplements

86. Diarrhea – Chronic, with Weight Loss

Diarrhea is considered chronic when it last longer than 14 days. Weight loss with diarrhea should always be concerning and deserves thorough investigation. Collectively the malabsorption syndromes are the most common etiologic factors.

Differential Diagnosis

- Allergic enteritis: Typically cow's milk or soy in infants
- Inflammatory bowel disease (IBD)
- Cystic fibrosis (CF)
  - –Chronic diarrhea may be the only sign
  - –90% have pancreatic insufficiency (PI)
- Celiac disease (CD): Gluten sensitivity, increased incidence in selective IgA deficiency, DM, and Down syndrome
- Immune deficiency (e.g., hypogammaglobulinemia)
- Sucrase-isomaltase deficiency: Autosomal recessive, symptoms with starting sucrose or glucose polymer-containing diet
- Microvillus inclusion disease: Most common cause of persistent diarrhea in the neonatal period
- Schwachman-Diamond syndrome
  - –Pancreatic insufficiency, neutropenia, short stature, skeletal abnormalitics
- Johannson-Blizzard syndrome
  - –Pancreatic insufficiency, scalp defects, agenesis of nasal cartilage, deafness, imperforate anus
- Whipple disease:
  - –*Tropheryma whippelii* (actinomycete)
  - –Diagnosed mainly in adults
  - –Weight loss, diarrhea, and arthropathy
- Tropical sprue: Common in developing countries; folate deficiency and diarrhea
- Neural crest tumors: Pheochromocytoma, VIPoma, Zollinger-Ellison syndrome, carcinoid tumors
- Mastocytoma
- Neuroblastoma
- Abetalipoproteinemia
- Giardiasis, *Strongyloides*, coccidia
- AIDS
- Acrodermatitis enteropathica: Zinc deficiency, acral perioral and perianal rashes, consider underlying cystic fibrosis
- Mutational defects in ion transport proteins
  - –Chloride-losing diarrhea: Rare, ileal chloride transport defect, maternal polyhydramnios
  - –Congenital sodium diarrhea
- Tufting enteropathy (epithelial dysplasia)
- Enterokinase deficiency

Workup and Diagnosis

- History and physical exam
  - –Diet history and nutritional assessment, onset, frequency, and consistency, history of foreign travel
  - –Associated symptoms: Vomiting, irritability, and rashes (dermatitis herpetiformis) with CD; frequent infections in CF and Schwachman-Diamond; digital clubbing in CF, CD, and IBD
  - –Hypertension, tachycardia, anxiety, flushing, and sweating with pheochromocytoma; peptic ulcers with Zollinger-Ellison; wheezing, abdominal pain, flushing with carcinoid tumors; pruritus, flushing, and apnea with mastocytoma
- Stool examination: Oily, bulky, and foul-smelling with fat malabsorption; massive watery stools with secretory diarrhea; blood and mucus seen with colitis; stool for ova and parasites or antigen test for *Giardia;* WBC, eosinophils in allergic disease; occult blood test, stool pH, electrolytes, osmolarity, reducing substances
- PI proven by 72-hour fecal fat, stool elastase, secretin stimulation test, fat-soluble vitamin deficiency (ADEK)
- CBC, ESR, electrolytes, LFT, albumin (low in CD or IBD)
- Sucrose breath test for sucrase-isomaltase deficiency
- Sweat test to rule out CF
- Endoscopic biopsy: CD, IBD, Whipple diagnosis, microvillus inclusion (abetalipoproteinemia)
- Hormonal assay: Gastrin, vasocative intestinal peptide
- Anti-tissue transglutaminase IgA antibodies for CD

Treatment

- Correct malnourished states
- IBD: Anti-inflammatories (e.g., steroids, 6MP, 5ASA)
- CD: Lifelong gluten-free diet
- CF: Pancreatic enzyme and nutritional supplements including fat-soluble vitamins (ADEK)
- Allergy: Food antigen avoidance
- Sucrase-isomaltase deficiency: "Sucraid" enzyme
- Neural crest tumors: Surgical resections
- VIPoma: Somatostatin
- Gastrinoma: Proton pump inhibitors
- Whipple disease: Trimethoprim-sulfamethoxazole
- Abetalipoprotenemia: No specific treatment
  - –Supplements of fat-soluble vitamins and MCT oil
- Acrodermatitis enteropathica: Zinc supplements
- Giardiasis: Metronidazole or nitazoxamide
- Hyperalimentation: Parenteral nutrition may be needed for familial enteropathies

87. Encopresis

Encopresis refers to the repeated voluntary or involuntary passage of quantitative normal feces into inappropriate places (usually clothing or floor) after the age of 4 years. Subtypes include encopresis with constipation and overflow incontinence, defective neuromuscular control, and functional nonretentive fecal soiling. Encopresis affects about 1% of school-age children, and it is more common in males in this age group.

Differential Diagnosis

- Functional constipation (accounts for 66%)
  - –Chronic constipation with fecal impaction results in a functional megacolon and overflow incontinence
  - –Repeated soiling of underpants
  - –Involuntary passage of loose feces around large balls of impacted feces
  - –Child is unaware of "accidents" and odor
- Functional nonretentive fecal soiling
  - –Rome II criteria: Inappropriate defecation in the absence of constipation and structural or inflammatory disease
  - –May be the manifestation of an emotional disturbance in a child
  - –Affects 2% of school-age children
  - –Male-to-female ratio of 4:1
- Spina bifida
  - –Incidence is 1/1,000 live births
  - –Myelomeningocele is the most common
  - –Bladder and bowel dysfunction is usual
- Anorectal malformations
  - –Incidence is 1/4,000 live births
  - –Anal stenosis with overflow incontinence
  - –Imperforate anus with perineal fistula
  - –Vestibular fistula: Most frequent defect seen in females, rectum opens into the vaginal vestibule
  - –Rectovaginal fistula: Can result from pressure necrosis with obstructed labor
  - –Persistent cloaca: The rectum, vagina, and urinary tract meet and fuse into a single common channel
- Postsurgical repair
  - –Common sequela of the repair of high imperforate anus and Hirschsprung
- Inflammatory bowel disease (IBD)
  - –Perianal fistulas or sinuses (Crohn disease)
- Diarrheal disease: Transient fecal soiling resolves with cessation of diarrhea
- Intestinal neuronal dysplasia
- Spinal tumors
- Tethered cord
- Diastematomyelia
  - –Difficulty in walking, dribbling of urine, and fecal incontinence
- Organic constipation
  - –Hypothyroidism, celiac disease, amyloid neuropathy, and endocrine disorders

Workup and Diagnosis

- Encopresis is often a clinical diagnosis
- History
  - –Age of onset, duration, frequency
  - –Stool-withholding behavior
  - –Chronic abdominal pain, anorexia
  - –Passive-aggressive relationship with caregiver
  - –Chronic constipation
  - –Prior anorectal malformations and corrective surgeries
  - –Growth failure, developmental delay
  - –History of depression and low self-esteem
  - –Urinary incontinence and frequent urinary infections
- Physical exam
  - –Abdominal distension
  - –Bimanual abdominal palpation for fecal mass
  - –Rectal examination to palpate fecal mass
  - –Signs of spinal dysraphism: Motor and sensory deficit, absent cremasteric reflex, patulous anus, urinary incontinence, hair tufts in sacrococcygeal region
- KUB demonstrates fecal mass in the uncooperative child
- Labs: In non-straightforward cases
  - –Serologic assay for celiac, thyroid function tests, serum electrolytes, calcium, and lead
- Colonic manometry
  - –Differentiates between neuropathy and myopathy
- Spinal MRI for sacral anomalies

Treatment

- Functional constipation
  - –Disimpaction (manual or with laxatives/enemas)
  - –Maintenance therapy (stool softeners and laxatives)
  - –Dietary manipulation (increase fluid and fiber)
- Surgical correction of anorectal anomalies
- Spina bifida
  - –Behavioral modification techniques
  - –Biofeedback training
  - –Large-volume enemas with enema incontinence catheter
  - –Continent appendicostomy (Malone procedure): Appendix is connected to the umbilicus, an antegrade colonic enema is given while the patient is sitting on the toilet
  - –Cecostomy tube inserted percutaneously via interventional radiology or endoscopically; can also be used for antegrade colonic enema
- Bowel management program

88. Hematochezia

Hematochezia refers to bright red blood per rectum (BRBPR). When the blood is maroon, the bleeding source is usually colonic. Massive upper GI bleed may rarely present with BRBPR because blood is a cathartic and children have a short intestinal transit time. Milk protein allergy is the commonest etiological factor, followed by anorectal fissure in infants. In the neonatal period, NEC must be ruled out. Infectious colitis, followed by anorectal fissures, are the most common in childhood. IBD should be considered in the older child and adolescent.

Differential Diagnosis

- Milk or soy protein allergy (colitis)
- Anorectal fissure: passage of hard stool causing rectal trauma
- Nectrotizing enterocolitis (NEC): Vast majority occur in premature infants
- Infectious colitis
  - –Bacterial: *Salmonella, Shigella, Campylobacter, Yersinia, Clostridium difficile,* and *E. coli* (O157:H7)
  - –Parasitic: *Entamoeba histolytica*
- Immunocompromised host
  - –CMV enterocolitis
  - –Disseminated aspergillosis
  - –*Mycobacterium avium* complex
  - –Typhlitis: Polymicrobial inflammation of the cecum associated with neutropenia
- AIDS
  - –Aphthous ulcerations of the intestine
- Juvenile polyps
  - –Most common source of significant rectal bleeding in childhood
  - –Pathologically benign inflammatory polyps
- Inflammatory bowel disease
- Meckel diverticulum: Ectopic gastric mucosa, 2% of population
- Intestinal duplication
- Henoch-Schönlein purpura (HSP)
- Lymphonodular hyperplasia
- Solitary rectal ulcer
- Ischemic injury
  - –Malrotation with volvulus
  - –Intussusception
  - –Postoperative (colonic watershed regions)
  - –Acute drug-induced ischemia (cocaine)
- Hirschprung enterocolitis
- Foreign body injury: Ingested glass, broken glass thermometer, other sharp objects
- Munchausen syndrome by proxy
- Vascular lesions
  - –Hemangiomas (rare)
  - –Arteriovenous, venous malformation
  - –Klippel-Trenaunay syndrome
  - –Blue rubber bleb nevus syndrome
  - –Hereditary hemorrhagic telangiectasia
- Hemorrhoids and colorectal varices from portal hypertension
  - –Hemorrhoids rarely bleed in children

Workup and Diagnosis

- History and physical exam
  - –Painless rectal bleeding is typical of juvenile polyp, vascular lesions, Meckel, or ulcerated duplication
  - –Crampy abdominal pain, bloody/mucoid stool, with or without fever suggest infectious, inflammatory, or ischemic process in the colon
  - –History of constipation and blood streaked stool points toward anorectal fissure
  - –Skin examination for vascular lesions
  - –Anal inspection and rectal examination may reveal markers of IBD, such as a skin tag, fistula, or fissures
- Stool examination: Currant-jelly stool is a late sign in intussusception; maroon-colored stool may represent blood from a distal small bowel lesion (e.g., Meckel); bacterial culture, *C. difficile* toxin assay, O&P
- CBC, blood smear, urinalysis, BUN, and Cr to evaluate for HUS
- Endoscopy
  - –Colonoscopy is the most valuable tool after infections have been ruled out
  - –May offer both diagnosis and therapy (polypectomy)
- X-rays: Obstructive series useful when pain or vomiting is present; thumb printing seen with bowel wall edema; pneumoperitoneum with perforation
- Ultrasound: Can detect intussusception
- Meckel scan (Tc-petichnitate)
- Angiography, scintigraphy, push enteroscopy, or capsule endoscopy for vascular lesions

Treatment

- Treatment is directed at the underlying cause
- Correct hemodynamic instability with volume expansion, pressure support, and blood transfusion
- Milk protein allergy: Protein hydrolysate formulas
- NEC: Antibiotics and supportive therapy, surgery for perforation
- IBD: Anti-inflammatory (e.g. steroids, 6MP, 5ASA)
- Hemangiomas: Corticosteroids or alpha-interferon
- Infectious colitis: Antibiotics for *Shigella, Campylobacter, C. difficile,* and amebiasis; treat *Salmonella* only in very young or febrile infants
- Endoscopic therapy: Polypectomy for juvenile polyp, elastic band ligation, sclerotherapy, and/or electrotherapy for vascular anomalies.
- Surgery: Indicated for failure of radiographic reduction of intussusception, volvulus, or other ischemic injuries; Meckel diverticulum, and vascular anomalies
- Stool softeners for anorectal fissures

89. Hematemesis

Hematemesis or blood in emesis can occur as recent or ongoing hemorrhage proximal to the ligament of Treitz. Hematemesis is relatively uncommon in the pediatric population, and its overall occurrence in an ambulatory setting has not been reported. The most common diagnoses vary based on the age of presentation of the patient.

Differential Diagnosis

- Gastritis
  - –More common in pediatrics than ulcers
  - –Medications (e.g., NSAIDs, aspirin)
  - –Infections (e.g., *Helicobacter pylori*, CMV, herpes)
  - –Crohn disease
- Esophagitis
  - –Gastroesophageal reflux disease
  - –Crohn disease
  - –Infection (e.g., *Candida, Aspergillus,* CMV, HSV)
  - –Medications (e.g., tetracycline, aspirin, NSAIDs, potassium chloride)
- Peptic ulcer disease
- Zollinger-Ellison syndrome
  - –Gastrinoma
  - –Results in multiple small bowel ulcers
- Milk protein allergy
- Eosinophilic enteropathy
- Portal hypertension
  - –Esophageal varices
  - –Gastric varices
  - –Hypertensive gastropathy
- Traumatic
  - –Mallory-Weiss tear (located at LES)
  - –Prolapsing gastropathy
  - –Foreign body ingestion
  - –Direct abdominal trauma
- Vascular malformations
  - –Hemangiomas
  - –Aortoenteric fistulas
  - –Dieulafoy lesion
  - –Osler-Weber-Rendu syndrome
  - –Watermelon stomach
  - –Hemorrhagic telangiectasia
  - –Blue rubber bleb nevus syndrome
- Tumors
  - –Polyps
  - –Lipomas
  - –Adenocarcinoma
  - –Lymphoma
- Miscellaneous
  - –Hemosuccus pancreaticus
  - –Hemobilia
  - –Swallowed maternal blood
  - –Gastric duplication
  - –Munchausen by proxy syndrome
  - –Coagulopathy
  - –Epistaxis (initially swallowed blood)
  - –Hemoptysis

Workup and Diagnosis

- History
  - –Quantity, frequency, type of blood (bright red vs "coffee grounds"); abdominal pain
  - –Dysphagia/odynophagia, chest pain/burning, hematochezia, melena, bruising, bleeding
  - –Birth history: Stressors, medications before delivery, medications in delivery room (vitamin K), lines placed (umbilical lines can result in clotting of portal vein)
  - –Past history: History of liver disease, ingestions, history of pancreatitis, GI surgeries
  - –Medications: NSAID use, aspirin use, recent meds
  - –Diet history: Formula intolerance, food allergies
- Physical exam
  - –Vital signs (tachycardia, tachypnea, hypotension), blood in nares, conjunctival/palatal pallor, flow murmur, hepatosplenomegaly, abdominal tenderness, abdominal bruising, petechiae
- Diagnostics
  - –Limited labs: CBC, liver function tests, coagulation studies, type and screen/cross
  - –Upper endoscopy most sensitive and specific for diagnosis and provides therapeutic options
  - –Ultrasound with Doppler to assess liver disease and portal hypertension
  - –Reserve nuclear medicine studies (e.g., tagged red cell study, angiography) as second line and for brisk bleeding

Treatment

- Large bleeds require two large-bore IVs and volume support with normal saline or packed red blood cells
- Closely monitor vital signs
- Acid blockade with histamine receptor antagonist or proton pump inhibitor
- Endoscopic therapy including
  - –Heater probe and bipolar coagulation for ulcers
  - –Band ligation or sclerotherapy for varices
- Octreotide or vasopressin to reduce splanchnic blood flow for variceal bleeding
- Selective embolization
- Surgical repair rarely indicated
- Treat infections including triple therapy (antibiotics and proton pump inhibitor) for *H. pylori*
- Remove allergen in case of allergy

90. Hepatomegaly

Hepatomegaly represents the clinical appearance of liver enlargement and can occur via five mechanisms, including inflammation, excessive storage, infiltration, congestion, and obstruction. The presence of a palpable liver does not always represent hepatomegaly and is determined on the basis of liver span and degree of extension below the right costal margin. Normal liver spans range from 5 to 9 cm depending on age.

Differential Diagnosis

- Inflammation
  - –Most common infections: EBV; hepatitis A, B, C; CMV; TORCH
  - –Less common infections: HIV, malaria, amebiasis, tuberculosis, toxocariasis, *Borrelia burgdorferi*
  - –Drugs: Acetaminophen (commonly used in overdoses among adolescents), NSAIDs, isoniazid, sodium valproate, propothiouracil, halothane
  - –Toxins: Tyrosinemia, galactosemia, vitamin A toxicity
  - –Autoimmune hepatitis
  - –Systemic lupus erythematosus
- Inappropriate storage
  - –Glycogen storage diseases I–V
  - –Lipids: Gaucher disease, Wolman disease, Niemann-Pick disease
  - –Fat: Fatty acid oxidation defects, mucopolysaccharidoses
  - –Metals: Wilson disease (copper), hemochromatosis (iron)
  - –Abnormal proteins: α-1 antitrypsin deficiency (store abnormal protein product)
  - –Peroxisomal disease: Zellweger
  - –Mucopolysaccharidoses, types I–IV
- Infiltration
  - –Hepatoblastoma
  - –Hepatocellular carcinoma
  - –Hemangioma
  - –Histiocytosis
  - –Extramedullary hematopoiesis
  - –Chronic granulomatous disease
- Vascular congestion
  - –Congestive heart failure
  - –Budd-Chiari syndrome
  - –Veno-occlusive disease
  - –Suprahepatic web
- Biliary obstruction
  - –Biliary atresia represents the most common cause of pediatric liver transplantation
  - –Alagille syndrome
  - –Cystic fibrosis
  - –Primary sclerosing cholangitis
  - –Inspissated bile syndrome
- Miscellaneous
  - –Reye syndrome, bile acid synthetic disorder

Workup and Diagnosis

- History
  - –Abdominal pain, fever, melena, weight loss, medications, age at onset, diarrhea, vomiting, hematemesis, bleeding, bruising, fatigue
  - –Exposure to blood products
  - –Nutrition history (neonatal formula)
  - –Travel history to endemic infectious areas
  - –Family history of liver disease, maternal HBV, HCV
- Physical exam
  - –Height, weight
  - –Liver size, margin, firmness, nodularity, tenderness
  - –Ascites, jaundice/scleral icterus
  - –Cataracts; Kayser-Fleischer rings (Wilson); posterior embryotoxin (Alagille)
  - –Cardiac exam for murmurs; splenomegaly; tone and strength development; hemangiomas/xanthomas
- Labs
  - –CBC, ALT, AST, fractionated bilirubin, alkaline phosphatase, total protein, albumin, globulin fraction, PT, U/A
  - –Hepatitis serologies, EBV, TORCH titers, plasma amino acids/urine organic acids for metabolic disease
  - –Serum AAT with protease inhibitor typing
  - –Ceruloplasmin (decreased in Wilson disease)
  - –ANA/anti-smooth muscle antibody/anti-liver kidney microsomal antibody, IgG for autoimmune hepatitis
- Ultrasound for echotexture and masses
  - –Consider nuclear study/CT for obstruction
- Liver biopsy in chronic disease (>3 months) or to elucidate etiology

Treatment

- Geared towards specific disease
- Cholestasis
  - –Ursodeoxycholic acid
  - –Supplemental fat soluble vitamins A, D, E, K
- Infections
  - –Consider interferon for hepatitis B
  - –Consider interferon and ribaviron for hepatitis C
- Toxins
  - –Use of NTBC for tyrosinemia
- Metabolic disease
  - –Metabolism consultation
  - –Often requires specific restricted formulas
- Surgical repair for biliary atresia
  - –Kasai portoenterostomy has better outcome if done before 60 days of age
- Mucomyst for acute acetaminophen toxicity
- Immune suppression for autoimmune hepatitis

91. Splenomegaly

The spleen is the largest lymphoid organ in the body. One of its primary functions is to filter defective and/or foreign cells. Splenomegaly is usually caused by systemic disease and not by primary splenic disease. Splenomegaly is usually caused by infection (excessive antigen stimulation), autoimmune disorders (disordered immunoregulation), or hemolysis (excessive destruction of abnormal blood components). Because of exposure below the protective rib cage, splenomegaly results in increased risk of splenic injury or rupture.

Differential Diagnosis

- Normal variants
  - –Palpable spleen tip due to thinner abdominal musculature
  - –15–30% of neonates
  - –10% of healthy children
  - –5% of adolescents
- Infection/inflammation
  - –Acute hepatitis (B or C)
  - –Viral (EBV, CMV, HIV)
  - –Bacterial (SBE, cat-scratch disease, TB, histoplasmosis, toxoplasmosis, *Salmonella*)
  - –Systemic lupus erythematosus (SLE)
  - –Rheumatoid arthritis
  - –Inflammatory bowel disease
  - –Celiac disease
  - –Acidosis
  - –Chronic granulomatous disease
  - –Serum sickness
  - –Protozoal infection (malaria and schistosomiasis are rare in the U.S.)
- Hemolytic anemias
  - –Hereditary spherocytosis
  - –Hemoglobinopathies
  - –Thalassemia major
  - –Nonspherocytic hemolytic anemias (pyruvate kinase deficiency)
- Malignancy
  - –Leukemia, 50% of children with ALL
  - –Hodgkin disease, non-Hodgkin lymphoma
  - –Metastatic disease
- Extramedullary hematopoiesis
  - –Thalassemia major
  - –Osteopetrosis (rare)
  - –Myelofibrosis
- Storage/infiltrative disorders
  - –Histiocytosis
  - –Lipidoses (e.g., Niemann-Pick, Gaucher)
  - –Mucopolysaccharidoses (e.g., Hurler, Hunter)
- Congestive
  - –Chronic congestive heart failure
  - –Portal hypertension
    - –Portal or splenic venous thrombosis
  - –Hepatic fibrosis
  - –Cirrhosis
- Structural
  - –Hematoma (trauma)
  - –Cysts or pseudocysts
- Wandering spleen

Workup and Diagnosis

- History
  - –Fever, LUQ pain, abdominal trauma
  - –Ingestion of hepatotoxic substances
  - –Acute illness, dyspnea, fatigue, diarrhea
  - –Signs of malignancy
  - –Pruritus, travel, sexual history
  - –Developmental milestones
  - –Medical history: NICU stay, umbilical catheter, jaundice, failure to thrive, anemia, heart disease
  - –Family history: Early cholecystectomy, gallstones, anemias, ethnic heritage
- Physical exam
  - –Vitals, growth parameters
  - –Pallor, jaundice, purpura, petechiae, ecchymoses, excoriated skin, rashes
  - –Scleral icterus, cherry red retinal spots, uveitis/iritis
  - –New murmur, edema
  - –Abdominal distension, ascites, prominent veins, spleen size, tenderness, liver size and texture
  - –Lymph node, joint pain or swelling
- Labs
  - –CBC/peripheral smear, ESR or CRP, LFT, PT/PTT
  - –EBV/CMV, viral titers, blood culture
  - –Autoimmune or rheumatologic tests (ANA, RF)
  - –CXR, bone marrow exam
  - –immunodeficiency workup, thrombophilia screen
- Ultrasound: Exclude retroperitoneal tumors or masses, evaluate portal vein flow with Doppler

Treatment

- Therapy is directed at treatment of underlying disease
- Splenectomy benefits need to be balanced with risk of postsplenectomy sepsis
- If splenectomy is performed, immunize at least 10 days prior
  - –Pneumococci
  - –*Haemophilus influenzae,* if under 5
  - –Meningococcal vaccine
  - –Postsurgical penicillin prophylaxis required
- Febrile illness in patients postsplenectomy is a life-threatening emergency
  - –Major risk is overwhelming sepsis from encapsulated bacteria (*Streptococcus pneumoniae, H. influenzae, Neisseria meningitidis*)
- Sepsis most frequent in first 5 years after splenectomy

92. Umbilicus – Delayed Separation

Umbilical cord separation usually occurs between 7 and 14 days of life. Delayed cord separation occurs after 2 weeks of life. Separation of the cord that occurs after 3 weeks of life is considered abnormal. The process of cord separation is chiefly due to the migration of neutrophils into the area, with digestion and necrosis of the umbilical cord.

Differential Diagnosis

- Vigorous use of antiseptics to clean the umbilical cord
  - –Probably the most common etiology
  - –Inhibits normal colonization of the umbilicus, which otherwise would allow chemotactic infiltration of neutrophils to mediate cord separation
- Immunodeficiencies
  - –Leukocyte adhesion defects affecting chemotaxis (LAD I/II)
  - –LAD is usually associated with significant systemic (sepsis) or local (omphalitis) infection, recurrent infections, or failure to thrive
  - –Sialyl Lewis X antigen deficiency
  - –Neonatal alloimmune neutropenia
  - –Defective immune (gamma) interferon
- Prematurity
  - –Gestational age less than 37 weeks
- Birth via cesarean section
  - –Associated with delayed separation, possibly due to decreased bacterial colonization from delivery through a sterile surgical field, resulting in decreased infiltration of neutrophils, which is essential for cord separation
- Neonatal sepsis
- Urachal anomalies
  - –More likely to be seen in otherwise healthy infants without signs of local or systemic infection
- Histiocytosis X

Workup and Diagnosis

- History
  - –Duration of umbilical cord attachment
  - –Risk factors for sepsis
  - –Recurrent or severe infections, especially without pus formation or resistance to antibiotic therapy
  - –Cleaning techniques for cord care and use of water vs antiseptics (e.g., alcohol, triple dye)
  - –Gestational age at birth
  - –Vaginal birth vs cesarean section
  - –Family history, consanguinity of parents
- Physical exam
  - –Signs of generalized neonatal infection/sepsis
  - –Omphalitis or other signs of local umbilical infection
  - –Drainage from the umbilical stump (seen in urachal anomalies)
- Labs
  - –Total and differential white blood cell counts (LADs are characterized by leukocytosis)
  - –T and B cell subset determination
  - –Testing for leukocyte adhesion molecules; look for abnormal expression of CD18, CD11a, b, and c molecules
  - –Functional tests for oxidative burst (zymosan-induced assay)
- Studies
  - –Ultrasound, CT, or VCUG to search for urachal or genitourinary anomalies

Treatment

- Decreased use of antiseptics (alcohol) along with the implementation of simple cleaning of the cord with water decreases the length of time to umbilical cord separation without increasing the risk of infection
- Surgical excision of umbilical cord
- Treatment of sepsis and infection with antibiotics
- Transplantation of bone marrow or umbilical blood hematopoietic stem cells to correct LADs
- Surgical repair of any urachal anomalies
- Prevention of transmission of autosomal recessive, inherited conditions (such as LAD) by genetic counseling and testing

93. Umbilicus – Herniation

Umbilical hernias are a common pediatric condition, with an estimated incidence of 1/6 children. Umbilical hernias are 10 times more common in black as compared to white children. Umbilical hernias are also seen more frequently in low birth weight infants. The majority of umbilical hernias spontaneously resolve by 5 years of age.

Differential Diagnosis

- Normal variant
- Diastasis recti abdominis
  - –Very common
  - –Supraumbilical rectus muscles separated laterally
- Athyrotic hypothyroidism sequence
  - –Primary defect in thyroid gland development
  - –58% have associated umbilical hernias
- Omphalocele
  - –Herniation of abdominal contents into umbilical cord, covered only by peritoneum not by skin
  - –Often associated with genetic syndromes
- Gastroschisis
  - –Intact umbilical cord
  - –Evisceration of bowel through a defect in the abdominal wall, usually found on the right side of the cord without an overlying membrane
- Genetic syndromes
  - –Beckwith-Wiedemann syndrome
    - –Exomph alos-macroglossia-gigantism
    - –May be associated with umbilical hernia or omphalocele
  - –Pentalogy of Cantrell: Omphalocele, pericardial defect, sternal defect, cardiac defect (commonly tetralogy of Fallot), diaphragmatic hernia

Workup and Diagnosis

- History and physical exam
- Umbilical hernia is covered by skin
  - –Presents as a swelling or bulge that increases with any Valsalva maneuver
  - –Easily reduced
  - –Fascial defect 1–5 cm in diameter
  - –May contain omentum or small intestine
- Most usually appear by 6 months of age and resolve by 1 year of age spontaneously
  - –Almost all disappear by 5–6 years of age
- If child is not black, assess for possible associated syndromes
- Labs may include T4 or thyroid stimulating hormone levels, karyotype

Treatment

- Observation is often all that is needed
- Covering the hernia or "strapping" is not useful
- Surgery is indicated only if:
  - –The defect enlarges after 1–2 years of age
  - –Symptomatic
  - –Incarceration or strangulation
  - –Persistent at 3–5 years of age
- Umbilical hernias are less likely to close if defect >1.5 cm or if it is a large proboscoid umbilical hernia with excessive overlying skin
- Incarceration of an umbilical hernia is rare, occurring in only 1/1,500 hernias
  - –Occurs more frequently if fascial defect >1.5 cm
  - –Usually only contains omentum and not intestine

94. Umbilicus – Single Umbilical Artery

A normal umbilical cord consists of one umbilical vein, which later becomes the ligamentum teres, and two umbilical arteries, which become the lateral umbilical ligaments. Single umbilical artery (SUA or 2-vessel umbilical cord) has an estimated incidence of approximately 5–10/1,000 births and 35–70/1,000 twin births. One-third of infants with SUA have associated congenital anomalies.

Differential Diagnosis

- Developmental agenesis or hypoplasia
  - No clear sex ratio
  - Males more likely to have associated malformations
  - Increased incidence in twins, either mono- or dizygotic
  - Increased incidence of placental anomalies
  - More common in low birth weight infants
  - More common in premature infants
- Associated maternal factors
  - Maternal diabetes
  - Maternal epilepsy
  - Toxemia
- Intrauterine thrombosis of other umbilical artery
- Malformations are associated with SUA in 45% of cases
  - Genitourinary (33%): Renal agenesis, dysgenesis, hypoplasia; ambiguous genitalia
  - Musculoskeletal (37%): Clubfoot, vertebral anomalies
  - Cardiovascular (30%): Patent ductus arteriosus, ventricular septal defect, dextrocardia
  - Gastrointestinal (28%): Imperforate anus, tracheoesophageal fistula
  - Respiratory (9%): Pulmonary hypoplasia (malformations due to disruption of blood flow), sirenomelia
- Chromosomal anomalies
  - Trisomy 18

Workup and Diagnosis

- History
  - Prenatal tests such as amniocentesis with karyotype
  - Twinning
- Physical exam
  - Dysmorphic facial features
  - Anomalies with genitourinary, gastrointestinal, cardiac, musculoskeletal organ systems
  - Neurologic signs associated with stroke (e.g., seizures)
- Level II prenatal ultrasound with Doppler examination of umbilical cord
- Examination of placenta and cord at delivery
  - Examine closer to umbilical end of cord since vessels may merge close to placental insertion
- Karyotype
- Genetics consultation
- Thrombophilia evaluation
  - Factor V Leiden or antithrombin III deficiency
  - Anticardiolipin or lupus anticoagulant

Treatment

- No treatment if anomaly is isolated
- Treat GI obstruction or urologic anomalies accordingly
- Many infants with chromosomal anomalies are stillborn or die soon after birth
- Genetic counseling regarding possible future risk associated with chromosomal anomalies

95. Vomiting

Vomiting is the forceful expulsion of gastric contents through the mouth that involves an integrated and largely somatic motor response. It represents a protective reflex in the body's defense system. Vomiting may be an initial symptom of an underlying condition or a symptom complex preceded by nausea and retching. The differential diagnosis varies with age, although each diagnosis should be entertained when seeing a patient who presents with vomiting.

Differential Diagnosis

- Infections
  - –Gastroenteritis is the most common cause among all pediatric age groups; may be viral, bacterial, or parasitic
  - –Urinary tract infection/pyelonephritis
  - –Sepsis
  - –Meningitis
  - –Viral hepatitis: e.g., Hepatitis A
  - –*Helicobacter pylori*-related ulcer
- Anatomic
  - –Esophageal: Tracheoesophageal atresia, esophageal ring/web/stricture, achalasia
  - –Gastric: Pyloric stenosis, volvulus
  - –Small intestine: Duodenal atresia, malrotation, meconium ileus, duodenal hematoma, SMA syndrome, duplication, intussusception, hernia
  - –Colon: Hirschprung, imperforate anus
- Gastrointestinal
  - –Gastroesophageal reflux disease
  - –Allergy (e.g., celiac disease, milk protein)
  - –Peptic ulcer disease
  - –Appendicitis
  - –Foreign body
  - –Pancreatitis
  - –Cholecystitis
  - –Eosinophilic enteropathy
  - –Pseudo-obstruction
- Neurologic
  - –Intracranial mass
  - –Hydrocephalus
  - –Pseudotumor cerebri
  - –Migraines
- Renal
  - –Obstructive uropathy
  - –Nephrolithiasis
  - –Glomerulonephritis
  - –Renal tubular acidosis
- Toxins/drugs
  - –Aspirin, theophylline, digoxin, lead
  - –Chemotherapeutics
- Pregnancy
- Inborn errors of metabolism
- Endocrine
  - –Diabetic ketoacidosis
  - –Adrenal insufficiency
  - –Congenital adrenal hyperplasia
- Respiratory
  - –Pneumonia
  - –Post-tussive

Workup and Diagnosis

- History and physical crucial because of large differential
- History
  - –Duration, frequency, bilious material, abdominal pain, diarrhea, hematemesis, hematochezia, melena, headache, fever, dysuria, weight loss, urine output
  - –Sick contacts, cough, rhinorrhea, neck stiffness
- Birth history: Polyhydramnios, passage of meconium
- Family history: Genetic disease, early childhood deaths
- Physical exam
  - –Vitals, weight, mucous membranes, nasal discharge, breath sounds, rashes, meningismus
  - –Abdominal pain/distension, hepatosplenomegaly, abdominal masses, Murphy/obturator/psoas sign
  - –Skin turgor, capillary refill
  - –Neuro exam including funduscopy for papilledema
- Labs: Initial screen based on physical exam
  - –Consider electrolytes, LFTs, amylase, lipase
  - –U/A and culture; lactate and pyruvate
  - –Serum amino acids/urine organic acids, ammonia for metabolic diseases; blood gas for acidosis
  - –CBC for infections, lumbar puncture
- KUB or obstruction series as initial X-ray
- Contrast study with upper GI series with or without small bowel follow-through or BE for anatomic problem
- Abdominal ultrasound for pyloric stenosis
- Head imaging including CT/MRI
- Upper endoscopy and colonoscopy for mucosal inflammation

Treatment

- Stabilize patient and fluid resuscitation as initial therapy with electrolyte correction
- Surgical consultation if obstruction suspected
- Oral rehydration with small amounts of liquids if tolerated
- If signs of obstruction, nasogastric tube decompression and bowel rest
- Treat infections if indicated
- Remove toxins and allergens
- Surgical interventions for volvulus, Hirschprung, intracranial masses, pyloric stenosis, other anatomic causes
- Correct metabolic derangements
- Lifelong gluten-free diet for celiac disease
- Rare use of antiemetics/promotility agents for chemotherapy, motion sickness, postsurgery, gastroesophageal reflux disease

96. Vomiting – Projectile

Projectile vomiting is the forceful expulsion of stomach contents classically associated with pyloric stenosis. Although pyloric stenosis is one cause, there are many other causes inside and outside the GI tract.

Differential Diagnosis

- Anatomic/obstructive
  - Pyloric stenosis: Classic description of progressive projectile vomiting; more common among first-born males and typically presents in weeks 4–8 of life; may see hypochloremic, hypokalemic metabolic alkalosis
  - Hiatal hernia
  - Pyloric atresia
  - Gastric volvulus
  - Gastric outlet obstruction due to chronic granulomatous disease, peptic ulceration near the pyloris, or gastric tumors
  - Duodenal web
  - Duodenal atresia
  - Duodenal stenosis
  - Superior mesenteric artery syndrome: Typically due to weight loss, postsurgical correction of scoliosis, or immobilization with body cast
  - Urinary tract obstruction: Ureteropelvic junction obstruction (abdominal pain and vomiting known as Dietl crisis); nephrolithiasis
- Inflammatory
  - Gastroesophageal reflux disease
  - Peptic ulcer disease
  - Pyelonephritis
  - Meningitis
  - Encephalitis
  - Eosinophilic enteropathy
- Central nervous system
  - Brain tumor
  - Trauma
  - Lead encephalopathy
  - Acute intracranial hemorrhage
  - Hydrocephalus
- Metabolic/endocrine
  - Congenital adrenal hyperplasia
  - Hypercalcemia
  - Wolman disease
  - Phenylketonuria

Workup and Diagnosis

- Differentiating vomiting from projectile vomiting is often difficult when obtaining history
- History: Age at presentation, frequency and amount of emesis, time after feeding until emesis, bilious or nonbilious, hematemesis, weight loss, fever, diarrhea, abdominal pain, melena, hematochezia, activity level, dysuria, menses, pica, recent trauma
- Birth history: Meconium in nursery, oligohydramnios, polyhydramnios, newborn screen, birth weight
- Family history: First born
- Diet history: Formula intolerance
- Surgical history: Previous abdominal surgeries
- Social history: House built before 1965 (lead paint)
- Physical exam: Weight, height, head cirumference, vital signs, mucous membranes, fontanelle, papilledema, equal breath sounds, abdominal distension, abdominal mass (palpable olive in pyloric stenosis), bowel sounds, skin turgor, capillary refill, reflexes, tone, strength
- Chemistry panel with focus on chloride, CO_2, potassium, calcium; CBC with differential for signs of infection, consider urine analysis and culture
- Abdominal films for obstruction
- Ultrasound a sensitive and specific method for pyloric stenosis; findings of elongation of pyloric channel and thickening of pyloric muscle; U/S for pelvic obstruction
- Upper GI series for malrotation, atresia, superior mesenteric artery
- CT scan for head or abdominal mass

Treatment

- Maintain fluid balance
- Correct electrolytes
- Surgical correction
  - Pyloroplasty for pyloric stenosis
  - Ladd procedure for malrotation
- Treat infections
- Superior mesenteric artery syndrome
  - May require nasojejunal feeds/TPN
- Acid blockers for gastroesophageal reflux
- Amino acid or hydrolysate formula for milk allergy
- PKU
  - Avoid phenylalanine (requires special formula, dietary restrictions until maturation, possibly lifelong)

Section 12

Back

KATHLEEN O. DeANTONIS, MD
DON LUJAN, MD, MS

97. Back Pain

Back pain is an uncommon complaint in children, but relatively more common in adolescents. Although relatively benign causes (such as muscular strain in adolescents) account for the majority of cases, some more severe causes should not be overlooked, especially in younger children. Back pain may be manifested by a refusal to walk in toddlers.

Differential Diagnosis

- Muscular strain, disk herniation
  - Most common in adolescents who are involved in competitive or contact sports; may be occupational
- Spondyloarthropathy
  - Ankylosing spondylitis is found primarily in boys, characterized by sacroiliitis, LE oligoarthritis, and may be associated with IBD
- Malalignment
  - Scoliosis: Idiopathic form is most common in girls, may be familial, may be secondary to neurologic disorder
  - Hyperlordosis
- Infectious
  - Diskitis: Characterized by spine stiffness and muscular spasm, *Staphylococcus aureus* is the usual pathogen, blood culture may be positive
  - Vertebral osteomyelitis: Exquisite point tenderness, pathogen may be *S. aureus, Streptococcus pneumoniae*, or others such as tuberculosis or brucellosis
  - Acute transverse myelopathy: Generally follows an upper respiratory tract infection; characterized by back pain, distal weakness and paresthesias at the midthoracic level
- Urinary tract
  - Urinary tract infection: Most common in postpubertal girls, occurrence in boys or prepubertal girls may require evaluation for urinary tract anomalies, especially if recurrent
  - Urolithiasis: Associated with hypercalcuria, cystinuria, Lesch-Nyhan; characterized by intense flank pain and hematuria
- Malignancy
  - Primary spinal cord or column tumors (osteogenic sarcoma, neuroblastoma)
  - Metastatic tumors (neuroblastoma)
  - Bone marrow infiltration (leukemia, lymphoma)
- Gynecologic
  - Menstrual cramps
  - PID
  - Endometriosis

Workup and Diagnosis

- History
  - Onset, duration, location of symptoms
  - History of trauma, heavy lifting, overuse, athletics
  - Systemic symptoms such as fever, irritability
  - Menstrual and sexual history
  - Past medical history of similar complaints, orthopedic conditions, general medical conditions
  - Family history of scoliosis, rheumatic disease
- Physical exam
  - General appearance, fever, irritability
  - Spinal contour, symmetry
  - Gait, posture
  - Range of motion limitations
  - Point tenderness, SI tenderness
  - Associated neurologic findings (sensation, strength, DTRs)
- Labs
  - If rheumatologic condition is suspected, consider CBC, ESR, ANA, RF, HLA typing
  - If infectious process is suspected, obtain CBC, ESR
  - Urine microscopy and culture
- Studies
  - Plain films can reveal fractures such as spinal compression fractures, disk space abnormalities, and sacroiliac abnormalities associated with spondyloarthrosis
  - MRI may be required to discover disk herniation, disk space infection, tumors

Treatment

- Muscular strain: Muscle relaxants, NSAIDs, rest, and reduction of exacerbating activities
- Disk herniation: Physical therapy, surgery is rarely indicated in children and adolescents
- Spondyloarthropathy: NSAIDs, exercise
- Scoliosis: Conservative management with observation, NSAIDs, bracing or surgery if more severe
- Gynocologic etiologies
  - Menstrual cramps: NSAIDs, OCPs for severe cases
  - PID: Appropriate cultures, treatment with antibiotics
  - Endometriosis: hormonal therapy such as OCPs may be effective, surgical ablation is rarely required
- UTI: Antibiotics
- Urolithiasis: Pain management followed by high fluid intake
- Infection: Diskitis requires 4–6 weeks of IV antibiotics
- Tumors: Referral to oncologist

98. Scoliosis

Idiopathic scoliosis often does not progress enough to require treatment and observation is sufficient. Painful scoliosis is a serious complaint, as an underlying condition may be the nidus of the curvature. Surgery is performed to fuse progressive curves greater than 50°, but surgical complications may occur, such as postoperative neurologic deficit.

Differential Diagnosis

- Idiopathic scoliosis
  - –Lateral deviation or curvature of either the thoracic or lumbar spine greater than 10°
  - –Right thoracic curves are most common
  - –Usually presents in early adolescence
  - –Girls > boys
- Risk factors for progression
  - –Curve >20°
  - –Age less than 12
  - –Skeletal maturity, Risser stage 0–1
- Infantile idiopathic scoliosis
  - –Presents at 0–3 years old
  - –Left thoracic curve more common
  - –Boys > girls
  - –85% spontaneously resolve
  - –Must rule out spinal cord disease or congenital cause of scoliosis
- Juvenile idiopathic scoliosis presents at 3–10 years old and is similar to adolescent (idiopathic) scoliosis
- Neuromuscular scoliosis
  - –Related to cerebral palsy, muscular dystrophy, myotonic myopathy, and spinal muscular atrophy
  - –Tends to progress more rapidly and even continues after maturity, as compared to idiopathic scoliosis
  - –Pulmonary complications seen with severe curves >90°
- Congenital scoliosis
  - –Failure of formation or segmentation of spinal vertebra
  - –Rapid progression and worse prognosis is associated with unilateral unsegmented bar with contralateral hemivertebra
- Other causes
  - –Tumor, infection, neurofibromatosis, metabolic bone disorders, and Marfan syndrome

Workup and Diagnosis

- Generally patients are referred after either school screening for scoliosis or well-child check
- History
  - –Painful symptoms in the history should be a red flag to rule out infection, tumor, or spinal cord anomaly
  - –There is often a positive family history
- Clinical examination
  - –Careful neurologic examination
  - –Moderate to severe curves demonstrate shoulder and waist asymmetry, trunk shift, and limb length inequality
  - –Forward bending test: Examiner stands behind patient while patient bends forward from the waist, hands hanging down, feet together and knees straight, evaluating for rib hump or depression or asymmetric paravertebral muscles
  - –Scoliometer may be used to measure rotational deformity (>7° requires radiographic evaluation)
- Radiographic studies
  - –X-ray: Standing AP and lateral radiographs allow measurement of curves by Cobb method (Cobb angle is made by line drawn along superior endplate of uppermost tilted vertebra and a line drawn along inferior endplate of lowest vertebra in curve)
  - –MRI indicated for neurologic compromise, excessive kyphosis, onset of scoliosis after age 11 years, rapid curve progression, structural abnormalities noted on plain X-ray, and left thoracic or thoracolumbar curves

Treatment

- Treatment options include observation while child is growing, bracing, and surgery
  - –Many curves do not progress enough to require treatment
  - –Spinal curve progression may occur despite bracing; however, for idiopathic scoliosis, response to brace wearing is dose-related and many patients do not like to wear the brace
- Exercise and electrical stimulation have not been shown to alter natural progression of curve
- Bracing for curves in 20–40° degree range may slow curve progression but does not reduce the magnitude of curve despite a well-made brace and compliance
- Surgery is reserved for progressive curves >40° in skeletally immature (Risser scale 0–1) and >50° in skeletally mature patients

Section 13

Genitourinary

KATHERINE MACRAE DELL, MD
KARI A. DRAPER, MD
ADDA GRIMBERG, MD
ROY J. KIM, MD
NADER SHAIKH, MD, MPH

99. Abnormal Vaginal Bleeding

Age of the patient is important when considering the differential diagnosis of abnormal vaginal bleeding. Pregnancy should always be ruled out despite a negative history of sexual activity. Bleeding that occurs before pubertal development of normal menarche should raise suspicion of nonendocrine causes.

Differential Diagnosis

- Dysfunctional uterine bleeding (DUB)
  - –Physiologic anovulation is normal for up to 2 years after menarche
  - –Androgen excess
  - –Functional ovarian hyperandrogenism, or polycystic ovary syndrome, is common in adolescence
  - –Estrogen excess
  - –Hyperprolactinemia
  - –Hypothyroidism
  - –Early premature ovarian failure
- Luteal phase defects
- Pregnancy disorders
  - –Spontaneous abortion (threatened, missed, incomplete)
  - –Molar pregnancy
  - –Ectopic pregnancy
- True vaginal bleeding
  - –Trauma (including sexual abuse)
  - –Vaginal sarcoma (sarcoma botyroides)
  - –Foreign body (more common in the younger child)
- Menorrhagia
  - –Idiopathic: Most common cause of menorrhagia in adolescents
  - –Coagulopathy/bleeding disorder (e.g., thrombocytopenia, von Willebrand disease, factor IX deficiency)
  - –Uterine polyp or neoplasm
- Hematuria mistaken for vaginal bleeding
  - –Urethral prolapse
  - –Urinary tract infection
- Excoriations due to pruritus
- Vulvovaginitis
  - –*Trichomonas*
  - –*Chlamydia*
  - –Gonorrhea
  - –Pinworms (rare)
- Cervical lesions
  - –Cervical polyp
  - –Hemangioma
  - –Cervical friability

Workup and Diagnosis

- History
  - –Age at onset of bleeding
  - –Quantity, duration, and frequency of bleeding
  - –Associated pain or discomfort
  - –Age at onset of puberty
  - –First day of last menstrual period
  - –Other symptoms: Dysuria, symptoms of hypothyroidism (fatigue, cold intolerance, constipation), symptoms of hyperprolactinemia (headaches, nipple discharge/galactorrhea)
  - –Sexual abuse; sexual activity
  - –Family history of irregular periods/infertility
- Physical exam
  - –Inspection of external genitalia (anatomy, evidence of trauma, source of bleeding)
  - –Evidence of puberty (breast development, estrogenization of vaginal mucosa)
  - –Signs of virilization (hirsutism)
  - –Nipple discharge
  - –Signs of hypothyroidism (bradycardia, dry skin, coarse hair, short stature, delayed reflexes)
- Labs
  - –LH, FSH, estradiol (E_2), hCG
  - –T4, TSH, prolactin
  - –Platelet count, PT, PTT, bleeding time, vWF
  - –Urine analysis
- Pelvic US to detect ovarian and uterine abnormalities
- MRI of pituitary to detect abnormalities of the gland

Treatment

- Physiologic anovulation does not usually need to be treated unless it persists beyond 2 years past menarche
- Polycystic ovary syndrome treat with: Oral contraceptives, androgen inhibitors (spironolactone) as adjunct, insulin sensitizing medications (metformin)
- Hyperprolactinemia: Treat with bromocriptine
- Hypothyroidism: Treat with L-thyroxine replacement
- Coagulopathy: Referral to hematologist for management
- Gynecologic tumor or foreign body: Surgical exploration and resection
- Intracranial mass (pituitary tumor): Referral to oncologist, endocrinologist
- Menorrhagia
  - –Oral estrogen is required to stop an acute episode
  - –Patient with very heavy bleeding may require hospitalization for IV fluid/blood products (correction of hypovolemia) and IV Premarin
  - –OCPs or progestins are useful to prevent recurrences

100. Amenorrhea – Primary

Menarche occurs at an average age of 12.7 years in the U.S. Primary amenorrhea occurs when menarche remains absent at age 16, or if 5 years have passed since the onset of puberty and menarche has not begun.

Differential Diagnosis

- Constitutional delay of puberty
  - –Most common cause
- Anatomic causes
  - –Uterine aplasia (Mayer-Rokitansky syndrome)
  - –Vaginal aplasia
  - –Imperforate hymen
- Hypogonadotropic hypogonadism
  - –Decreased FSH
  - –Congenital and acquired etiologies
- Congenital hypogonadotropic hypogonadism
  - –Kallmann syndrome
  - –Panhypopituitarism
- Aquired hypogonadotropic hypogonadism
  - –Malnutrition
  - –Stress
  - –Anorexia nervosa
  - –Inflammatory bowel disease
  - –Celiac disease
  - –Excessive exercise
  - –Pituitary tumor (e.g., prolactinoma or craniopharyngioma)
- Hypergonadotropic hypogonadism
  - –Increased FSH
  - –Gonadal dysgenesis (Turner syndrome is the most common)
  - –Ovarian failure: Autoimmune oophoritis, galactosemia, effects of chemotherapy or radiation, FSH or LH receptor mutations (rare)
- Abnormal thyroid function
- Androgen insensitivity syndrome
- Congenital adrenal hyperplasia and other causes of hyperandrogenism
- Medications
- Pregnancy

Workup and Diagnosis

- History
  - –Screen for eating disorders, weight change, colitis, excessive exercise, chronic illnesses, medications
  - –Family history: Age of menarche, puberty onset, autoimmune disorders, fertility issues
  - –Puberty history: Age of thelarche (breast development) and pubarche (pubic hair growth); lack of breast development suggests insufficient estrogen (e.g., lack of gonadotropins or ovarian insufficiency/absence)
  - –Abdominal pain, especially cyclic (imperforate hymen)
  - –Anosmia or hyposmia (seen with Kallmann syndrome)
  - –Headaches or visual changes (with pituitary tumors)
  - –Galactorrhea (with prolactinoma)
  - –Hirsutism, excessive weight, acne may result from hyperandrogenism
- Physical exam
  - –Height, weight, Tanner staging
  - –Features of Turner syndrome: Short stature, ptosis, high palate, webbed neck, shield chest, cubitus valgus, heart murmur, sexual infantilism
  - –Signs of virilization: Acne and facial hair
  - –Visual fields and optic discs, goiter
  - –Striae, galactorrhea, inguinal masses
- Labs: FSH, LH, thyroid function tests, prolactin, testosterone, 17-hydroxyprogesterone, urine hCG
- Karyotype: Turner syndrome, gonadal dysgenesis, or androgen insensitivity syndrome
- Pelvic US, MRI of brain/pituitary for suspicion of pituitary mass or if hypogonadotropic hypogonadism is present with no clear precipitating factor

Treatment

- Underlying chronic illnesses, malnourished states, or hypothyroidism should be treated
- Stop medications causing hyperprolactinemia (e.g., antidepressants, phenothiazines) if safe to do so
- Prolactinomas can be treated medically with a dopamine agonist
- Other pituitary tumors will need treatment according to their specific type
- Patients with ovarian insufficiency or hypogonadotropic hypogonadism need estrogen therapy for breast development, and then should cycle estrogens and progestins to establish menses

101. Amenorrhea – Secondary

Secondary amenorrhea is the absence of menses for 6 months in a woman with previously regular menstrual cycles, or 12 months in a woman whose periods had been irregular.

Differential Diagnosis

- Pregnancy
  - Most common cause
- Anovulatory cycles
  - Common during first few years after menarche
- Hyperandrogenism
  - Polycystic ovary syndrome: Problems with fertility are common, LH/FSH ratio is greater than 2.5/1
  - Some adrenal tumors
  - Congenital adrenal hyperplasia
  - Exposure to anabolic steroids
- Major illness or stress
- Large changes in weight
  - Anorexia nervosa
- Hypothyroidism
- Prolactinoma
- Other causes of hyperprolactinemia
  - Marijuana
  - Opioids
  - Antidepressants
  - Phenothiazines
- Hypothalamic-pituitary failure
  - Pituitary tumor
  - Sheehan syndrome
  - Cranial irradiation
- Ovarian failure
  - Autoimmune destruction
  - Infarction due to gonadal torsion
  - Chemotherapy or radiation
  - Idiopathic
- Oral contraceptives
  - May delay return to regular menses
- Cushing syndrome
- Uterine synechiae (Asherman syndrome)
- Chiari-Frommel syndrome

Workup and Diagnosis

- History
  - Major illness, thyroid disease, malnutrition, eating disorder, excessive weight gain or loss
  - Intensive exercise
  - Previous uterine procedures
  - Prior pregnancy with failure of lactation
  - Sexual activity
- Review of systems
  - Virilization (e.g. facial hair, acne)
  - Symptoms of hypothyroidism
  - Headache or visual changes (for intracranial tumors)
  - Breast discharge, decreased breast size
- Physical exam
  - Height, weight, acne, facial hair, acanthosis nigricans, striae, galactorrhea
  - Visual fields and optic discs (for intracranial tumors)
  - Palpate thyroid for goiter
  - Underestrogenized vaginal mucosa is reddish, thin, and atrophic
- Labs
  - Pregnancy test
  - Thyroid function tests, FSH, LH, estradiol, prolactin, total and free testosterone, dehydroepiandrostenedione sulfate (DHEA-s), 17-hydroxyprogesterone
  - 3-day progesterone "challenge" that induces withdrawal bleeding suggests adequate estrogen
- MRI of the brain/pituitary to evaluate for pituitary pathology

Treatment

- Correction of systemic illness, malnutrition, eating disorder, or other stress
- Hyperprolactinemia
  - Prolactinoma: Treat with dopamine agonist
  - Medication-induced: Cessation of the offending agent
- Polycystic ovary syndrome
  - Weight loss
  - Oral contraceptives
  - Antiandrogen agents such as spironolactone
  - Insulin sensitizers such as metformin
- Ovarian failure
  - Treat with estrogen-progestin replacement
- Asherman syndrome
  - Treat by surgical excision of adhesions

102. Congenital Penile Anomalies

For male genital anomalies, the most important consideration is detection of the anomaly before circumcision. A surgical consultation must take place before circumcision, because the treatment plan may involve the use of the foreskin in reconstruction.

Differential Diagnosis

- Hypospadias
  - –Most common penile anomaly
  - –Incidence of 1/500
  - –Urethral meatus is typically located on the ventral surface of the glans penis
  - –The meatus may also be located on the ventral surface of the penile shaft, the scrotum, or the perineum
  - –Frequently associated with a ventral curvature of the penis (chordee) and/or a hooded prepuce
  - –Less commonly associated with undescended testes or inguinal hernia
- Epispadias
  - –Less common than hypospadias
  - –Urethral meatus on dorsal surface of the penis
- Chordee
  - –Ventral curvature of the penis
  - –Most often associated with hypospadias
  - –May occur without hypospadias when the ventral tissue is hypoplastic or fibrotic
- Dorsal hood
  - –Incomplete formation of the ventral foreskin
  - –May occur with hypospadias
- Micropenis (microphallus)
  - –Defined as stretched penis length shorter than 2 standard deviations below the mean for gestational age
  - –Associated with Prader-Willi, Kallmann Laurence-Moon-Biedl syndrome, and growth hormone deficiency

Workup and Diagnosis

- History
  - –Prenatal exposure to sex steroids
  - –Associated anomalies or syndromic findings
  - –Family history
- Physical exam
  - –Careful examination of the glans penis, the penile shaft, the scrotum, and the perineum
  - –Examination for syndromic features (e.g., hypotonia, small hands and feet, almond-shaped eyes in Prader-Willi)
- Labs
  - –Micropenis: Gonadotropin-releasing hormone, anterior pituitary function studies
- Radiology
  - –Hypospadias: VCUG is indicated if hypospadias is severe to rule out other anomalies of the urinary tract
  - –Micropenis: MRI of the hypothalamus and anterior pituitary
- Studies
  - –Genetics consultation if features of Prader-Willi, Kallmann or Laurence-Moon-Biedl syndrome are present
  - –Karyotype for patients in whom the genitalia are at all ambiguous

Treatment

- Routine circumcision should be avoided as the foreskin may ultimately be used in the repair
- Surgical revision is usually performed for cosmetic and functional reasons
- Hypospadias and epispadias
  - –Canalization of the penis improves urinary flow, erectile function, and fertility
  - –Optimally, a skin flap is created using the foreskin
- Chordee
  - –Ventral release and urethroplasty at age 6–12 months
- Dorsal hood
  - –May not require treatment, or a modified routine circumcision may restore expected appearance
- Micropenis
  - –Androgen stimulation before puberty has been used but is controversial because it may impair penile growth during puberty

103. Dysuria

Dysuria is defined as pain with urination and is a very common complaint in female children. It is commonly due to either urinary tract infection or perineal irritation from a variety of causes.

Differential Diagnosis

- Urinary tract infection (UTI)
  - –Common cause of dysuria in children
  - –Common pathogens: bacteria including *E. coli* (85%), *Klebsiella pneumoniae, Proteus vulgaris, Pseudomonas aeruginosa* and other gram negatives
- Sexually transmitted disease (STD)
  - –Gonorrhea, *Chlamydia, Trichomonas*
  - –Very common in sexually active patients
  - –More common in girls
- Bacterial vaginosis
  - –*Gardnerella* or *Mobiluncus* spp, may be sexually or nonsexually transmitted
- Candidal vaginitis
  - –Common after antibiotic treatment
- Local urethral irritation
  - –Pinworms
  - –Irritative dermatitis (e.g., bubble bath)
  - –Diarrhea
- Hemorrhagic cystitis
  - –Typically viral in origin
  - –Sudden in onset
- Macroscopic blood in the urine from any cause, causing urethral irritation
- Periurethral herpes simplex
- Periurethral varicella
- Hypercalciuria
  - –Dysuria and urinary frequency
- Kidney stone (within the urethra)
- Renal tuberculosis (rare)
  - –Typically asymptomatic
  - –Sterile pyuria
- Prostatitis (uncommon)
  - –Can affect adolescent boys
  - –Gonorrhea is the most common cause
- Trauma to the perineum
  - –Sexual abuse
  - –Masturbation
- Meatal ulceration
  - –In boys, may occur from contact with diapers
- Pelvic abscess, including appendicitis
- Drugs
  - –Amitriptyline hydrochloride (antidepressant)
- Reiter disease
  - –Uncommon in children
  - –Triad of arthritis, urethritis, and conjunctivitis

Workup and Diagnosis

- History
  - –UTI, STD, sexual activity, recent antibiotic exposure
  - –Instrumentation/irritation (urinary catheters, bubble baths, creams, masturbation)
  - –Fever, abdominal pain, flank pain, vaginal discharge
  - –Enuresis (especially new-onset), macroscopic hematuria, frequency, urgency
  - –Family history of kidney stones (increased likelihood of hypercalciuria)
- Physical exam
  - –Fever, CVA tenderness
  - –Exam of the urethra/periurethral area for irritation
  - –Pelvic exam (if done) for cervical motion tenderness, cervicitis, or vaginal discharge
- Labs
  - –Urinalysis, urine culture
  - –STD screening if sexually active
  - –Urine spot calcium and creatinine if evidence of microscopic hematuria
- Additional studies based on clinical situation
  - –Pelvic ultrasound if PID suspected
  - –Renal ultrasound/voiding cystourethrogram if history of previous UTI (in girls <7 and boys of any age), or if macroscopic hematuria is present
  - –High-resolution CT without contrast (kidney stones)
  - –24-hour urine calcium (hypercalciuria, kidney stones)

Treatment

- UTI: Empiric antibiotics (e.g., co-trimoxazole) pending culture; adjust antibiotics based on bacterial sensitivities
- STD
  - –Simple cervicitis: Treat with IM ceftriaxone and PO azithromycin, metronidazole if *Trichomonas* present
  - –For an ill patient with signs of PID, consider hospital admission, give IV cefoxitin and PO doxycycline
- Candidal vaginitis: Topical antifungal agents or oral fluconazole
- Hypercalciuria/kidney stones
  - –Increase fluid intake, decrease sodium intake (increases urinary calcium excretion), do not restrict calcium intake
  - –Treat with thiazide diuretics (decrease urinary calcium excretion) if patient is persistently symptomatic and/or has urinary calculi
- Avoid instrumentation/local irritants (e.g., bubble baths)

104. Enuresis

Enuresis is defined as urinary incontinence. The age of achieving daytime or night-time continence can vary considerably. Nocturnal enuresis (night-time bedwetting) can be normal in children up to age 8. Daytime continence is usually achieved by age 4. Enuresis can be primary (i.e., the patient has never been dry) or secondary (develops after a period of dryness). Primary enuresis (particularly nocturnal enuresis) is usually a developmental issue, whereas secondary enuresis is more likely due to a pathogenic, identifiable cause.

Differential Diagnosis

- Urinary tract infection (UTI)
  - –Most common cause of new onset, secondary enuresis
  - –Common pathogens: *E. coli* (85%), *Klebsiella pneumoniae, Proteus vulgaris, Pseudomonas aeruginosa,* and other gram-negatives
- Primary nocturnal enuresis
  - –Normal in children up to 8 years
  - –Often there is a strong family history
  - –Affected family members may not achieve night-time continence until adolescence
- Dysfunctional voiding
  - –Unstable (uninhibited) bladder of childhood
  - –Infrequent voiding
  - –Neurogenic bladder
- Psychosocial stress
- Chronic constipation
  - –Often associated with encopresis
- Chronic kidney disease
- Nephrogenic diabetes insipidus (DI)
- Central DI
- Diabetes mellitus (DM)
- Ectopic ureter
- Posterior urethral valves
- Urethral stricture
- Developmental delay
- Neurologic disease
  - –Tethered cord
  - –Spina bifida
  - –Spinal tumors
  - –Spinal dysraphism
- Sexual abuse
- Prostatic tumor or abscess
- Hydrocolpos or hematocolpos
- Osteomyelitis of vertebral body with compression of the spinal cord
- Spinal epidural abscess
- Obstructive sleep apnea
- Giggle micturition

Workup and Diagnosis

- History
  - –Primary vs secondary; daytime vs night-time
  - –Previous urinary tract infection or renal disease
  - –Poor growth, recurrent dehydration
  - –"Curtsying" or urinary withholding/delay maneuvers
  - –Stooling frequency
  - –Psychosocial stressors, social withdrawal, poor performance in school (depression or sexual abuse)
  - –Developmental delay
- Family history: Primary nocturnal enuresis, polyuria; early infant death (suggests nephrogenic DI)
- Symptoms
  - –Fever, flank pain (UTI), dysuria, urgency, frequency (cystitis or dysfunctional voiding)
  - –Fatigue and polyuria (renal disease)
  - –Headache or vision changes (intracranial process)
- Physical exam
  - –Affect, developmental assessment, growth parameters (height/weight), blood pressure
  - –Pallor (e.g., due to anemia of renal failure)
  - –Neuro: Reflexes, anal wink, sensation, strength
  - –Spinal exam (hair tufts, clefts suggest spina bifida)
  - –GU exam
- Labs: Urinalysis, urine culture, chemistry panel
- Additional evaluation based on the clinical situation
  - –Spinal MRI for sacral dimple or hair cleft
  - –Ultrasound/VCUG for UTI or other kidney /bladder disease

Treatment

- UTI
  - –Empiric antibiotics (e.g., co-trimoxazole) after culture
  - –Adjust antibiotics based on bacterial sensitivities
- Primary nocturnal enuresis
  - –Behavioral measures (limit fluids at night, enuresis alarms, reward system)
  - –Consider pharmacologic treatments (i.e., DDAVP) for short-term use (e.g., vacations, sleepovers)
- Dysfunctional voiding
  - –Unstable bladder of childhood
  - –Treat with anticholinergic agents (e.g., oxybutynin)
  - –Other causes are treated with behavior interventions (e.g., timed voiding and positive reinforcements)
  - –Manage constipation, if present
- Nephrogenic DI: Treat with large volumes of fluid intake, close attention to fluid status during acute illnesses
- Central DI: Treat with DDAVP

105. Hematuria

Hematuria is defined as >5 red blood cells per high-power field in a freshly voided, spun urine specimen. Macroscopic (gross) hematuria is less common, is more likely to be attributed to an identified cause, and is always "pathologic." Cola-colored urine, hematuria with proteinuria, hypertension, or dysmorphic urinary RBCs suggest "upper tract" disease (involving the kidney itself). "Lower tract" (ureter/bladder) findings include terminal hematuria, visible clots, or absence of proteinuria.

Differential Diagnosis

- Transient (fever, dehydration, exercise)
- Urinary tract infection
  - –Most common cause of gross hematuria
- Hypercalciuria (common)
- Primary glomerulonephritis (GN)
  - –Acute poststreptococcal GN: Gross hematuria +/− hypertension, oliguria; 5 days to several weeks after Group A strep pharyngitis or pyoderma; can also occur after other infections
  - –IgA nephropathy (Berger disease): recurrent gross hematuria occurs at or near onset of a URI
  - –Membranoproliferative GN
- GN associated with systemic disease
  - –HSP
  - –SLE
  - –Other vasculitis (rare) e.g.,Wegener
- Other glomerular disease
  - –Benign familial hematuria
  - –Alport syndrome: Usually X linked, high-frequency deafness, progression to renal failure
  - –Glomerular disease (e.g., FSGS) usually presents as nephrotic syndrome
- Tubulointerstitial disease
  - –Polycystic kidney disease, interstitial nephritis, papillary necrosis, ATN
- Urinary pelvic junction obstruction
- Urolithiasis/nephrolithiasis
  - –Painless in up to 50% of children
- Urethrorrhagia
  - –Recurrent gross hematuria (spotting on the underwear)
  - –Most common in peripubertal males
- Malignancies (e.g., Wilms tumor)
- Vascular (e.g., renal vein thrombosis)
- Trauma
- Non-urinary tract blood
  - –Menses, perineal irritation, pinworms, masturbation, STDs, sexual abuse
- Munchausen/Munchausen by proxy (rare)

Workup and Diagnosis

- History
  - –Antecedent illness (including timing)
  - –Prior episodes, medication/food exposure
  - –Quality of gross hematuria (if present): Color, terminal vs present throughout stream, clots
  - –Symptoms: Fever, flank pain, dysuria, rash, hemoptysis, breathing difficulty, joint complaints
  - –Family history: Kidney stones, kidney disease, deafness (Alport)
- Physical exam
  - –Blood pressure, growth parameters, skin or pharyngeal lesions, cardiac gallop, rales, edema, CVAT, genitourinary exam (external)
- Labs/studies
  - –U/A (dipstick and microscopy), urine culture
  - –Dipstick negative = foods, medications
  - –Dipstick positive, no RBCs = myoglobin, hemoglobin
  - –Dipstick positive, with RBCs = hematuria
  - –Macroscopic or microscopic with symptoms (e.g., HTN): Serum chemistries, CBC, ASO, C3, ANA, sickle prep, spot urine calcium/creatinine, STD screen (if sexually active), renal/bladder ultrasound, consider noncontrast helical CT if kidney stones suspected
  - –Microscopic hematuria, no symptoms: Repeat U/A two times, 1 week apart; if persists, check serum chemistries, urine culture, sickle prep, spot urine calcium/creatinine and U/As of parents/siblings

Treatment

- UTI: Empiric antibiotic (e.g., co-trimoxazole)
- Manage hypertension
  - –ACE inhibitors or calcium channel blockers
  - –Consider diuretics if edematous
- Suspected acute glomerulonephritis
  - –Low C3, evidence of recent strep or other infection
  - –Monitor urine output, weight, BP closely
  - –Daily outpatient visits until stable
  - –Inpatient admission if oliguria/edema is severe
  - –Once acute phase is over, monitor every 1–2 weeks and recheck C3 in 6–8 weeks
- Nephrolithiasis: Increase fluid intake
  - –Sodium-restrict (do not calcium-restrict)
  - –Consult urology for severe pain or obstruction
- Consult nephrology if hematuria persists or is associated with proteinuria, hypertension, persistently decreased C3, or abnormal creatinine

106. Precocious Puberty

Precocious puberty is early sexual development or onset of puberty before 8 years in girls and 9 years in boys by traditional standards (recent survey suggested definition may be changing to 7 years in white girls and 6 years in black girls). The first sign of puberty in males is testicular enlargement; in girls, it is breast development.

Differential Diagnosis

- True central precious puberty (TCPP)
  - –Normal puberty as a result of activation of hypothalamus with anterior pituitary release of LH and FSH
  - –No identifiable cause in 95% (idiopathic)
  - –Most cases sporadic, not familial
  - –Any type of neurologic disturbance can be the cause: Tumor, cerebral palsy, head trauma, hydrocephalus, cranial irradiation
  - –Rare in boys; must search for underlying cause as less likely to be idiopathic
  - –Onset can be triggered or primed by exposure to androgens
- Precocious pseudopuberty
  - –Maturation due to peripheral gland activity; hypothalamic-pituitary unit not activated for puberty
  - –Enzyme defects (congenital adrenal hyperplasia)
  - –Tumors
  - –McCune-Albright syndrome
  - –Ovarian cysts
  - –Anabolic steroid exposure
  - –May advance the bone age
- Premature adrenarche
  - –Development of pubic hair without other signs of puberty
  - –May be accompanied by the development of body odor, greasy skin and hair
  - –May have advanced bone age
  - –More common in girls
  - –Androgen-secreting tumor
  - –Simple virilizing and nonclassical congenital adrenal hyperplasia (most commonly 21-hydroxylase deficiency; also 3-β-hydroxysteroid dehydrogenase deficiency)
- Benign premature thelarche
  - –Development of breast tissue without pubic hair
  - –Common between ages of 6–24 months
  - –May be present since birth
  - –Normal height velocity
  - –Appropriate skeletal maturation (bone age)
  - –Normal hormone studies and pelvic ultrasound

Workup and Diagnosis

- History
  - –Puberty age of onset, progression
  - –Height velocity
  - –Greasy hair and skin, acne, body odor, mood swings
  - –Pubic hair, axillary hair, breast development
  - –Cyclic vaginal bleeding, muscle bulk
  - –Headache, vomiting, visual changes (intracranial mass)
  - –Perinatal problems leading to intraventricular hemorrhage and hydrocephalus
  - –Cerebral palsy, head trauma, prior cranial irradiation
  - –Steroid creams, estrogens, anabolic steroids
  - –Family history of early puberty
- Physical exam
  - –Weight, height, BP, funduscopic examination, thyroid, Tanner staging, dermatologic exam for café-au-lait (McCune-Albright syndrome or neurofibromatosis)
- Labs/studies
  - –LH, FSH, estradiol, testosterone
  - –17-hydroxyprogesterone, 17-hydroxypregnenolone
  - –Androstenedione, DHEA
  - –Thyroid function tests
  - –hCG in boys (screen for tumors)
  - –Provocative testing with GnRH (hypothalamic-pituitary axis) to assess central activation
  - –Bone age: Degree of skeletal maturation
  - –Abdominal and pelvic ultrasound: Adrenal or ovarian/testicular masses
  - –MRI of head/pituitary to assess for intracranial mass

Treatment

- Idiopathic TCPP
  - –No treatment is required if there are no psychological issues and patient is close to pubertal age
  - –Short stature and psychosocial issues are the potential consequences of withholding treatment
- TCPP can be treated with GnRH analog
- Premature adrenarche and thelarche warrant close follow-up
- Removal of adrenal or ovarian/testicular mass if detected
- Treatment of intracranial lesion if diagnosed
- Gonadotropin-independent McCune-Albright syndrome
  - –Aromatase inhibitors (testolactone) have been tried with some success
- Psychological support if indicated

107. Proteinuria

Proteinuria in children is defined as a quantitative 24-hour urine collection with >4 mg/m^2/hour (>100 mg/m^2/day) of protein. Semiquantitative definitions include urine dipstick ≥1+ (30 mg/dL) for specific gravity (SG) ≤1.015, or 2+ (100 mg/dL) for SG >1.015, or a random urine protein:creatinine ratio >0.2 (0.5 for age<2 years). Nephrotic syndrome (NS) has four components: (1) Nephrotic range proteinuria (>40 mg/m^2/hour or >1,000 mg/m^2/day); (2) edema; (3) hypoalbuminemia; and (4) hyperlipidemia.

Differential Diagnosis

- Transient proteinuria
  - With fever, dehydration, exercise, seizures, cold exposure, or stress
  - Rarely >2+ on dipstick
  - Usually remits within 1–2 weeks
- Orthostatic (postural) proteinuria
  - Occurs mostly in adolescence
  - First morning U/A is negative for protein
- Primary glomerular disease
  - MCNS: Most common cause of nephrotic syndrome (NS) in younger children, usually presents in ages 2–6, more common in boys; etiology possibly immune-mediated, typically responds to corticosteroids
  - Mesangial proliferative GN: Intermediate lesion between MCNS and FSGS
  - FSGS: Progressive disease of glomerular scarring, more common in blacks and adolescents, presents as NS or asymptomatic proteinuria, frequently resistant to corticosteroid therapy
  - Membranous nephropathy
  - Any primary GN (e.g., APSGN) can present with hematuria and proteinuria
- Systemic lupus erythematosus nephritis
- Henoch-Schönlein purpura (HSP)
- Wegener granulomatosis
- Tubulointerstitial disease: Proteinuria is less than with primary glomerular diseases
  - Reflux nephropathy
  - Renal dysplasia
  - Interstitial nephritis (especially NSAIDs)
  - Polycystic kidney disease
- Infectious disease
  - Bacterial (e.g., poststrep, shunt nephritis, leprosy, syphilis, infective endocarditis)
  - Viral (e.g., HBV, CMV, EBV, VZV, HIV)
  - Protozoal (e.g., malaria, toxoplasmosis)
  - Parasitic (e.g., schistosomiasis, filariasis)
- Neoplasm (e.g., lymphoma, leukemia, Wilms tumor, pheochromocytoma)
- Alport syndrome
- Fabry disease
- Nail-patella syndrome
- Medications (e.g. gold, mercurials)
- Constrictive pericarditis

Workup and Diagnosis

- History
  - Renal disease
  - Recurrent UTIs
  - HIV infection
  - Edema (periorbital or extremity)
  - Fatigue
  - Weight loss or gain
  - Pallor (seen with anemia of chronic disease)
  - Gross hematuria
  - "Foamy" urine
- Physical exam
  - Blood pressure, growth parameters
  - Edema (periorbital or extremity), ascites
  - Rashes or joint abnormalities
- Labs
  - Serum chemistries including albumin and triglycerides
  - U/A, 24-hour urine collection for protein
  - C3, C4
- If asymptomatic proteinuria, obtain "first morning" void, preferably prior to ambulation, to rule out orthostatic proteinuria before performing extensive lab workup
  - If U/A is negative for protein, additional diagnostic testing is not necessary
- Additional tests as indicated by the history
  - ANCA, ANA, HIV
- Renal ultrasound

Treatment

- All patients with persistent proteinuria should be referred to a pediatric nephrologist for evaluation
- Younger children with the typical presentation of MCNS are treated with an empiric course of corticosteroids (4–6 weeks of high dose followed by a gradual taper)
- Patients with atypical features (e.g., renal insufficiency, older age at presentation), asymptomatic proteinuria, or suspected systemic disease undergo renal biopsy with treatment directed at the underlying cause
- Patient with "steroid-dependent" or steroid-resistant forms of NS may be treated with alternative immunosuppressant agents (e.g., cyclosporine, mycophenolate)
- ACE inhibitors are an important adjunct therapy for proteinuric renal diseases, because they not only control hypertension if present, but also have direct antiproteinuric/antifibrotic effects

108. Pubertal Delay

Pubertal delay for a boy is defined as not beginning secondary sexual development by age 14 years (more than 2.5 standard deviations [SD] older than the mean). For a girl, lack of breast or pubic hair development by age 13 years and absence of menarche by age 16 years are considered abnormal. If pubertal changes are not complete in 4 years in females, possible hormone deficiency should be investigated

Differential Diagnosis

- Constitutional delay of puberty
  - Most common cause, explaining 90–95% of pubertal delay, often familial
  - Delay in the onset of puberty (and associated linear growth spurt)
  - Once puberty begins, progression and final height and development are normal
  - Frequently called "late bloomers"
  - Bone age is delayed and growth velocity is normal for bone age
- Chronic disease
  - All can cause delay of growth and puberty
  - Associated with delayed bone age
- Hypogonadotropic hypogonadism
  - Isolated gonadotropin deficiency (Kallmann syndrome)
  - Congenital hypopituitarism
  - Congenital CNS abnormalities: Septo-optic dysplasia, hydrocephalus, holoprosencephaly
  - Acquired CNS abnormalities: Tumors (e.g., craniopharyngioma), infection (e.g., meningitis), trauma, histiocytosis X
  - Radiation treatment for brain tumor (hypothalamus/pituitary dysfunction)
  - Hyperprolactinemia (sometimes with microadenoma)
  - Thalassemia major (iron deposition in anterior pituitary)
  - Prader-Willi syndrome
  - Laurence-Moon-Bardet-Biedl syndrome
  - Anorexia nervosa
- Congenital hypergonadotropic hypogonadism
  - Turner syndrome in girls (most common cause of primary hypogonadism in girls)
  - Klinefelter syndrome in boys
  - Noonan syndrome
- Acquired hypergonadotropic hypogonadism
  - Autoimmune disease
  - Infection (e.g., mumps causing orchitis in males)
  - Radiation or chemotherapy
  - Ischemic (e.g., after gonadal torsion)
  - Surgical resection

Workup and Diagnosis

- History
  - Growth history, age of development of secondary sexual characteristics
  - Sense of smell; visual or other neurologic problems
  - Signs/symptoms of hypopituitarism (hypoglycemia and jaundice in infancy, midline defects, micropenis)
  - Headaches, autoimmune history, galactorrhea, medications, radiation
  - Prior infections such as mumps; trauma
- Family history: Age of puberty; growth pattern, congenital problems or genetic syndromes; anosmia
- Physical exam
  - Vitals, height, weight, dysmorphic features, midline defects (e.g., cleft palate), test of smell; neuro (disconjugate gaze, visual field defect, etc.)
  - Galactorrhea, axillary hair; Tanner staging; acne
  - Hirsutism in girls; webbed neck, increased carrying angle of the arms, low posterior hairline, shield chest, pectus excavatum, lymphedema (Turner, Noonan)
- Workup
  - Bone age, FSH, LH, testosterone (males), prolactin, thyroid tests
  - Systemic disease: ESR, CBC with differential, comprehensive metabolic panel
  - If central (hypogonadotropic): Morning cortisol and growth factors, GnRH stimulation testing, MRI of brain and pituitary, FISH for Prader-Willi
  - If peripheral (hypergonadotropic): Karyotype, pelvic ultrasound, MIF = marker for testicular tissue

Treatment

- Constitutional delay of puberty
  - Support and reassurance, sometimes brief testosterone treatment to stimulate puberty in males
- Treatment of underlying chronic disease
- Hypopituitarism: Replace all hormone deficiencies
  - Sex hormones, replacement during adolescence
  - Congenital hypopituitarism in males, brief course of testosterone during infancy to enlarge penis
- Prolactinoma: Treat with dopaminergic agonist
- Turner syndrome
  - Growth hormone therapy then estrogen replacement
- Hormone replacement
  - Increase the doses to mimic normal puberty
  - Eventually cycle estrogen and progesterone in girls
  - Testosterone in males (via injection, patch, or gel)
- hCG and pulsatile GnRH for fertility in adults with hypogonadotropic hypogonadism (hormonal treatment cannot overcome injury to oocytes and spermatogenesis in hypergonadotropic)

109. Pyuria

Pyuria is defined as the presence of white blood cells in the urine. This condition is commonly caused by urinary tract infection, asymptomatic bacteriuria, or vaginal contamination of the urine specimen.

Differential Diagnosis

- Urinary tract infection
- Asymptomatic bacteriuria
  - –Relatively common in school-age girls
  - –Urine cultures are repeatedly positive
  - –Patients remain asymptomatic
- Sexually transmitted disease (STD)
  - –Gonorrhea, *Chlamydia, Trichomonas*
  - –Bacterial vaginitis (can be nonsexually transmitted)
- Other causes of vaginal discharge/perineal irritation (e.g., candidal vaginitis)
- Acute interstitial nephritis
  - –"Allergic" tubulointerstitial process
  - –Occurs 7–14 days after exposure to inciting agent (e.g., antibiotics or NSAIDs)
  - –May have polyuria, fever, and rash, and elevated serum creatinine of unclear etiology
  - –Urinalysis is otherwise unremarkable
- Inherited cystic diseases
  - –PKD: Occurs in both autosomal dominant and autosomal recessive forms
  - –Juvenile nephronophthisis: Rare cause of inherited chronic tubulointerstitial nephritis, steady progression to kidney failure in the first two decades of life, autosomal recessive inheritance
- Appendicitis
  - –May present with symptoms suggestive of acute pyelonephritis (fever, flank or abdominal pain)
  - –Urine culture is negative
  - –Symptoms are progressive
- Renal tuberculosis
  - –Routine urine culture negative
- Gastroenteritis (typically viral)
- Lupus nephritis
- Alport syndrome
- Nail-patella syndrome
- Urethritis
- Kawasaki disease
  - –Most common vasculitis of childhood
  - –Characterized by high fever, irritability, mucous membrane changes, edema of the hands and feet, lymphadenopathy
  - –Coronary vasculitis and aneurysms may result
  - –Treated with aspirin and IVIG

Workup and Diagnosis

- History
  - –Previous UTI or positive urine culture
  - –Unprotected sexual activity, previous STD
  - –Recent antibiotic or other medication exposure
  - –Poor growth (seen in chronic kidney disease)
  - –Dysuria, urgency, frequency, fever, flank pain
  - –Polyuria, polydipsia
  - –Abdominal pain (particularly right lower quadrant)
  - –Family history of polycystic kidney disease or other inherited kidney disease
- Physical exam
  - –Temperature, BP, height, and weight
  - –Rashes
  - –Pelvic exam (if patient sexually active)
  - –Exam of the external genitalia
  - –Abdominal masses
  - –Costovertebral angle tenderness
- Labs
- Urinalysis (including microscopy), urine culture
  - –STD screen if sexually active: GC culture, *Chlamydia* DNA probe or ligase chain test, wet prep for *Trichomonas*
  - –Chemistry panel to screen for renal disease
- Additional studies depend on the clinical situation
  - –Abdominal CT scan or ultrasound for appendicitis
  - –Renal ultrasound if inherited cystic diseases are suspected

Treatment

- Suspected UTI: Empiric oral antibiotics after culture (e.g., co-trimoxazole); if acutely ill, consider intravenous antibiotics
- Asymptomatic bacteriuria: Should not be treated unless patient develops symptoms or has a previous history of symptomatic UTI, because treatment of asymptomatic patients promotes antibiotic resistance
- STDs
  - –Simple cervicitis, treat with IM ceftriaxone and PO azithromycin; add metronidazole for *Trichomonas*
  - –Ill patients or PID: Consider hospital admission, IV cefoxitin and oral doxycycline
- Suspected acute interstitial nephritis
  - –Discontinue any potential causative agents
  - –Ensure adequate hydration
  - –Monitor serum creatinine and electrolytes daily
  - –Treat sequelae of acute renal failure (hyperkalemia)

110. Scrotal Pain

Acute scrotal pain demands immediate attention. Although not every cause constitutes an emergency, testicular torsion must be discovered immediately to save the testicle. Testicular pain should be triaged to an emergency center with access to Doppler evaluation and a surgery consult.

Differential Diagnosis

- Testicular torsion
  - –Twisting of the spermatic cord and vessels, resulting in testicular ischemia
  - –Patients present with an excruciatingly painful swollen testicle with or without a history of previous milder episodes (intermittent torsion)
  - –May occur at any age (including in utero)
- Torsion of the appendix testis
  - –May be difficult to distinguish clinically from testicular torsion
  - –Typically, pain is less severe and the onset less acute (over several days as opposed to several hours)
  - –Most common ages 7–12 years
- Testicular trauma
  - –Blunt trauma occurs as saddle injuries, in sports such as soccer and baseball, and during altercations
- Epididymitis
  - –Inflammation of the epididymis usually secondary to bacteria
  - –Rare before puberty and often seen in sexually active young men with acutely swollen and painful testis
  - –Pain is usually less acute in onset than torsion
- Inguinal hernia
  - –Incarcerated inguinal hernia may present as a painful, edematous scrotum
- Orchitis
  - –Inflammation of the testes due to viral infection; classically mumps
  - –Patient presents with an acutely swollen, red testicle(s)
  - –Uncommon since widespread vaccination
- Henoch-Schönlein purpura
  - –Vasculitis characterized by palpable purpura usually in the lower half of the body
  - –Painful testicular swelling can be a sign of this disorder
- Varicocele
  - –A collection of dilated veins in the scrotum
  - –Usually painless, but occasionally patients may complain of chronic nagging pain and discomfort (especially during physical activity)
  - –Presents after puberty

Workup and Diagnosis

- History
  - –History of trauma, viral symptoms, rash
  - –Sexual history and history of STDs
  - –Past medical history of similar episodes
- Physical exam
  - –With testicular torsion, the absence of the cremasteric reflex is one of the most characteristic features; the affected testis is also often higher and more horizontal than the contralateral testis
  - –In epididymitis and orchitis, elevation of the testis improves the pain, and the cremasteric reflex is usually preserved
  - –In torsion of the appendix testis, a bluish dot may be seen in the superior portion of the affected testis
  - –A hernia often can be felt extending from the inguinal area into the scrotum
  - –A varicocele is described as feeling like a "bag of worms," and is best examined with the patient standing
- Urinalysis
  - –Normal in patients with torsion
  - –Pyuria is a feature of epididymitis
- Doppler ultrasound is indicated for patients in whom the physical exam is not diagnostic; it may be bypassed by the surgeon in the interest of time when the exam is very specific for testicular torsion

Treatment

- Torsion
  - –To salvage the testis, detorsion must take place within 6 hours of the onset of symptoms
  - –Surgical exploration and detorsion is the approach of choice for children with suspected testicular torsion
  - –With torsion of one testicle, the surgeon may elect to surgically fix the contralateral testicle to prevent future torsion
- Torsion of the appendix testis is treated conservatively
- Antibiotics, typically doxycycline, are used to treat epididymitis
- Inguinal hernias are reduced surgically; surgical exploration of the contralateral side is often performed
- Orchitis is treated supportively
- HSP is treated supportively and sometimes with systemic corticosteroids
- Varicoceles may not require treatment, but may interfere with fertility

111. Scrotal Swelling

A scrotal mass may or may not be detected by the patient or the patient's parent. Many are discovered by the clinician during routine physical examinations. Most scrotal masses seen in infants are hydroceles and inguinal hernias; both are more common in premature infants. Hernia is the most common cause in teenagers.

Differential Diagnosis

- Hydrocele
  - –Fluid surrounding the testicle
  - –Typically seen in infancy
  - –Results from remnant of testicular descent from the abdomen through the inguinal canal into the scrotum
  - –May be communicating or noncommunicating; communicating hydroceles have retained patency of the tract of descent, and noncommunicating hydroceles do not
  - –Communicating hydroceles may be reducible and are likely to fluctuate in size depending on the amount of fluid within the scrotal sac; crying or any increase in intra-abdominal pressure results in an increase in size
  - –Usually is noncommunicating; i.e., not reducible, and does not change in size with crying
  - –Testes may be difficult to palpate because surrounded by the hydrocele
- Hernia
  - –Protrusion of a loop of bowel into the scrotum
  - –Direct hernias represent a channel directly through the musculature of the pelvic floor; indirect hernias have proceeded through the inguinal canal
  - –Usually painless unless incarcerated
  - –Usually reducible and changes in size with changes in intra-abdominal pressure
  - –Testes usually palpable below the hernia
- Varicocele
  - –A collection of dilated veins in the scrotum
  - –Usually painless, but patients may complain of heaviness
- Edema
  - –Generalized edema often is accompanied by scrotal edema
- Tumor
  - –Presents as painless nodule on testes
  - –May be accompanied by sexual precocity or gynecomastia secondary to hormone production by the tumor
- Leukemia
  - –Patients may present with unilateral scrotal swelling (common site for relapse)

Workup and Diagnosis

- History
  - –Onset, duration of symptoms
  - –Unilateral or bilateral
  - –Associated systemic symptoms
- Physical exam
  - –General state of health, including growth parameters and weight loss
  - –Unilateral or bilateral lesions
  - –Reducibility of scrotal mass or enlargement
  - –Palpation of testes: Tenseness, nodules
  - –Hydroceles can sometimes be transilluminated
  - –Patent defects can usually be palpated when there is a hernia, particularly if the patient performs a Valsalva maneuver ("turn your head and cough")
  - –Varicocele is usually left sided and feels like "a bag of worms"
- Labs
  - –CBC and differential, LDH, ESR if malignancy is suspected
- Radiology
  - –Ultrasound may be helpful confirming hernia, hydrocele, or varicocele
  - –PET scans are used to detect malignant metastasis or relapse
- Studies
  - –A testicular nodule usually must be biopsied to rule out malignancy

Treatment

- Hydrocele
  - –Usually resolves spontaneously by 1 year of age
  - –Surgery is indicated at 6–12 months if stable, sooner if hydrocele is tense or progressively enlarging
- Hernia
  - –Inguinal hernias must be repaired surgically to avoid incarceration
  - –Contralateral side is frequently explored surgically and closed if necessary
- Varicocele: Can be associated with infertility and may need to be surgically repaired
- Edema: Treatment of the cause of generalized edema
- Tumor and leukemia: Management by pediatric oncologist
- Men and teenage boys should be taught testicular self-examination to assist with early detection of testicular cancer

112. Vaginal Discharge

The pubertal vaginal flora is primarily lactobacillus, and the vagina has an acidic pH with a thick, estrogenized epithelium acting as a protective mechanism. The prepubertal vagina is less estrogenized and has a thinner epithelium, predisposing it to irritation. Any complaint of a vaginal discharge must be taken seriously as it may be a sign of an infection, underlying medical disorder, or sexual abuse.

Differential Diagnosis

- Physiologic leukorrhea
  - –In newborns for 2–3 weeks, due to maternal estrogen effect, and in pubertal girls
  - –Discharge typically clear to white, sticky, and nonirritating
  - –Newborns may have withdrawal bleeding
- Infections
  - –Bacterial vaginosis: Previously known as nonspecific vaginitis; polymicrobial in etiology (coliforms, streptococci, *Gardnerella*); discharge may be gray and malodorous (fishy smell) but generally nonirritating
  - –*Candida:* Discharge may be cheesy and white with erythematous, pruritic, irritated vulva; typical discharge is rarely seen in prepubertal children; discharge typically has no odor
  - –*Trichomonas:* Discharge may be frothy, malodorous, creamy, green, bloody, or pruritic (or asymptomatic)
  - –*Chlamydia:* Commonly asymptomatic or a nonspecific discharge
  - –Gonorrhea: Infection is commonly asymptomatic or has a gray-white, thick, purulent discharge
  - –Group A β-hemolytic streptococci: Discharge may be bloody
  - –*Shigella:* Discharge may be bloody
- Irritation/hygiene
  - –Due to bubble baths and other chemical irritants, tight clothing, obesity, poor wiping
- Foreign body
  - –Commonly includes toilet paper, forgotten tampon
  - –Discharge is often bloody and malodorous
- Anatomic
  - –Ectopic urethra
  - –Rectovaginal fistula
  - –Urethral prolapse
- Urinary tract infection
- Masturbation
- Sarcoma botyroides
- Oral contraceptives (estrogen effect)

Workup and Diagnosis

- History
  - –Age of girl (pubertal vs prepubertal)
  - –Sexual activity and number of partners
  - –Possibility of sexual abuse
  - –Medications (e.g., steroid, oral contraceptive, antibiotic)
  - –PMH of diabetes mellitus or immunocompromised
  - –Type of discharge and duration of symptoms
  - –Hygiene practices including feminine hygiene products, soaps, wiping techniques
  - –Therapy tried at home
- Physical exam
  - –Frog-leg or lithotomy position; examine external genitalia for abnormalities; speculum exam in sexually active adolescents
  - –Amount, odor, color, consistency of discharge
- Labs
  - –pH: Normal in the pubertal female is 3.8–4.4; if >5, consider bacterial vaginosis or *Trichomonas*
  - –Vaginal gram stain and culture
  - –Cultures for gonorrhea and *Chlamydia* (DNA amplification may not hold up in court for abuse cases)
  - –Wet prep: *Trichomonas* has motile trichomonads; bacterial vaginosis has clue cells (vaginal epithelial cells coated with bacteria)
  - –KOH for *Candida*
  - –Whiff test (KOH added to discharge yields a fishy smell in *Trichomonas*)
- Urine culture and pregnancy test as indicated by history

Treatment

- Physiologic leukorrhea: Provide reassurance
- Irritative vaginal discharge: Educate on proper wiping techniques, avoidance of tight clothing and irritants
- Foreign bodies such as toilet paper can usually be removed with gentle vaginal lavage, sitz baths
- Treatments for infectious causes of vaginal discharge:
  - –Bacterial vaginosis: Metronidazole or topical clindamycin
  - –*Candida* can be treated with topical or oral antifungals
  - –*Trichomonas* is treated with metronidazole
  - –Group A β-hemolytic streptococci: Penicillin
  - –*Chlamydia* is treated with doxycycline or azithromycin
  - –Gonorrhea: Ceftriaxone, ciprofloxacin, or ofloxacin
  - –*Shigella* is treated with trimethoprim-sulfamethoxazole
- Encourage barrier contraception in sexually active adolescents

Section 14

Extremities

KATHLEEN O. DeANTONIS, MD
FATMA DEDEOGLU, MD
VLAD D. IANUȘ, MD, MPH
DON LUJAN, MD, MS
MUSTAFA SAHIN, MD, PhD
NICOLE J. ULLRICH, MD, PhD

113. Arthritis – Multiple Joints

Clinical history and physical examination is a fundamental diagnostic tool in polyarthritis. Laboratory findings of inflammation include anemia, elevated ESR, CRP, and thrombocytosis. Normal or low platelet count, elevated LDH and uric acid levels raise the possibility of a malignancy. Establishment of methotrexate therapy in arthritis of many rheumatologic conditions has started a new era in treatment of childhood arthritides, and newer treatments under investigation may enable the prevention of long-term disability.

Differential Diagnosis

- Infectious
  - –Reactive arthritis (postenteric or genital including Reiter syndrome, postviral, poststreptococcal)
  - –Acute rheumatic fever (ARF): Migratory, painful; usually affects large joints; diagnosis is based on Jones criteria, which includes five major (arthritis, carditis, Sydenham chorea, erythema marginatum, subcutaneous nodules) and several minor (fever, arthralgia, elevated ESR or CRP, prolonged P-R interval) manifestations
  - –Lyme disease: Arthritis is monoarticular or oligoarticular, is rarely symmetric, and is the second most common manifestation of Lyme disease after erythema migrans
  - –SBE-related arthritis
  - –Septic polyarthritis (unusual)
- Rheumatic
  - –Polyarticular JRA: Arthritis in five or more joints in first 6 months of disease, insidious onset, symmetric involvement, may be RF+ (erosive, similar to adult RA) or RF−
  - –Systemic-onset JRA: Presents with severe systemic involvement (fever, rash, serositis), which may precede the arthritis, usually oligoarticular
  - –Juvenile ankylosing spondylitis (JAS): Initially affects lower extremity joints; later affects axial skeleton, also affects tendons
  - –Psoriatic arthritis
  - –Arthritis of IBD: Usually more transient than JRA
  - –SLE: May present only with arthritis, may be misdiagnosed as JRA
  - –Other connective tissue diseases (scleroderma)
  - –Vasculitis (HSP, Kawasaki disease)
- Malignancy such as leukemia
- Other systemic disorders: Serum sickness, sarcoidosis, Behçet disease, Ehler-Danlos syndrome, mucopolysaccharidoses, Noonan syndrome, Turner syndrome
- Medications (minocyline, carbamazapine)
- Sickle cell disease

Workup and Diagnosis

- History
  - –Acute or chronic; persistent or intermittent; degree of pain, night-time symptoms
  - –Systemic symptoms such as fever, weight loss, rash, and fatigue
  - –Mouth and/or genital ulcers, abdominal pain, vomiting, diarrhea, bloody stools
  - –Past medical history: Birth history, existing medical conditions, surgeries, broken bones, growth and development, any recent URI, genital infection or strep infection, unusual exposures such as tick bites
- Physical exam
  - –Vital signs including growth parameters
  - –Musculoskeletal exam for swelling, tenderness, warmth, redness over the joints, range of motion of the joints; asymmetry, muscle strength
  - –Lympadenopathy, organomegaly, rash, dysmorphic features, presence of bone pain and neurologic exam (tone, sensory, and reflexes)
- Labs: CBC, ESR or CRP, RF and ANA; Lyme titers, lupus panel, complement (C3, C4) levels; viral titers (HCV, EBV, parvovirus), LDH, U/A, LFTs
- Radiology: CXR, X-ray of involved joints, US, MRI, and bone scan to rule out infection, malignancy, and to confirm effusion and tenosynovitis
- Studies: ECG, echocardiogram, angiogram, UGI/SBF, endoscopy when clinically indicated

Treatment

- Even though unlikely, if septic arthritis (such as with *Neisseria gonorrhoeae*) is a possibility, antibiotic treatment should be started immediately
- Appropriate treatment of malignancy
- NSAIDs for JRA and spondyloarthropathies as an initial therapy; disease-modifying antirheumatic drugs (DMARDs) such as sulfasalazine and methotrexate, and biologics (e.g., TNF blockers) are added depending on clinical response
- Specific treatments of other mixed connective tissue diseases depending on their severity
- Corrective and/or supportive medical/surgical interventions
- Supportive therapy such as PT and OT to increase range of motion and strength; insoles to correct leg length discrepancy
- Psychosocial support especially with chronic diseases

114. Arthritis – Single Joint

Arthritis in a single joint, or monoarthritis, is a difficult diagnostic challenge, because any disorder affecting joints may initially present as monoarthritis. After establishing that the arthritis is truly monoarticular, the most important considerations are septic joint and trauma. Joint pain may arise not only from joint itself but from adjacent bone, ligaments, tendons, bursae, or soft tissues. Presence of effusion usually indicates intra-articular pathology, although osteomyelitis, fractures, or tumors may cause effusion as well.

Differential Diagnosis

- Septic arthritis
  - –Rapid diagnosis critical: Untreated septic arthritis causes irreversible joint and bone destruction
  - –Usually presents hyperacutely with very tender, swollen, warm, red joint with severely restricted range of motion
  - –Usual pathogens: *Haemophilus influenzae* type b, *Staphylococcus aureus*, group B strep in neonates, and *Neisseria gonorrhoeae* in adolescents; fungal and mycobacterial arthritis are seen rarely, may have chronic course
- Lyme arthritis
  - –Second most common manifestation of Lyme disease (after erythema migrans)
  - –Monoarthritis of a knee occurs in about two-thirds of children with Lyme disease
- Reactive arthritis
  - –Probably the most common etiology of childhood rheumatic diseases
  - –Transient sterile arthritis following a bacterial GI infection
  - –Usually full resolution, but a few children have a chronic course
- Trauma, overuse, fracture
  - –Often acute onset with significant pain
- Malignancy such as leukemia, neuroblastoma and osteogenic sarcoma
- Pauciarticular juvenile rheumatoid arthritis (JRA)
- Spondyloarthropathies (SpA)
- Congenital hip dysplasia
- Slipped capital femoral epiphysis (SCFE)
  - –Most common adolescent hip disorder
  - –Separation of the femoral growth plate
  - –More common in obese males
- Spontaneous osteonecrosis of the joint
  - –Mostly in hip (Legg-Calvé-Perthes disease), shoulder, and knee
  - –More common in males
- Internal structural abnormality
  - –Discoid meniscus, osteochondritis dissecans, synovial chondromatosis
- Hemarthrosis due to trauma, bleeding disorder such as hemophilia, or benign tumors such as hemangiomas and pigmented villonodular synovitis
- Periodic fever syndromes such as familial Mediterranean fever

Workup and Diagnosis

- History
  - –Acute or chronic
  - –Mechanical (pain worsens with activities, improves with rest, and usually involves weight-bearing joints)
  - –Inflammatory (waxing and waning, symptoms unrelated to use, morning stiffness)
  - –History of trauma
  - –Night-time symptoms
  - –Attempted treatments
  - –Systemic symptoms: Fever, rash, pain, fatigue
  - –Past medical history: Birth history, existing medical conditions, surgeries, broken bones, growth and development, medications
  - –Unusual exposures such as tick bites
- Physical exam
  - –Vital signs, including growth parameters
  - –Musculoskeletal exam for swelling, tenderness, warmth, redness, range of motion, asymmetry
  - –Muscle strength and neurologic exam (tone, sensory and reflexes)
  - –Lympadenopathy, organomegaly, rash, systemic symptoms
- Radiologic evaluation may include X-ray, US, MRI, and bone scan to evaluate for fracture, infection, tenosynovitis, or internal derangements
- Lab investigation may include CBC, ESR, CRP, examination of synovial fluid, viral titers (parvovirus), Lyme titers, RF, and ANA

Treatment

- If septic arthritis is a possibility, broad-spectrum antibiotic treatment should be started immediately
- Fractures and most internal derangements require orthopedics involvement
- Appropriate referral and treatment for malignancy
- JRA and SpA are usually treated with NSAIDs initially, DMARDs (e.g., sulfasalazine and methotrexate) and biologics (e.g., TNF blockers) are added depending on the degree of inflammation and the response of individual patient
- Supportive therapy such as PT and OT to increase range of motion and strength; insoles to correct leg length discrepancy
- Psychosocial support, especially with chronic arthritis

115. Asymmetric Limbs

With asymmetry of body parts, it can be difficult to differentiate whether one side is hypertrophic or the other side is atrophic. One of the most common asymmetries seen in children is leg-length discrepancy. Growth disturbances around the knee have a substantial effect on leg length, because distal femur (37%) and proximal tibia (28%) contribute the most to the growth of entire lower extremity.

Differential Diagnosis

- Physiologic: Left leg is often longer than right, and right arm is longer than left, though it is usually not noticeable
- Disturbances of bone
  - –Increased blood flow such as occurs in arthritis (infectious, inflammatory), neoplasms, or AVM
  - –Premature closure of epiphysis occurs with infection, fracture, radiation therapy, JRA
  - –Fracture may also result in malposition or malunion
  - –Diaphyseal operations (bone grafts, osteotomy)
  - –Developmental dysplasia of the hip
  - –Coxa vara, tibia vara (Blount disease)
  - –Hypoplastic bones (short femur)
  - –Legg-Calvé-Perthes disease
  - –SCFE
  - –Syndromes such as Albright; Ollier disease; neurofibromatosis
  - –Rickets
- Hemihypertrophy
  - –Idiopathic: May be associated with other anomalies involving GU tract, hemangiomas, mental retardation, and pigmented skin lesions
  - –Associated with tumors: Wilms, adrenocortical, hepatoblastoma
  - –Associated with dysmorphogenic syndromes: Beckwith-Wiedemann, Russell-Silver, *Proteus*
  - –Associated with soft tissue abnormalities: Lymphedema, Klippel-Trenaunay-Weber syndrome
- Neuromuscular disorders
  - –Cerebral palsy
  - –Poliomyelitis
  - –Myelomeningocele
  - –Peripheral neuropathy
  - –Focal cerebral lesions (Sturge-Weber syndrome)
  - –Stroke (due to coagulopathies, sickle cell disease)
- Hemophilia (bleeding into a joint)
- Reflex sympathetic dystrophy (RSD)
- Congenital syphilis
- Absence or hypoplasia of thumb and radius (Holt-Oram syndrome, TAR syndrome)

Workup and Diagnosis

- History
  - –Past medical and surgical history
  - –Constitutional symptoms (fever, fatigue, weight loss)
  - –Family history of similar disorder
- Physical exam
  - –Joint exam should include erythema, warmth, swelling, hyperflexibility, decreased range of motion, tenderness including pain localized to bone
  - –Leg-length discrepancy can be measured from symphysis pubis to lateral malleoli while patient is supine or by putting blocks of various thickness under the short leg until pelvis is leveled
  - –Dysmorpic features, skin lesions
  - –Neurologic exam for muscle weakness, decreased tone, reflexes, mental status
- Labs
  - –Infectious and inflammatory markers such as CBC, ESR, CRP, viral or bacterial titers and/or cultures; tumor markers; chromosomal analysis and genetic markers
  - –Radiologic evaluation as indicated by history and physical exam to find abnormalities in any part of musculoskeletal system (lytic lesions, soft tissue and joint swelling)
  - –Bone age
  - –Leg lengths measured by teleoroentgenogram, orthoradiograph, scanogram, or CT

Treatment

- Since underlying cause of an asymmetric limb is very broad, treatment varies depending on the etiology
- In certain cases, especially in those in which specific treatment would make a difference (DDH, SCFE, infection, inflammation malignancy), diagnosis must be made as soon as possible to prevent permanent damage
- Consider surgical (shortening or lengthening procedures, prostheses) and nonsurgical (orthotics, pressure stockings)
- Angular deformity should be looked at carefully and corrected before or at the same time of length equalization to avoid joint dislocation

116. Genu Varum (Bowed Legs)

Physiologic bowlegs is the most common cause of genu varum. It is a physiologic condition that resolves by 2 years of age. However, Blount disease is becoming a more common disorder due to increasing obesity in children.

Differential Diagnosis

- Physiologic
  - At birth, normal alignment is 10–15° of varus
  - Remodeling of bone resulting in neutral alignment occurs by 2 years of age
- Tibia vara (Blount disease)
  - Osteochondrosis of the medial tibial physis, combined with early walking and obesity, leads to compression across the physis that prevents normal growth
  - Increased incidence in males, blacks, and obese children
  - Infantile tibia vara (1–3 years old) is the most common form, is usually bilateral
  - Juvenile (4–10) and adolescent (>11) forms also exist, differing mainly in age at onset, remaining growth, and amount of compressive forces across posterior tibial medial physis
- Rickets
  - Growing bone is inadequately mineralized due to vitamin D deficiency (nutritional rickets) or a defect in mineral metabolism (X-linked hypophosphatemia)
- Skeletal dysplasias
  - Achondroplasia
  - Enchondromatosis
  - Metaphyseal dysplasia
- Trauma
  - Injury to proximal tibia physis may lead to growth arrest of physeal bar

Workup and Diagnosis

- History
  - Parental concern is often the presenting complaint
  - Past medical history and associated symptoms may aid in diagnosis of an underlying cause for bowlegs
- Physical exam
  - Plot the child's height on a nomogram
  - With patient standing in feet-together position, measure each femoral-tibial angle with a goniometer to quantify the genu varum
  - Measurement of the distance between the femoral medial condyles can aid in demonstrating progression or resolution
  - Assess tibial torsion (see Intoeing)
- Radiographic evaluation
  - In children younger than 2 years of age, plain X-ray may show proximal medial tibial metaphyseal beaking or fragmentation
  - In older children, standing, weight-bearing, full-length AP, and lateral X-rays allow for measurement of the metaphyseal-diaphyseal angle
  - Measurement of <10° correlates with physiologic bowing, and >16° correlates with Blount disease
- Langinskiold's I–VI stages are used to quantify degree of deformity

Treatment

- Treatment is based on age and severity
- Nonoperative
  - Bracing is effective in children <3 years old
  - 50% of patients have a mild form that responds to bracing
  - Trial time 9–12 months before considering surgery
- Operative
  - Operative treatment is more likely to be indicated for late-onset tibia vara
  - Proximal tibiofibular corrective osteotomy is performed in patients age >4 years old with progressive changes, and age <4 years old who have failed conservative treatment
  - Adolescent tibia vara can be corrected with osteotomy or hemiepiphysiodesis to restore normal mechanical axis

117. Clubbing

Clubbing (also termed acropachy, Hippocratic or watch-glass nails, drumstick fingers), characterized by an increase of the transverse and longitudinal nail curvatures, is a feature unique to humans. In children it is frequently associated with cyanotic congenital heart disease, cystic fibrosis, and inflammatory bowel disease. The exact etiology—circulating growth factor vs hypoxia—is unclear. It can occur as early as 3 months of age.

Differential Diagnosis

- Pulmonary
  - –Cystic fibrosis
  - –Bronchiectasis
  - –Empyema
  - –Pulmonary abscess
  - –Tuberculosis, aspergillosis
  - –Asthma complicated by infections
  - –Pulmonary alveolar proteinosis
  - –Sarcoidosis
  - –Interstitial pneumonitis (lymphoid, chronic)
  - –Pulmonary fibrosis
- Cardiovascular
  - –Cyanotic congenital heart disease
  - –Congestive heart failure
  - –Myxoid tumor
  - –Subacute bacterial endocarditis
  - –Myxomas
- Gastrointestinal
  - –Inflammatory bowel disease
  - –Gardner syndrome
  - –Parasitosis
  - –Biliary cirrhosis or biliary atresia
  - –Chronic active hepatitis
  - –Celiac disease
- Other
  - –Diamond syndrome (myxedema, exophthalmos, clubbing)
  - –Thyrotoxicosis
  - –Hypervitaminosis A
  - –Malnutrition
- Acquired, one or more digits
  - –Aortic/subclavian aneurysm
  - –Brachial plexus injury
  - –Shoulder subluxation
  - –Trauma
  - –Maffucci syndrome
  - –Gout
  - –Sarcoidosis
  - –Severe herpetic whitlow
- Idiopathic
- Hereditary, familial (isolated)
  - –Pachydermoperiostosis
- Pseudoclubbing (broad distal phalanges with normally shaped nails)
  - –Apert syndrome
  - –Pfeiffer syndrome
  - –Rubinstein-Taybi syndrome

Workup and Diagnosis

- Physical exam is diagnostic
  - –Often begins in the thumb and index fingers; earliest signs are softening and loss of angle at the base of the nail; nail beds are excessively compressible and skin overlying the base of the nail is red and shiny
  - –The ungual-phalangeal angle (Lovibond angle): Measured by visualizing a "V," with the tip placed on the nail fold, one arm pointing toward the tip of the nail and the other arm oriented along the finger; with clubbing the angle is $\geq 180°$
  - –Opposition of the dorsum of two fingers from opposite hands in normal individuals delineates a diamond-shaped window at the base of the nail beds; in early clubbing, this window is obliterated
  - –The clubbing index (CI) is a ratio of distal phalangeal depth to interphalangeal depth; CI is equal or greater to 1.0 when clubbing is present; in cystic fibrosis patients, CI correlates negatively with PaO_2, FEV_1, $FEF_{25–75\%}$, and positively with the residual volume
  - –Painful clubbing is indicative of periostitis associated with hypertrophic pulmonary osteoarthropathy
  - –Toe clubbing can be seen in patent ductus arteriosus, reversed shunt, and pulmonary hypertension
- Histologic changes of the nail matrix include increased dermal fibroblasts, mucoid degeneration; and interstitial edema, infiltration with plasma cells, lymphocytes, and primitive fibroblasts

Treatment

- No specific treatment available
- In general, elimination or improvement in the associated condition is associated with a decrease in the degree of clubbing
- Reversible in cystic fibrosis patients who undergo lung transplantation
  - –Regression noted mostly during the first 3 months post transplantation
- Remission observed after sectioning the thoracic vagus nerve in patients with pulmonary malignancy (uncommon condition in the pediatric population), even without removing the tumor itself
- Colchicine can be used for the associated pain

118. Hip Pain

Hip pain encompasses a broad differential that relies on a focused and detailed history to determine the acute and emergent diagnoses from the less urgent hip problems. The most urgent diagnosis to make is septic arthritis, and the most challenging etiologies to manage are those that mimic septic arthritis.

Differential Diagnosis

- Septic arthritis
  - –Surgical emergency due to irreversible chondrolysis and epiphyseal injury
  - –Acute process leading to decreased hip range of motion, severe pain with passive range of motion
- Slipped capital femoral epiphysis (SCFE)
  - –Typically in obese, adolescent males with aching groin, hip, or knee
  - –May have externally rotated hip position and gait
- Legg-Calvé-Perthes
  - –Presents at younger age than SCFE (3–8 years old)
  - –Five times greater incidence in boys than girls
  - –Pain in hip or knee, decreased active and passive ROM, and Trendelenburg gait
- Developmental dysplasia of the hip (DDH)
  - –Early diagnosis with newborn exam finding of easily dislocatable hip
  - –Older infants have limited hip abduction
- Osteomyelitis
  - –Vague symptoms may make this a difficult diagnosis
  - –Limp, fever, pain in the proximal thigh or pseudoparalysis of an extremity in an infant may be the only sign
- Fracture
  - –Consider accidental and nonaccidental trauma
  - –Pain, limited ambulation, limited active and passive ROM, or inability to bear weight
- Transient monoarticular synovitis
  - –Often preceded 1–2 weeks by upper respiratory infection
  - –Antalgic gait, moderate pain in hip, groin, or knee, and uncomfortable range of motion
- Neoplasia
  - –Although primary bone disorders do not generally present with hip pain, other malignancies such as acute leukemia may initially present with bone or joint pain
- Vertebral osteomyelitis/diskitis
  - –Referred pain from lumbrosacral region may present as hip pain

Workup and Diagnosis

- Despite urgency of surgical emergencies, a thorough history is essential
  - –Onset and duration of symptoms, location, and character of pain
  - –Previous trauma, preceding illness, or associated symptoms
  - –Past medical history/family history: Bone, hematologic, and metabolic disorders
- Labs
  - –CBC with differential, platelets, PT/INR, ESR, CRP
- Radiographic evaluation
  - –Plain X-ray: AP pelvis and frog-leg lateral of the pelvis, full length femur, and knee films
  - –CT scan: Helps define bony anatomy especially with 3D reconstruction images
  - –MRI may demonstate joint effusion in synovitis and infection, marrow edema in osteomyelitis, physeal widening in SCFE, or occult fracture such as femoral neck stress fracture
  - –Ultrasound for newborn DDH
- Nuclear medicine
  - –Triple-phase bone scan may be helpful when the diagnosis is questionable, or if differentiating between bone and joint infections
- Interventional radiology
  - –Joint aspiration to evaluate for septic arthritis

Treatment

- Septic arthritis, femoral neck fracture, and irreducible traumatic hip dislocation require immediate surgical intervention
- Infectious disease consult for septic joint
- Once surgical emergencies are ruled out, keeping the patient non-weight bearing on the affected extremity will allow continued investigation without further injury
- SCFE: Prevent further slippage by percutaneous pinning or screw fixation
- Legg-Calvé-Perthes: Treatment goals include restoring ROM, improving symptoms, and containing the femoral epiphysis during reossification phase; accomplished by limiting activity, traction, Petrie casting, and surgical procedures for containment
- DDH: Pavlik harness, closed reduction and casting, open reduction for irreducible hip dislocation, or femoral and/or pelvic osteotomy depending on status and age of developing hip

119. Knee Pain

Knee pain is a common complaint that is readily evaluated by focusing on the anatomic structures. A focused history and exam will often give the diagnosis. Because hip pain can radiate to the knee, a thorough lower extremity exam should always be performed.

Differential Diagnosis

- Septic arthritis
  - –Characterized by redness, swelling or effusion, warmth, pain with active and passive ROM, fever or chills
  - –Requires urgent evaluation and diagnosis
- Osgood-Schlatter disease (OSD)
  - –Repetitive microtrauma to the bone-tendon junction where patellar tendon inserts into the secondary ossification center of the tibial tubercle
  - –Onset at early adolescence, more often in athletes
- Sinding-Larsen-Johansson disease
  - –Similar to OSD, except localized to distal pole of the patella
- Meniscal pathology
  - –Meniscal tears are usually associated with acute trauma, and involve pain and swelling with mechanical symptoms such as popping, clicking, or locking
  - –Discoid meniscus: Mechanical symptoms and plain X-rays show squaring, widening, and cupping
- Ligamentous injury
  - –Medial collateral ligament sprain via overuse injury or valgus force to knee
  - –Anterior cruciate ligament tear associated with sport noncontact pivoting injury, associated with a "pop" and immediate swelling
  - –Posterior cruciate tear associated with direct trauma to anterior tibia or hyperflexion with plantar flexed foot
  - –Lateral collateral ligament injury is rare
- Osteochondritis dissecans
  - –Trauma resulting in separation of subchondral bone and cartilage at lateral aspect of medial femoral condyle
- Patellar subluxation/dislocation
  - –Lateral displacement of patella associated with increased Q angle, genu valgum, and femoral anteversion (more common in women)
- Bursitis
  - –Chronic friction over pes anserine, iliotibial band, or capsular bursa leads to inflammation and thickening of the bursa
- Bipartite patella
  - –Common variant of patellar ossification

Workup and Diagnosis

- History
  - –Specific location, duration, onset, aggravating or alleviating factors, and pain characteristics
  - –Previous trauma, preceding illness, or associated symptoms
  - –Past medical history and family history including bone, hematologic, or metabolic disorders
- Physical exam
  - –Bilateral hip, knee, and ankle exam
  - –Redness, warmth, effusion, active and passive ROM
  - –Palpate joint line, patella, tibial tubercle, pes anserine, and medial/lateral ligaments
  - –Patella tracking or apprehension, varus/valgus stress, Lachman, and anterior posterior drawer tests
  - –Crepitus along the flexion arc and McMurray test
- Labs
  - –Often not needed unless concerned about infection
  - –CBC with differential, platelets, PT/INR, ESR, CRP
  - –Knee aspirate for cell count and differential with Gram stain, culture, and crystals
- Radiography
  - –Plain X-ray: Screening knee films include AP, lateral, Merchant views
  - –AP pelvis and frog-leg lateral of the pelvis or femur films if indicated by exam findings
- MRI to show soft tissues such as meniscus and ligaments
  - –May demonstate joint effusion in synovitis/infection, marrow edema in osteomyelitis, ligament rupture

Treatment

- Septic arthritis requires immediate surgical intervention and, unlike hip sepsis, the knee may be easily ruled out by aspiration in either emergency room or clinic
- Generally rest, ice, NSAID therapy, and short course of physical therapy to improve strength is the treatment of choice for many of the more common ailments, including bipartite patella, bursitis, patella subluxation, small osteochondritis dissecans lesions, ligament sprain, Osgood-Schlatter and Sinding-Larsen-Johanssen disorders
- Knee immobilization is warranted in acute injuries and non-weight bearing when fracture or ligament injury is suspected, to allow time for diagnostic evaluation to be performed while keeping the patient comfortable and protected from further injury
- Knee arthroscopy is minimally invasive and helpful with diagnosis or treatment in case of ligament repair, Osteochondritis dissecans repair and realignment procedures

120. Limp

Evaluation of limp in a child can be very difficult. The differential is very wide, and the history is often nonspecific. Physical examination may likewise be unremarkable or nonspecific. Limp may be the herald sign of a systemic condition, so treatment may be directed at the underlying cause rather than at the affected extremity.

Differential Diagnosis

- Transient synovitis: Etiology unknown; may be viral, postviral, or traumatic; occurs in preschool children, M>F; presents with limp or refusal to walk
- Malignancy: Neuroblastoma, leukemia, sarcoma (Ewing, osteogenic), rhabdomyosarcoma
- Osteochondritis dissecans: Necrosis of the articular surfaces due to repetitive stress
- Fracture
  - –Stress fracture of foot, subtle ankle, foot fractures, patellar avulsion fracture, toddler's fracture of the tibia
- Musculoskeletal injury
  - –Knee and ankle injuries are most common in school-age and adolescents during athletics or vigorous activity
  - –Meniscal and ligamentous injuries to the knee are increasingly common
- Spine: Compression fracture, herniated disc, diskitis
- Rheumatologic: JRA, ankylosing spondylitis, SLE
- Legg-Calvé-Perthes disease (LCP): Vascular insult to the proximal femoral epiphysis leading to osteonecrosis
- Slipped capital femoral epiphysis (SCFE): Result of weakness of the perichondral ring, leading to slippage through the hypertrophic zone in the growth plate of the proximal femoral epiphysis
- Osgood-Schlatter (OSD): Repetitive small avulsion injuries at the tibial tuberosity
- Infectious
  - –Septic arthritis of hip: Fever, hip pain, refusal to walk, limp
  - –Septic arthritis of knee: Swelling, usually fever, well-localized pain
  - –Lyme arthritis
  - –Cellulitis
  - –Soft-tissue abscess
  - –Osteomyelitis (pelvis, femur, knee, foot, ankle)
- Duchenne muscular dystrophy
- Charcot-Marie-Tooth disease (CMT)
- Non-accidental trauma (NAT)
  - –Musculoskeletal injury in a child who is not developmentally capable of an action that would cause such an injury is very suspicious

Workup and Diagnosis

- History
  - –Pain: Musculoskeletal is worse in the evening and after activity; malignancy may present with pain at night, early morning pain may be transient synovitis or JRA
  - –Duration of symptoms: Long-term is more alarming
  - –Malaise, fever, activity
  - –Exposure to STD, ticks
  - –Location of pain
- Physical exam
  - –Areas of tenderness, muscle weakness or atrophy
  - –ROM of spine, extremities
  - –Spine abnormalities, tenderness, SI joint
  - –Symmetry
- Labs
  - –ESR, CBC
  - –Blood culture if osteomyelitis or septic joint is suspected
- Studies
  - –Plain films, including special views as directed by H&P; tunnel view for osteochondritis dissecans; frog-leg view to evaluate the joint space of the hip
  - –Bone scan is best for osteomyelitis, may be positive in malignancy
  - –CT for benign bony lesions
  - –MRI for soft-tissue lesions and sarcomas

Treatment

- Transient synovitis: Resolves with supportive care
- Malignancy: Referral to oncologist
- Osteochondritis dissecans: Rest, immobilization, or surgical debridement and fixation
- Musculoskeletal injury: Variable depending on degree and location of injury; options include supportive care, physical therapy, surgical reconstruction
- Fractures: Variable depending on degree and location of injury: options include traction, casting, surgical pins
- Rheumatologic: Generally treated with NSAIDs, steroids, immunosuppressives
- LCP: Rest, traction, bracing, surgery
- SCFE: Non-weight bearing, percutaneous pinning
- Infectious: Appropriate antibiotics for cellulitis, septic arthritis, osteomyelitis, diskitis
- OSD: Resolves with decreased activity, rest, NSAIDs
- Duchenne MD and CMT: Progressive neurologic deterioration; physical therapy may help

121. Muscle Weakness – Distal

Distal weakness is most likely secondary to neuropathy, and is often associated with loss of deep tendon reflexes (DTRs) either with or without sensory abnormalities. In contrast, increased DTRs or extensor plantor responses raise the concern for "central" causes of weakness (stroke, neoplasm, demyelinating disease, etc.).

Differential Diagnosis

- Guillain-Barré syndrome (GBS)
  - –Acute, acquired, or monophasic
  - –Ascending weakness and parasthesias
- Chronic inflammatory demyelinating polyradiculoneuropathy (CIDP)
- Compression neuropathy
  - –Trauma
  - –Neoplasm (e.g., plexiform neurofibroma in neurofibromatosis type 1)
- Charcot-Marie-Tooth
  - –Defect in peripheral myelin protein
  - –Causes distal segmental demyelination
  - –Manifested by distal muscle atrophy and weakness
- Drug-induced
  - –Phenytoin
  - –Isoniazid
  - –Nitrofurantoin
  - –Vincristine
  - –Zidovudine
- Spinal muscular atrophy
- Juvenile segmental spinal muscular atrophy
- Miller-Fisher syndrome
  - –Clinical triad of ataxia, ophthalmoplegia, and areflexia
- Tick paralysis
- Juvenile amyotrophic lateral sclerosis
- Giant axonal neuropathy
- Vitamin B12 deficiency
- Toxic neuropathy
  - –Arsenic
  - –Lead
  - –Mercury
  - –Thallium
  - –Glue sniffing
- Uremic neuropathy
- Idiopathic axonal neuropathy
- Hereditary distal myopathy
- Inclusion body myopathy
- Rheumatoid arthritis
- Refsum disease
- Metachromatic leukodystrophy
- Krabbe disease
- Cockayne syndrome
- Conversion reaction
  - –Usually fluctuating and unpredictable

Workup and Diagnosis

- History
  - –Acute vs chronic, associated sensory findings, associated systemic/neurologic abnormalities
  - –Family history (family members may not be affected to same degree)
  - –Toxic exposures
- Physical exam
  - –Abnormal gait can be the presenting symptom of either proximal or distal leg weakness
  - –Stumbling, especially with foot eversion or dorsiflexion
  - –Weakness of the hand muscles (e.g., difficulty writing, opening jars, or working with tools)
  - –Inspect muscle for atropy, hypertrophy, fasciculations, myotonia, cogwheeling
  - –Palpate muscles for tenderness
  - –Mirror movements, hypotonia, spasticity/rigidity
  - –Assess strength and power with push/pull testing, functional hop in place, knee bends, posture
  - –Pronator drift, standing on toes/heels, symmetry
- Labs
  - –Serum CK
  - –In neuropathic disorders, CK is usually normal or mildly increased; moderate to severe elevation of CK suggests myopathy
- Electromyogram/nerve conduction studies
  - –Demonstrate the extent, chronicity, and categorization
- Muscle biopsy
  - –Histochemistry, EM, enzymatic/genetic testing

Treatment

- Acute demyelinating disorders (GBS, CIDP)
  - –Often respond to intravenous gamma-globulin
- Medication/chemotherapy-induced neuropathies
  - –Often improved after cessation of the offending medication
  - –Response is time-dependent; may take up to months
- Toxic exposures
  - –Often difficult to detect, unless resulting from acute overdose
- Metabolic neuropathies are treated supportively
- Braces often assist with foot drop for both acquired and congenital neuropathies

122. Muscle Weakness – Proximal

Proximal weakness is usually due to dysfunction of the lower motor unit; that is, anterior horn cells in the spinal cord, neuromuscular junction (NMJ), or the muscle itself. The neurologic examination, EMG, and nerve conduction studies, and finally the muscle enzymes and biopsy, guide the diagnosis.

Differential Diagnosis

- Duchenne and Becker muscular dystrophy
- Spinal muscular atrophy
- Spinal cord disorders
  - –Trauma
  - –Myelitis
  - –Neoplasm
  - –AVM
  - –Hemorrhage
  - –Tansverse myelitis
- Limb-girdle myasthenia
- Dermatomyositis
- Congenital myopathies
  - –Central core disease
  - –Myotubular
  - –Nemaline (rod)
  - –Congenital fiber-type disproportion
- Facioscapulohumeral syndrome
- Limb-girdle muscular dystrophies
- Glycogen storage myopathies
- Endocrine myopathies
  - –Hypo- and hyperthyroidism
  - –Hyperparathyroidism
  - –Adrenalism
- Polymyositis
- GM2 gangliosidosis
- Pompe disease
  - –Glycogen storage disease type II
  - –Acid maltase deficiency
- McArdle disease
- Carnitine deficiency
- Fatty acid oxidation defects
- Mitochondrial disorders
- Steroid-induced myopathy
- Slow channel syndrome
- Toxins
  - –Organophosphates
  - –Aminoglycosides
  - –Tetrodotoxin (pufferfish)
- Conversion reaction
- Myasthenia gravis

Workup and Diagnosis

- History: Age upon reaching developmental milestones, abnormal gait, toe walking, easy fatigability, muscle cramps, facial weakness, cardiac, respiratory, GI problems, dark urine
- Physical exam: Muscle mass, texture and tenderness, scoliosis, cardiac exam, skin rashes, joint contractures
- Neurologic exam
  - –Muscle strength and tone
  - –Gowers sign
  - –Mental status, eye movements
  - –Facial movements, tongue fasciculations
  - –Muscle stretch reflexes and sensory responses
  - –Stance and gait
  - –Spinal cord disorders, examine dermatomal sensory loss, anal wink, cremasteric reflex
- Labs: Muscle enzymes (CPK, aldolase); electrolytes, TSH, lactate, pyruvate, carnitine; ANA, RF, genetic testing for muscular dystrophy and spinal muscular atrophy; hexosaminidase, acetylcholine receptor antibodies, myoglobin in urine (muscle breakdown)
- EMG/nerve conduction studies
  - –Differentiates dysfunction of the anterior horn cell, muscle, or neuromuscular junction
- Muscle biopsy for metabolic, inflammatory, and congenital myopathies; distinguishes myopathy from anterior horn cell disease
- MRI of the spine for spinal cord disorder
- Tensilon test for myasthenia

Treatment

- Combination of physical therapy, bracing, and orthopedic surgical interventions can help patients maintain functional motor skills
- Duchenne muscular dystrophy
  - –Oral prednisone to increase and sustain muscle strength
- Endocrine myopathies
  - –Treating the underlying endocrine disease corrects the myopathy and weakness
- Dermatomyositis
  - –Oral prednisone
  - –If resistant to oral steroids, immunosuppression with high-dose intravenous steroids, methotrexate, cyclophosphamide or intravenous immunoglobulins
- Transverse myelitis
  - –Treat with high-dose intravenous steroids
- Myasthenia gravis
  - –Acetylcholinesterase inhibitors (pyridostigmine), immunosuppression, and thymectomy

123. Raynaud Phenomenon

Raynaud phenomenon is a periodic vasoconstrictor response to cold and physical or emotional stress. It was first described in 1862 by Raynaud, a French medical student. He attributed the color changes to exaggerated CNS response. Exact pathophysiology is still not understood, but several players, such as altered skin blood flow, platelet activation, locally secreted mediators of smooth muscle tone, and endothelial injury may be involved to various degrees depending on the form of Raynaud. The population prevalence is 5–10%.

Differential Diagnosis

- Raynaud phenomenon is triphasic
  - –Pallor (white): Decreased cutaneous blood flow
  - –Cyanosis (blue): Venous stasis
  - –Erythema (red): Reflex vasodilation
  - –Fingers are affected more than toes; earlobes, tip of nose, lips, and tongue may also be affected
  - –The presence of intense, painful episodes with ischemic skin lesions and clinical features (arthritis, rash) of a connective tissue disease suggests a secondary cause
  - –Idiopathic Raynaud is uncommon in children apart from familial benign type; however, if there are no clinical or laboratory signs in the 2 years after Raynaud develops, an underlying disease is unlikely
- Familial benign type
  - –Median age at onset is around 14 years
  - –Positive family history in a first-degree relative in 25%
  - –ESR is normal and ANA is negative
- Connective tissue disease
  - –Scleroderma: Almost 90% have Raynaud; it is the initial symptom in most cases
  - –May also be found in SLE and CREST syndrome
- Vascular diseases
  - –Takayasu arteritis
  - –Giant cell arteritis
  - –Arteriosclerosis
  - –Thromboangitis obliterans
  - –Thoracic outlet syndrome
- Environmental causes
  - –Frostbite
  - –Polyvinyl chloride disease
  - –Vibration disease
  - –Hypothenar hammer syndrome
- Neuropathy (e.g., carpal tunnel syndrome)
- Primary endocrine abnormalities
  - –Hypothyroidism
  - –GH excess/acromegaly
- Hormone-secreting tumors
  - –Pheochromocytoma
  - –Carcinoid syndrome

Workup and Diagnosis

- History
  - –Sensitivity to cold with color changes (white or blue)
  - –Medication and environmental/cold injury, toxins, digital ulcers, long-lasting wounds
  - –Signs and symptoms of a possible systemic disease (myalgias, arthralgias/arthritis, weakness, weight loss, fever, rash; respiratory, CV, and GI symptoms)
- Physical exam
  - –Vital signs (fever, tachypnea, tachycardia, absent pulses, asymmetric blood pressure)
  - –Skin exam for rashes and ulcers
  - –Nail fold capillary exam
  - –Arthritis
  - –Lymphadenopathy
  - –Organomegaly
- Labs
  - –Indicated for patients with signs and symptoms compatible with a systemic disease
  - –CBC with differential, ESR/CRP, chemistry, urinalysis
  - –ANA and disease-specific autoantibodies, C3, C4
  - –TFTs, serum protein electrophoresis, cryoglobulins
- Vascular studies
  - –Indicated for patients with history of asymmetric attacks, physical exam findings of absent pulses, blood pressure asymmetry, evidence of ischemia
  - –Doppler ultrasonography
  - –Plethysmography
  - –Angiography

Treatment

- Avoidance of cold temperature exposure
  - –Wear warm hats, socks, and gloves
- Stress management
  - –Biofeedback techniques
  - –Both temperature-related and other relaxation techniques
- Calcium-channel blockers (such as nifedipine)
  - –Clinical trials have shown significant benefit, thus they are widely used
- Other agents (frequently used but not well studied) Prazosin, losartan, pentoxifylline, fluoxetine, nitroglycerine, hydralazine, papavarine
- Promising experimental agents: Iloprost (prostacyclin analog); cilostazol and sildenafil (phosphodiesterase inhibitors); bosentan (endothelin-receptor inhibitor)
- Sympathectomy: Limited benefit, should be reserved for patients with severe ischemia unresponsive to medical treatment

124. Toeing In

Toeing in, or intoeing, is a commonly referred problem to orthopedic surgeons. The mainstay of treatment includes parental reassurance. Symtoms in the majority of patients resolve spontaneously by 8 years old.

Differential Diagnosis

- Femoral anteversion
  - –Most common cause of intoeing in children between 2 and 6 years old
  - –Incidence in females is twice that of males
  - –Femoral shaft internal alignment leads to entire lower limb to be inwardly rotated
- Internal tibial torsion
  - –Most common cause of intoeing in children less than 2 years of age
  - –Inward rotation of the tibia leads to intoeing
- Metatarsus adductus
  - –Forefoot is adducted, with a concave medial foot border with increased space between the first and second toes
  - –May be due to in utero packaging problems; thus is associated with a higher incidence of hip dysplasia
- Muscle force imbalance
  - –Neuromuscular disorders such as cerebral palsy have a higher incidence of lower extremity rotational abnormalities due to increased muscular tone and dynamic imbalance
- Pronated feet (flatfeet)
  - –Children typically stand with feet in valgus position, because this is unstable for walking; children toe in to shift the center of gravity to the center of the foot
- Knock knees
- Maldirection of the acetabulum
  - –If the acetabulum is directed anteriorly toeing in will stabilize the hip joint

Workup and Diagnosis

- History is generally limited
  - –Often the family gives a history that the child tends to stumble or fall more than other children
  - –Development and milestones are usually normal
- Physical exam consists of a rotational profile using four elements to help with diagnosis and monitoring the progression of intoeing
- First element: Hip rotation
  - –Measured with the patient prone, hips extended, and knees flexed 90°
  - –Lateral rotation; external rotation with <20° indicates femoral anteversion
  - –Medial rotation; internal rotation with >70° also indicates femoral anteversion
- Second element: Thigh-foot angle
  - –Measurement in prone position of long axis of foot relative to axis of thigh with knee flexed at 90°
  - –Neutral or foot pointed inward indicates internal tibial torsion
- Third element: Foot evaluation
  - –Foot alignment is assessed in prone position, and heel bisector line lines up with second metatarsal
- Fourth element: Foot progression angle (gait evaluation)
  - –When the child walks, estimate the angle of the foot relative to the line of progression
  - –If patella is inward, then the femur may be anteverted
  - –If patella points straight, then the tibia or foot is causing the deviation

Treatment

- Natural history of rotational variations is gradual normalization and is not altered by nonsurgical methods
- The use of orthotics, shoe modifications, or exercises is ineffective
- Femoral anteversion seen in children 2–6 years old usually corrects spontaneously by 10 years old
- Most cases of tibial torsion resolve spontaneously by 4–6 years old
- Surgical correction is reserved for severe gait deformity (patients who have persistent rotational abnormality into adolescence and find their gait appearance unacceptable)

125. Toeing Out

Toeing out, or out-toeing, is not as common as intoeing. Excessive out-toeing is considered a normal variant. Observation and parental reassurance are the mainstays of therapy.

Differential Diagnosis

- Femoral retroverson
  - Usually bilateral with excessive external and limited internal range of motion of both hips
- External tibial torsion
  - More common than femoral retroversion
  - May be related to in utero positioning and is sometimes associated with calcaneovalgus foot
- Slipped capital femoral epiphysis (SCFE)
  - Most common in obese adolescent boys
  - Unilateral out-toeing with painful hip
  - Pain and limited range of motion or antalgic externally rotated gait pattern
- Talipes calcaneovalgus
  - Positional deformity in which the foot is extremely dorseflexed and everted
- Everted flat feet
  - Children stand in a toe out position but toe in when walking
- Triceps surae muscle contracture
  - Can be seen with cerebral palsy
- Vertical talus (rocker-bottom foot)
- Congenital absence of the fibula
  - Shortening of the peroneal and triceps surae muscles result in bowing of the tibia and equinovalgus
- Maldirection of the acetabulum
  - If the acetabulum faces posteriorly, leg position is everted

Workup and Diagnosis

- History is generally limited
  - Development and milestones are generally normal
  - Hip pain and limp are red flags for SCFE
- Physical examination consists of a rotational profile using four elements to help with diagnosis and monitoring
- First element: Hip rotation
  - Measurement is performed in prone position, hips extended and knees flexed to 90°
  - Lateral rotation; external rotation with >70° indicates femoral retroversion
  - Medial rotation; internal rotation with <20° also indicates femoral retroversion
- Second element: Thigh-foot angle
  - Measurement is performed in prone position, hips extended, and knee flexed at 90°, evaluating long axis of foot relative to axis of thigh
  - Neutral or foot pointed outward >40° (normal 0–30°) indicates external tibial torsion
- Third element: Foot evaluation
  - Foot alignment is assessed in prone and standing position; heel bisector line should line up with second metatarsal
- Fourth element: Foot progression angle (gait evaluation)
  - When the child walks, estimate the angle of the foot relative to the line of progression
  - If patella is outward, then the femur may be retroverted
  - If patella points straight, then the tibia or foot is causing the deviation

Treatment

- Natural history of rotational variations is gradual normalization and is not altered by nonsurgical methods
- Out-toeing is generally self-limited and improves at 2–3 years old until 8 years old; reassurance that the condition will improve is the most important component of treatment
- The use of orthotics, shoe modifications, or exercises is ineffective
- Surgical correction is reserved for severe gait deformity or when related to SCFE
- Even after surgical intervention for SCFE, external rotational abnormality into adolescence may persist, and derotational osteotomy may be beneficial

Nervous System

Section 15

NICOLE J. ULLRICH, MD, PhD
MUSTAFA SAHIN, MD, PhD

126. Ataxia

Ataxia is due to dysfunction of the cerebellum or its connections. It can present as an acute or chronic/progressive illness. Associated signs and symptoms such as papilledema, myoclonus, and retinopathy help determine the underlying etiology.

Differential Diagnosis

- Infectious
  - –Postinfectious cerebellitis: Due to varicella, EBV, mumps, *Legionella*, hepatitis A
  - –Encephalitis, acute disseminated encephalomyelitis (ADEM)
  - –Cerebellar abscess
  - –Labyrinthitis
- Toxic/metabolic encephalopathy
  - –Phenytoin, carbamazepine, antihistamines, sedatives, and ethanol
- Posterior fossa tumor
  - –Medulloblastoma, glioma
- Opsoclonus/myoclonus syndrome: May be postinfectious or paraneoplastic (reaction most likely to neuroblastoma)
- Friedreich ataxia: Absent DTRs, positive Babinski sign, proprioceptive sensory loss, dysarthria, cardiomyopathy, diabetes
- Ataxia-telangiectasia
- Miller-Fisher variant of Guillain-Barré syndrome, with areflexia, ophthalmoparesis
- Basilar migraine
- Postconcusssion
- Seizure
- Arnold-Chiari, Dandy-Walker malformation
- Cerebellar hemorrhage or ischemia
- Multiple sclerosis
- Vitamin E (AVED), biotinidase deficiency
- Metabolic disorders
  - –Urea cycle disorders
  - –Organic acidurias (maple syrup urine disease)
  - –Carbohydrate-deficient glycoprotein syndrome
- Sphingolipidoses (GM2, Niemann-Pick type C, metachromatic leukodystrophy, Krabbe disease)
- Neuronal ceroid-lipofuscinosis
- Mitochondrial disease
  - –NARP, MERRF, Kearns-Sayre syndrome
- Spinocerebellar ataxias (SCA)
- Hartnup disease
- Refsum disease
- Episodic ataxia type I/II (channelopathy)
- Celiac disease
  - –Have cerebellar calcification
- Conversion disorder

Workup and Diagnosis

- History: Acute vs chronic, progression, episodicity, recent illness (especially varicella), ingestion of toxins or drugs, trauma, previous episode of ataxia, headaches, gait disturbance, family history of migraine or spinocerebellar ataxias
- Physical exam
  - –Skin (telangiectasias), ear, sinus examination
  - –Cardiac exam, abdominal masses (for neuroblastoma)
  - –Neurologic exam: Cranial nerve and cerebellar examinations, papilledema, extraocular eye movements and nystagmus, DTRs, Babinski sign, proprioceptive sense, Romberg sign
- Labs
  - –Toxicology screen
  - –LP (only after neuroimaging) for infection/GBS/MS
  - –HVA, VMA levels (for neuroblastoma)
  - –Thoracic and abdominal MRI for neuroblastoma
  - –EEG for seizures
- Metabolic testing: Serum amino acids, vitamin E, cholesterol and subtypes, lactate, pyruvate, ammonia, α-feto protein (for ataxia telangiectasia), lysosomal enzymes, transferrin eletrophoresis
  - –Electromicroscopy of lymphocytes for inclusion bodies
  - –Muscle biopsy for mitochondrial disease
- Genetic testing for Friedreich ataxia and SCA
- Imaging: CT or MRI for mass lesion or demyelination
  - –MRI is superior to CT for detection of posterior fossa

Treatment

- In most cases, the treatment will be supportive
- Exogenous toxins should be stopped and removed
- Neoplasms, abscesses, hemorrhage require neurosurgical evaluation and intervention
- Patients with Friedreich ataxia and mitochondrial disease need cardiac evaluation
- Miller-Fisher variant of Guillain-Barré syndrome
  - –Usually has a very good prognosis
  - –IV immunoglobulin or plasmaphoresis may be used
- Opsoclonus/myoclonus syndrome
  - –Treated with steroids, ACTH, or IVIG
  - –Neuroblastoma needs surgical evaluation
- ADEM: Treat with high-dose intravenous steroids
- AVED: Treat with vitamin E
- Biotinidase deficiency: Treat with biotinidase
- Hartnup disease: Treat with niacin
- Refsum disease: Dietary restriction of phytanic acid
- Epidosic ataxia: Treat with acetazolamide

127. Chorea

Chorea consists of brief, irregular, nonrhythmic, unsustained involuntary movements that flow from one part of the body to another. Chorea is often accompanied by athetosis, which are slow, writhing, involuntary movements. These movement disorders are thought to result from dysfunction of the basal ganglia.

Differential Diagnosis

- Toxins
  - –Neuroleptics, phenytoin, antiemetics, oral contraceptives, theophylline, L-dopa, stimulants, lithium, carbon monoxide, manganese
- Sydenham chorea (in rheumatic fever)
  - –Migratory chorea, hypotonia, dysarthria, emotional liability
  - –Usually 4 months after group A β-hemolytic *Streptococcus* infection
  - –Molecular mimicry between streptococcal and CNS antigens results in formation of cross-reactive antibodies that disrupt basal ganglia function
  - –Carditis is present in 80% of Sydenham chorea patients
- Inherited choreas
  - –Benign familial chorea
  - –Juvenile Huntington chorea (usually presents with rigidity)
  - –Familial paroxysmal choreoathetosis
- Postinfectious: Mycoplasma, HSV, EBV, echovirus 25, varicella
- Encephalitis: viral, mycoplasma, Lyme
- Post-cardiac surgery
  - –"Post-pump chorea"
  - –Usually 2 weeks after cardiac surgery
- Syndrome or disease associated
  - –Wilson disease
  - –Hallervorden-Spatz (disorder of iron metabolism with degeneration of globus pallidus)
  - –Fahr disease: Encephalopathy and progressive calcification of basal ganglia
  - –Lesch-Nyhan syndrome
  - –Ataxia-telangiectasia
- Endocrine: Hyperthyroidism, pregnancy (chorea gravidarum)
- Acquired brain disorders
  - –Multiple sclerosis, basal ganglia stroke, hypoxic ischemic encephalopathy, neoplasm
- Abetalipoproteinemia
- Glutaric aciduria type I
- Neuroacanthocytosis
- Systemic lupus erythematosus
- Kernicterus
- Antiphospholipid antibody syndrome
- Mitochondrial encephalopathies

Workup and Diagnosis

- History
  - –Fever, rash associated symptoms
  - –History of streptococcal infections, rheumatic fever, arthritis
  - –Birth history, family history, medications, ingestions
- Physical exam
  - –Eye exam: Kayser-Fleischer rings (Wilson disease)
  - –Cardiac, joint, and skin exam (for rheumatic fever)
  - –Neurologic exam should include eye movement, dysarthria, evaluation of tone, motor impersistence
- Labs
  - –Electrolytes, glucose, calcium, magnesium, LFTs, BUN/Cr, acetate, pyruvate
  - –TSH, parathyroid hormone, hCG
  - –CBC and blood smear (for acanthocytes)
  - –Throat culture, antistreptolysin O titer
  - –Ceruloplasmin (low in Wilson disease), amino acids
  - –Lyme titer
  - –Anti-nuclear, anti-cardiolipin, anti-phospholipid, anti-dsDNA antibodies
  - –Rheumatoid factor, lipid profile
  - –Huntington disease genetic testing
- Studies
  - –Cardiac evaluation with Echo, ECG
  - –LP useful in infectious or postinfectious cases
    - –Multiple sclerosis (find oligoclonal bands)
  - –Neuroimaging: CT or preferably MRI

Treatment

- Treatment should be reserved for patients in whom chorea severity interferes with function
  - –Simple measures such as rest and avoidance of stress often alleviate symptoms
  - –Anti-epilepsy medications are used for paroxysmal choreas
  - –Dopamine blockers such as haloperidol and pimozide are used to decrease the movement disorder
- Sydenham chorea
  - –May be treated with valproate or pimozide
  - –Immunosuppression with steroids, intravenous immunoglobulin or plasmapheresis have been used
  - –Secondary prophylaxis with penicillin is required
- Wilson disease: Treat with penicillamine, trientene chelation, or zinc
- In cases of toxin-induced chorea, removal of the offending agent is usually sufficient

128. Hyperreflexia

Deep tendon reflexes (DTRs) are routinely tested on neurologic examination and are nonspecific but helpful in localization. Increased DTRs often reflect a problem of the central nervous system and can be a localizing sign of focal injury. Upper motor neuron lesions are often associated with weakness, hyperreflexia, hypertonia, and extensor plantar responses.

Differential Diagnosis

- Normal variant (no other neurologic signs)
- Cerebral palsy
- Hypoxic ischemic encephalopathy
- Stroke
  - –Hypercoagulable state (e.g., protein C deficiency, factor V Leiden)
  - –Coagulation disorder (e.g., hemophilia)
  - –Mitochondrial disease (e.g., MELAS)
  - –Vascular malformation (e.g., Moya moya)
  - –Vasculitis
- Tumors of the central nervous system
  - –Cerebellar astrocytoma
  - –Medulloblastoma
  - –Ependymoma
  - –Astrocytoma
- Spinal cord tumors
  - –Neuroblastoma
  - –Ewing sarcoma
  - –Astrocytoma
  - –Ependymoma
- Tethered spinal cord
- Familial spastic paraplegia
- Transverse myelitis
- Multiple sclerosis
- Acute disseminated encephalomyelitis (ADEM)
- Hyperthyroidism (isolated or secondary to renal disease)
- Hyperparathyroidism
- Hypomagnesemia
- Pelizeus-Merzbacher
- Rett syndrome
- Rating of deep tendon reflexes
  - 0: Absent reflex
  - 1: Trace, or seen only with reinforcement
  - 2: Normal
  - 3: Brisk
  - 4: Nonsustained clonus
  - 5: Sustained clonus

Workup and Diagnosis

- History: Chronic vs. acute; other associated neurologic deficits, bladder or bowel compromise, spinal trauma
  - –Present with inappropriately preserved neonatal reflexes
- Physical exam
  - –Reflex assessment: Limbs should relaxed and symmetric; if reflex cannot be elicited, use reinforcement procedures (gritting teeth, pushing hands together), spinal tenderness
  - –Musculoskeletal exam: Contractures, increased tone, spasticity, deformity (suggestive of chronicity)
  - –Neurologic exam: Associated weakness, spinal cord sensory level, Babinski sign, signs of hyperreflexia (clonus, spread of reflexes to other muscle groups not being tested, crossed adduction of opposite limb)
  - –Main spinal nerve roots: Biceps (C5, C6), brachioradialis (C6), triceps (C7), patellar (L4), achilles tendon (S1), bulbocavernosus (S3–4), anal wink (S3–5)
- Labs
  - –Thyroid function studies
  - –Serum electrolytes, BUN, Cr, Ca, Mg, Ph
  - –Urine chemistry and microscopy
  - –PTH and vitamin D levels
- Studies
  - –Evaluation may include MR imaging of the brain and/or spine to evaluate for acute/chronic lesions and central causes of increased reflexes

Treatment

- Hyperreflexia itself does not require treatment
- Spasticity and hypertonicity
  - –Treated with a combination of physical therapy, stretching, bracing, and, occasionally, tendon releases
  - –Baclofen and botulinum toxin injections can help
- There is no treatment for many of the neurodegenerative and genetic conditions
- Management of treatable endocrine and neurologic disorders
- Acute spinal shock should be treated aggressively with corticosteroids
- Children with brain or spinal cord tumors should be referred to a neurosurgeon and oncologist for consideration of resection and further treatment

129. Hyporeflexia

Deep tendon reflexes (DTRs) can be decreased by any process that affects the reflex arc (lower motor neuron, muscle, sensory neuron), by acute upper motor neuron lesions, and by mechanical factors such as joint disease. DTRs are routinely tested on neurologic examination and are nonspecific but helpful in localization. Lower motor neuron lesions are often associated with weakness, muscle atrophy, fasciculations (visible contractions), and hypotonia in addition to hyporeflexia.

Differential Diagnosis

- Normal variant (no other abnormal neurologic signs)
- Acute spinal cord injury
  - –Spinal cord compression/infarction
  - –Disc herniation
  - –Transverse myelitis
  - –Occult spina bifida
- Toxins
  - –Antineoplastic agents
  - –Antiretroviral drugs
  - –Isoniazid
  - –Metronidazole
  - –Phenytoin
  - –Pyridoxine
- Neuropathy
  - –Diabetes mellitus associated
  - –Giant axonal neuropathy
  - –Hereditary neuropathy with liability to pressure palsies (tomaculous neuropathy)
  - –Chronic inflammatory demyelinating polyneuropathy (CIDP)
- Structural lesion/tumor affecting nerve roots, peripheral nerves (e.g., plexiform neurofibroma in NF1)
- Chromosome abnormality (trisomy 21, trisomy 18)
- Spinal muscular atrophy (SMA)
- Charcot-Marie-Tooth (CMT) disease
- Guillain-Barré syndrome (GBS)
- Muscle disease
  - –Muscular dystrophy
  - –Myotonic dystrophy
- Pompe disease
  - –Glycogen storage disease type II
  - –Acid maltase deficiency
- Hypothyroidism
- Hypokalemia
- Hypoparathyroidism
- Miller-Fisher syndrome
- Tick paralysis
- Friedreich ataxia
- Acute stroke
- Familial dysautonomia (Riley-Day syndrome)
- Metachromatic leukodystrophy
- Xeroderma pigmentosa
- Vitamin B12, vitamin E deficiency
- Poliomyelitis

Workup and Diagnosis

- History
  - –Other associated neurologic deficits
  - –PMH, medication use
  - –Chronic versus acute
  - –Muscle weakness, tenderness (suggests infection)
- Family history
  - –Myopathy, muscle diseases
  - –Neuropathies or mitochondrial disease
- Physical exam
  - –Musculoskeletal exam: Muscle bulk, consistency, tenderness, tone
  - –Neurologic exam: Associated weakness, spinal cord sensory level, Babinski sign
  - –DTRs: Limbs should be in a relaxed and symmetric position; if reflex cannot be elicited, use reinforcement procedures (gritting teeth, pressing hands together)
  - –Main spinal nerve roots: Biceps (C5, C6), brachioradialis (C6), triceps (C7), patellar (L4), achilles tendon (S1), bulbocavernosus (S3–4), anal wink (S3–5)
- Labs
  - –Electrolytes, CK, aldolase, lactate, pyruvate
- Studies
  - –Consider genetic studies
  - –Consider muscle biopsy and/or nerve biopsy
  - –Nerve conduction studies and electromyography
  - –Cardiac evaluation (cardiomyopathy may coexist)

Treatment

- Hyporeflexia alone is not an indication for treatment
- Weakness and hypotonia require intervention by physical therapy and bracing
- There is no treatment for many of the genetic conditions
- Guillain-Barré syndrome
  - –Treated with plasmapheresis or IV immunoglobulin
  - –Frequent respiratory checks with vital capacity
  - –If the vital capacity falls below 12–15 cc/kg, patient needs endotracheal intubation and ventilatory support
- Infantile botulism
  - –Support respiratory insuffiency or bulbar dysfunction
  - –Botulinum immune globulin is beneficial if given within the first 3 days of illness
- Tick paralysis—spontaneous resolution after removal of the tick

130. Hypotonia

Hypotonia can present as decreased resistance to passive movement and increased range of motion of joints. Etiology may be abnormalities of the brain, anterior horn cells of the spinal cord, peripheral nerve, neuromuscular junction, or muscle. Neurologic examination and the ancillary tests help narrow the possible etiologies.

Differential Diagnosis

- Benign congenital hypotonia
- Chromosome abnormalities: Trisomy 21, trisomy 13, Prader-Willi, cri-du-chat
- Hypoxic ischemic encephalopathy
- Spinal muscular atrophy (SMA)
- Infantile botulism
- Hypothyroidism
- Spinal cord injury
- Cerebral malformations
- Toxins: Organophosphates, aminoglycosides, antineoplastic agents, chloroquine, glue-sniffing
- Myasthenia gravis
  - –Transient neonatal myasthenia
  - –Congenital myasthenia
  - –Familial infantile myasthenia
- Guillain-Barré syndrome (GBS) or chronic inflammatory demyelinating polyneuropathy (CIDP)
- Muscular dystrophy: Duchenne, Becker, facioscapulohumeral, Fuluyama, merosin-deficient congenital muscular dystrophy
- Congenital myotonic dystrophy
- Hereditary motor-sensory neuropathy
- Metachromatic leukodystrophy
- Globoid cell leukodystrophy
- Congenital myopathies: Central core disease, myotubular, nemaline (rod), congenital fiber-type disproportion
- Peroxisomal disorders
  - –Neonatal adrenoleukodystrophy, Zellweger
- Hypermagnesimia
- Myositis
- Lipid storage muscular disorders
- Mitochondrial encephalomyopathy
- Pompe disease (glycogen storage disease type II, acid maltase deficiency)
- McArdle disease
- Walker-Warburg syndrome
- Lowe syndrome (oculocerebrorenal)
- Werdnig-Hoffman Disease
- Familial dysautonomia
- Tick paralysis
- Poliomyelitis

Workup and Diagnosis

- History
  - –Birth history, fetal motion, oligo-polyhydramnios
  - –Feeding, head control, gross/fine motor milestones
  - –Seizures, family history, constipation, tick bite
- Physical exam
  - –Deformities, dermatoglyphics, contractures, scoliosis, spinal dimple, hernias, corneal opacities, high or cleft palate, muscle mass
  - –Cardiac size, hip dislocation, flat occiput
  - –Muscle mass, strength and tone, facial movements, fasiculations, DTRs, sensory responses
  - –Newborns: Posture, spontaneous movements, plantar response, primary neonatal reflexes (Moro, palmar grasp, tonic neck response)
  - –Older child: Gowers sign, mental status, eye movements, stance and gait
- Labs
  - –Muscle enzymes (CPK, aldolase)
  - –Electrolytes, TSH, lactate, pyruvate
  - –Carnitine, acylcarnitine, very long chain fatty acids
  - –Stool botulinum toxin
  - –LP for GBS
- Studies
  - –EMG/nerve conduction studies
  - –Muscle biopsy for metabolic, congenital myopathies
  - –MRI for cerebral malformations, spinal cord lesions
  - –Specific genetic testing
  - –SMA, muscular dystrophy, myotonic dystrophy

Treatment

- Treatment is tailored for each patient and is mostly supportive for genetic diseases, metabolic disorders, and myopathies
- Combination of physical therapy, bracing, and orthopedic surgical interventions can give patients longer life expectancy
  - –Efficacy of the physical therapy programs for most progressive diseases is limited
- Cardiomyopathy frequently coexists with neuromuscular conditions causing hypotonia
- Duchenne muscular dystrophy
  - –Oral prednisone is used to increase and sustain muscle strength
- Infantile botulism
  - –Supportive therapy for respiratory insuffiency or bulbar dysfunction
  - –Botulinum immune globulin is beneficial if given within the first 3 days of illness
- Synthoid for hypothyroidism

131. Paresthesias

Paresthesias are abnormal sensations in the extremities in the absence of stimuli. Sensation arises spontaneously and is not always painful. The patient may experience numb, cold, warm, or burning sensations, prickling, tingling or pins and needles, skin "crawling" sensation, or pruritus.

Differential Diagnosis

- Peripheral neuropathies (with or without pain)
  - –Entrapment neuropathies
  - –Carpal tunnel
  - –Lateral femoral cutaneous syndrome
  - –Pressure palsy
  - –Charcot-Marie-Tooth disease
  - –Amyloid neuropathy
  - –Symmetric peripheral neuropathy
- Central nervous system etiologies
  - –Stroke
  - –Brain tumor
  - –Head trauma
  - –Abscess
  - –Encephalitis
  - –Systemic lupus erythematosus (SLE)
  - –Multiple sclerosis
  - –Transverse myelitis
  - –Vitamin B12 deficiency
- Metabolic
  - –Diabetes
  - –Hypothyroidism
  - –Alcoholism
  - –Amyloidosis
  - –Uremia
- Hyperventilation causing respiratory alkalosis
- Connective tissue disorders
  - –Rheumatoid arthritis
  - –SLE
  - –Sjögren syndrome
- Toxins
  - –Chemotherapy
  - –Heavy metal poisoning (e.g., lead, arsenic, and other metals)
  - –Medications (e.g., HIV medications, metronidazole, vincristine)
- Neoplastic
  - –Multiple myeloma
  - –Monoclonal gammopathy
- Infectious
  - –HIV
  - –Lyme disease
  - –Syphilis

Workup and Diagnosis

- History
  - –Age of onset, frequency, duration
  - –Worsening with movement
  - –Recent trauma
  - –Exposure to heavy metals or toxins
  - –Medications (e.g., chemotherapy, antibiotics)
  - –Family history of neuropathy/muscle problems
- Associated symptoms
  - –Weakness, falls, pain (back pain, regional pain)
- Physical exam
  - –Vital signs (temperature, heart rate, blood pressure)
  - –Musculoskeletal exam (joint or muscle tenderness, spine tenderness, bony pain, neck stiffness)
  - –Neurologic examination: Detailed sensory examination (vibratory, pinprick, position sense) to evaluate for nerve root, spinal cord, or central etiology
- Initial labs
  - –CBC, chemistry panel, U/A, TSH, ESR
- Secondary evaluation
  - –Serum folate, serum B12, syphilis serology, ANA
  - –Electromyogram, nerve conduction velocities
  - –X-ray of the affected extremity
  - –CT or MRI of the brain
  - –Nerve biopsy
  - –Muscle biopsy
  - –Serum electrophoresis

Treatment

- Paresthesias emanating from peripheral neuropathy: Trial of amitriptyline, gabapentin, or carbamazepine
- Transverse myelitis and acute flares of multiple sclerosis are often treated with steroids
- Acute cerebrovascular events are treated according to the cause; anticoagulant therapy is sometimes indicated
- Entrapment neuropathies or pressure palsies
  - –Treated supportively with bracing
  - –Sometimes require release of tensor fascia
- Vitamin B12 deficiency
  - –Treated with exogenous administration of B12
- Uremic neuropathy responds to dialysis; may often be cured with renal transplantation
- Paresthesias resulting from connective tissue diseases or infectious etiologies often improve after treatment of the underlying disease
- Drug-induced and toxin-related paresthesias typically improve after cessation of the offending agent

132. Seizures – Neonatal

Seizures in the newborn are often difficult to diagnose, because there may only be subtle manifestations. Any insult that affects the brain in this age group can present with seizures, thus the differential diagnosis is quite extensive. One also has to rule out several mimics such as jitteriness, sleep myoclonus, and gastroesophageal reflux.

Differential Diagnosis

- Hypoxic ishemic encephalopathy
- Bacterial meningitis/sepsis
- Stroke
- Cerebral dysgenesis
- Electrolyte disturbances
  - –Hypoglycemia
  - –Hyponatremia
  - –Hypomagnesemia
  - –Hypocalcemia
- Maternal drug use
  - –Drug withdrawal after delivery
  - –Direct effect of drugs, such as cocaine
- Congenital infections (TORCH)
  - –Toxoplasmosis
  - –Syphilis
  - –Rubella
  - –CMV
  - –HSV
- HSV encephalitis
- Intracranial hemorrhage
  - –Subdural hemorrhage
  - –Intraparenchymal hemorrhage
  - –Intraventricular hemorrhage in the premature infant
  - –Subarachnoid hemorrhage
- Urea cycle disturbances
- Smith-Lemli-Opitz syndrome
- Nonketotic hyperglycinemia
- Pyridoxine deficiency
- Fructose dysmetabolism
- Amino acidurias
  - –Maple syrup urine disease
  - –Proprionic acidemia
- Molybdenum cofactor deficiency
- Mitochondrial encephalopathy
- Glucose transporter deficiency
- Benign etiologies
  - –Benign idiopathic neonatal seizures (fifth day fits)
  - –Benign familial neonatal seizures
- Movements commonly mistaken for seizures
  - –Benign neonatal sleep myoclonus
  - –Jitteriness (may be secondary to hypoglycemia, drug withdrawal, or idiopathic)
  - –Gastroesophageal reflux (arching, writhing)
  - –Breath-holding spell

Workup and Diagnosis

- History: Previous pregnancies, fetal movements, infections, blood pressure problems during pregnancy, maternal drug/medication use, family history, Apgar scores, nuchal cord, birth weight, feeding problems, association of the spells to feeding and sleep
- Physical exam
  - –Deformities, dermatoglyphics, skin lesions, hepatosplenomegaly, funduscopic exam, corneal opacities
  - –Mental status: Spontaneous level of activity of the infant; responsiveness to light, sound, and touch
  - –Muscle tone: Passive manipulation of limbs
  - –Primary neonatal reflexes (Moro, palmar grasp, tonic neck response) and muscle stretch reflexes
- Labs: Glucose, electrolytes, lactate, liver function tests, ammonia, TORCH titers, pyruvate, chromosomes, 17-hydroxycorticosteroid, serum amino acids, copper
- Neuroimaging: CT or MRI
- Lumbar puncture for meningitis and encephalitis, including HSV, glucose transporter deficiency, nonketotic hyperglycinemia
- EEG: Critical in making the diagnosis of seizures in the newborn; monitoring of the child during one of the spells is the best way to make the diagnosis of seizures
- If gastroesophageal reflux is suspected, pH/thermistor monitoring is helpful to document a temporal relation

Treatment

- Evaluate and secure airway, breathing, and circulation
  - –Benzodiazepines or phenobarbital infused intravenously can stop the seizures
- If there is reason to suspect hypoglycemia, even if blood glucose level cannot be quickly established, treat with glucose intravenously
- Treat hypocalcemia with calcium gluconate
- Treat hypomagnesemia with magnesium sulfate
- Meningitis and HSV encephalitis require intravenous antibiotics and acyclovir, respectively
- Depending on the etiology, the infant may stay on phenobarbital for varying duration of time
- Glucose transporter deficiency can be treated with ketogenic diet
- For pyridoxine deficiency, pyridoxine 50–100 mg injected intravenously during an EEG recording can be both diagnostic and therapeutic

133. Seizures – Childhood

Febrile seizures occur in 3–4% of all children; they often do not require long-term treatment. Each year, between 25,000 and 40,000 children in the U.S. have a first unprovoked afebrile seizure. Most of these children will not have a second seizure and do not require prophylaxis. The neurologic exam and the EEG help guide the evaluation and treatment.

Differential Diagnosis

- Febrile seizure
- Cerebral dysgenesis: Disorders of neuronal migration, heterotopias, lissencephaly
- Epilepsy syndromes
  - –Childhood absence
  - –Juvenile absence
  - –Juvenile myoclonic epilepsy (JME)
  - –Benign rolandic epilepsy (BRE)
- Meningitis/encephalitis (e.g., HSV)
- Cerebral abscess
- Postinfectious (e.g., ADEM)
- Hyponatremia
- Hypernatremia
- Hypocalcemia
- Hypoglycemia
- Toxins: Ingestions or sedative withdrawal
- Trauma
- Pyridoxine deficiency
- Neoplasm
- Degenerative
  - –Alpers disease
  - –Rett syndrome
  - –Unterricht-Lundborg disease
  - –Lafora disease
  - –Neuronal ceroid lipofuscinosis
- Genetic
  - –Angelman syndrome
  - –Aicardi syndrome
- Metabolic
  - –Medium chain acyl-CoA dehydrogenase deficiency (MCAD)
  - –Myoclonus epilepsy and ragged-red fibers syndrome (MERRF)
  - –Sialidosis
  - –Glucose transporter deficiency
  - –Urea cycle defects
- Vascular: Stroke, hemorrhage, vasculitis
- Hashimoto encephalitis
- Seizure mimics
  - –Breath-holding spells
  - –Syncope, convulsive syncope
  - –Gastroesophageal reflux
  - –Cardiac arrhythmia
  - –Movement disorder
  - –Migraine
  - –Benign paroxysmal vertigo
  - –Parasomnia
  - –Pseudo-seizure
  - –Rage attack

Workup and Diagnosis

- History: Detailed description of the spell, loss of consciousness, eye deviation, time of onset, other suspicious spells (jerking, staring, day-dreaming), birth and developmental history, previous history of head trauma, encephalitis, febrile seizures, medications at home, recent infections
- Physical exam: Dysmorphic features, skin rash, retinal exam for cherry-red spot, macular degeneration, hepatosplenomegaly, meningismus
- Full neurologic examination: Postictal weakness can provide clues to the focus of seizures (Todd paralysis)
- Labs: Glucose, electrolytes, calcium, toxicology screen, ammonia, lactate, pyruvate, genetic testing for specific disorders (MECP2 mutation for Rett, FISH on chromosome 15 for Angelman)
- Lumbar puncture to rule out infection (including HSV PCR), glucose transporter deficiency
- EEG can help make the diagnosis of focal vs generalized epilepsy
  - –Crucial for decisions of treatment choices
- MRI can help determine any structural abnormalities, including cerebral dysgenesis, abscess, neoplasm, temporal lobe sclerosis
- For other specific etiologies, one can follow up with skin biopsy, CSF amino acids, biotinidase level, TSH, anti-thyroglobulin antibodies, rheumatologic workup

Treatment

- In the acute setting: First evaluate and secure airway, breathing, and circulation
  - –IV benzodiazepines (lorazepam) is first line of treatment; in the absence of IV access, rectal diazepam may be used
  - –IV fosphenytoin is the second line of treatment and provides longer seizure suppression
  - –If not sufficient, phenobarbital can be added
  - –Constant evaluation of the airway during treatment, and, if necessary, intubation is critically important
- If the seizure continues despite these medications, anesthesia with pentobarbital, midazolam, or propofol may be used to suppress the refractory seizures
- Long-term prophylaxis can be obtained by one or a combination of anti-epileptic medications
  - –Focal seizures: Carbamazepine, oxcarbazepine, gabapentin, levetiracetam, or valproate
  - –Absence seizures: Ethosuximide or valproate

134. Vertigo

Vertigo is an illusion of movement (usually rotatory) due to an acute imbalance of tonic vestibular activity. Symptoms of vertigo are nonspecific and occur when there is a disturbance anywhere in the peripheral or central vestibular system. Determining the site of the lesion is important, as central causes can be life threatening and require immediate intervention. Vertigo should be differentiated from other causes of dizziness such as disequilibrium, presyncope, and anxiety.

Differential Diagnosis

- Benign paroxysmal positional vertigo (BPPV)
  - Each episode lasts seconds to minutes
- Vestibular neuritis
  - Viral infection of the vestibular nerve
- Otitis media
- Migraine
  - Vertigo may precede, follow, or present with the headache and aura
- Acute labyrinthitis
  - Acute onset with nausea and vomiting
  - Lasts for days and slowly resolves
  - 45% cluster with viral infections
- Posttraumatic
  - Perilymphatic fistula
  - Labyrinthine concussion
  - Associated with postconcussive syndrome
  - Worsened by change in head position, cough, sneeze, swallow, straining, and airplane travel
- Cerebellar tumors
  - Tumors may be associated with tinnitus, facial weakness, and nystagmus
- Toxins/drugs: Antibiotics (aminoglycosides), salicylates, alcohol, phenytoin, quinine, arsenic, tricyclic antidepressants
- Autoimmune: Collagen vascular disease, Wegener granulomatosis
- Posterior circulation dissection
  - Often associated with a history of neck extension or rotational injury
- Cerebellar hemorrhage: Acute onset of vertigo, headache, nausea, and vomiting
- Multiple sclerosis
  - Vertigo is the presenting symptom in 5%
  - Hearing loss rare
  - Most common in young women
- Temporal lobe or complex partial seizures
- Ménière disease
- Familial periodic ataxia syndromes
  - Recurrent bouts of vertigo brought on by emotional stress or physical exertion
- CNS infection: Syphilis, Lyme disease
- Motion sickness
- Vertigo mimics: Presyncope, disequilibrium from decreased vision or proprioception
- Psychogenic
  - Panic or anxiety disorder

Workup and Diagnosis

- History
  - Duration, headache, nausea, vomiting, worsening with activity or movement (postural hypotension, hyperventilation)
  - Nausea and vomiting are classically more prominent with peripheral vertigo
  - Associated neurologic deficits (extremity weakness, numbness, incoordination, dysarthria, diplopia, tinnitus, hearing loss, loss of consciousness)
  - Facial numbness/weakness
  - History of autoimmune disease, hyperlipidemia, stroke, migraine, seizure, cancer, prior ear surgery
- Physical exam may be normal in asymptomatic periods
- Cardiac and peripheral vascular examination for murmurs, arrhythmias, orthostatic changes in pulse and blood pressure (+/− ECG, Holter, Echo, Doppler)
- Nystagmus, truncal ataxia, and limb incoordination are sometimes found in cerebellar infarction or neoplasm
- Vertigo of a panic attack can sometimes be elicited by having the patient hyperventilate
- Dix-Hallpike maneuver: Rapidly lay the patient down from sitting allowing the head to hang over the side of the bed while turning to the left or right; positive test shows vertigo with rotatory nystagmus within 30 seconds; if the etiology is peripheral, the nystagmus shows extinction with positioning maneuvers
- MRI and MRA can help evaluate the posterior circulation

Treatment

- If the vertigo is accompanied by nausea and vomiting, supportive care with fluid and electrolyte replacement
- Migraine aura associated vertigo: Analgesics and vestibular suppressants such as sumatriptan, propranolol, amitriptyline, diazepam; avoid triggers
- Acute viral labyrinthitis: Bedrest, antiemetics, IV fluids, diazepam, antihistamines
- Control of hypertension, diabetes, cardiac arrhythmia
- Cerebellopontine angle tumors: Surgical resection
- BPPV/ Ménière disease: Positioning procedure; brief treatment with diazepam, meclizine, or dimenhydrinate
- Perilymph fistula: Pneumatic otoscopy reproduces symptoms; often heals spontaneously
- Vertebrobasilar stroke: Neurology consultation
- Cerebellar hemorrhage: Emergent neurosurgical consult for question of posterior fossa decompression

Section 16

Skin

KATHERINE MACRAE DELL, MD
SARAH FRIEBERT, MD
VLAD D. IANUȘ, MD, MPH
TOMISLAV IVSIC, MD
DOUGLAS A. JACOBSTEIN, MD
HEATHER KASTEN, MD
C. BECKET MAHNKE, MD

135. Alopecia

Alopecia (from Greek "alopekia" = a disease like fox mange; "alopex" = fox) represents a significant loss or absence of hair, affecting the scalp or any other hair-bearing part of the body. Human hair follicles have three distinct growth phases: anagen (active), catagen (regressive), and telogen (resting). The human scalp contains approximately 100,000 hairs, with an average growth rate of 2.5 mm/week. In healthy individuals, about 50–100 hairs are lost daily, and 25% must be shed before thinning becomes apparent.

Differential Diagnosis

Non-scarring alopecia

- Inflammatory/infectious disorders: Tinea capitis (*Trichophyton tonsurans, Microsporum canis*), kerion
- Alopecia areata
  - –Sudden localized loss of hair in round/oval patches; associated with Scotch plaid nails (transverse and longitudinal pitting rows) in 10–20% of the cases, and with autoimmune disorders
  - –Ophiasis alopecia starts the posterior occiput; extends anteriorly, bilaterally
  - –Other forms show loss of all scalp hair (alopecia totalis) or body hair (alopecia universalis)
- Trauma: Traction (trichotillomania, tight braiding, ponytails), pressure (prolonged bed rest, especially in infants [occiput])
- Telogen effluvium: Partial alopecia noted 3 months after a stressful event; reversible; rarely involves more than 50% of the hair
- Anagen effluvium: Sudden loss of the growing hairs (80% of the scalp), resulting from the interruption of the anagen phase of the hair cycle; follows chemotherapy (folic acid and purine antagonists, alkylating agents, alkaloids), irradiation, or intoxication (lead, thallium, arsenic, bismuth, coumadin)
- Hair shaft anomalies (moniletrix, trichothiodystrophy, pili torti)
- Seborrheic dermatitis
- Thyroid disease
- Male-pattern alopecia (in both sexes)
- Congenital triangular alopecia

Scarring alopecia (cicatricial)

- Dermatologic disorders and syndromes: Lichen planus, SLE, acrodermatitis enteropathica, sarcoidosis, scleroderma (localized/systemic), keratosis pilaris, folliculitis decalvans
- Infectious (prolonged scalp infections, tuberculosis, syphilis, herpes zoster)
- Physical trauma (chronic irradiation, trichotillomania, thermic/caustic burns)
- Developmental defects (aplasia cutis) and genetic syndromes (Hallerman-Streiff, Treacher Collins, Marie-Unna hypotrichosis, trisomy 13, etc.)

Workup and Diagnosis

- History
  - –Duration, drugs used
  - –Stressful events (febrile illness, surgery, shock, diet, injury, emotional stress) preceding the alopecia by 2–4 months
  - –Family history for inherited forms; family members or close contacts with scalp infections
- Physical exam
  - –Examination of hair root and shaft: "Exclamation point hairs" (hair shaft narrows just near the follicle) are pathognomonic for alopecia areata; telogen hairs have a club-shaped tip; hair is broken in various lengths in trichotillomania or child abuse
  - –Examination of the scalp skin: Inflammation, atrophy, scales; "salt-and-pepper" appearance in tinea capitis; Wood lamp examination detects *Microsporum*, but misses *Trichophyton*
- Labs
  - –Microscopic examination of the hairs with KOH for hyphae
  - –Dermatophyte test medium innoculation
  - –Fungal cultures from skin scrapings, brushings, hairs
  - –Thyroid function tests, especially in patients with alopecia areata (25% have thyroid abnormalities)
- Scalp biopsy to determine cause of scarring alopecia
- Consider presence of trichobezoars and obsessive-complusive disorders in trichotillomania

Treatment

- Elimination of the precipitating factor/agent
- Tinea capitis: Oral griseofulvin for 4–6 weeks; oral itraconazole, terbinafine, or fluconazole can also be used; selenium sulfide shampoo decreases fungal shedding and hastens healing of lesions
- Alopecia areata: Topical steroids, PUVA, intradermal corticosteroid injections, very rarely systemic steroids
- Kerion is treated with griseofulvin and sometimes with corticosteroids; antimicrobials are not necessary unless secondary infection is suspected
- Use of cooling or a scalp tourniquet during the IV use of certain chemostatic agents (e.g., vincristine)
- Male pattern alopecia: Topical minoxidil, plastic surgery techniques, implantation of nylon filaments
- Psychological assistance; psychiatric evaluation should be considered in trichotillomania and in certain cases antidepressant treatment (fluoxetine, clomipramine)

136. Annular Rashes

Annular rashes (from Latin "annulus" = ring; syn. circinate) are ring-shaped lesions, although their morphology can vary and may also present as irregular, oval, semiannular, target-like, polycyclic, serpiginous, or reticular lesions.

Differential Diagnosis

- Infectious
  - –Dermatophytes: *Microsporum, Trichophyton, Epidermophyton* infections (tinea capitis, corporis, cruris, pedis)
  - –Tinea versicolor: Superficial infection, caused by *Malassezia furfur*
  - –Erythema migrans: Earliest sign in Lyme disease, at the site of the tick bite; typically 7–10 days after bite; initially an erythematous macule that expands to form a large, annular lesion (up to 70 cm, average 15 cm) if left untreated
  - –Erythema marginatum: In about 10% of the patients with rheumatic fever and occasionally in juvenile rheumatoid arthritis; associated with active carditis
  - –Pityriasis rosacea
  - –Secondary syphilis
  - –African trypanosomiasis: Circinate outline and normal central area
  - –Larva migrans cutanata: Can present with a serpiginous rash
  - –Lupus vulgaris (rare, chronic, progressive form of cutaneous tuberculosis)
- Numular eczema
- Pityriasis alba
- Seborrheic dermatitis
- Immune mediated
  - –SLE
  - –Urticaria
  - –Erythema multiforme, minor and major (including Stevens-Johnson syndrome): Hypersensitivity syndrome to a variety of etiologies (mostly infectious in children, notably *Mycoplasma*, and sulfonamides) and presentations; the hallmark is the target lesion (also occasionally seen in erythema annulare centrifugum and Kawasaki disease)
  - –Toxic epidermal necrolysis (Lyell disease)
- Granuloma annulare
- Sarcoidosis
- Drug eruptions
- Cutaneous T-cell lymphoma

Workup and Diagnosis

- History
  - –Age, diet, drugs, fever, tick bites
  - –History of maternal conditions (e.g., SLE)
  - –Association with other signs/symptoms, such as malaise, headache, myalgia, lymphadenitis, pharyngitis, cranial nerve palsies, subcutaneous nodules, arthritis, chorea, genital chancres
- Physical exam
  - –Pattern and distribution of the rash; duration, spread mode, crops formation, presence of pruritus, involvement of the mucosal surfaces
  - –Visualization of the pale or barely perceptible vascular reactive lesions can be enhanced by gentle warming of the skin
  - –Wood lamp examination identifies *Microsporum* spp in tinea capitis, but misses *Trichophyton*; also useful in tinea cruris and tinea versicolor
- Labs
  - –CBC with differential, ESR/CRP
  - –Serology for SLE, Lyme disease, syphilis
  - –Skin scrapings, KOH preparations, fungal cultures
  - –Skin biopsy is rarely needed
- ECG if carditis is suspected
  - –Prolonged PR interval
  - –Atrioventricular block

Treatment

- Some annular rashes may not require treatment, but the condition that it is associated with them usually does
- Avoidance of the triggering agent and treatment with antihistamines and corticosteroids (for recalcitrant cases) in urticaria
- Antifungals for dermatophyte infections (oral griseofulvin if hair and nails are involved, topical clotrimazole, miconazole, or haloprogin for the others)
- Topical steroids and wet dressings for eczema, antibiotics for secondary infection
- Antibiotics
  - –Lyme disease (doxycycline or ampicillin)
  - –Syphilis (penicillin G)
- Skin sunlight exposure until mild sunburn occurs hastens the disappearance of lesions in pityriasis rosea
- Intensive care unit admission and support for severe conditions such as Stevens-Johnson syndrome and toxic epidermal necrolysis

137. Cyanotic Newborn

By far the most common causes of cyanosis in the newborn are respiratory (pneumonia, newborn respiratory distress syndrome [NRDS], meconium aspiration, etc.). Babies with respiratory illness are frequently in respiratory distress (grunting, flaring, retracting, tachypneic), whereas patients with cardiac causes are not (the "happy blue baby"). This page focuses on cardiac causes.

Differential Diagnosis

- Transposition of the great vessels (TGV)
  - –The most common cardiac cause of cyanosis in the newborn
  - –Aorta connected to RV and pulmonary artery connected to LV
  - –PE, ECG normal
  - –CXR: Normal or egg-on-string
- Tetralogy of Fallot
  - –Most common cyanotic heart disease
  - –Right ventricular hypertrophy, pulmonary stenosis, VSD, and an overriding aorta
  - –Associated with 22q11 deletion
  - –Murmur; reduced PVM; R-axis deviation, RVH
- Critical pulmonary valve stenosis
  - –Thickened pulmonary valve
  - –Murmur; reduced PVM; RVH
- Pulmonary atresia
  - –No flow from RV to pulmonary artery, so pulmonary blood flow depends on ductus arteriosus
  - –PE normal; reduced PVM; reduced R-sided forces with normal axis
- Tricuspid atresia
  - –No inflow into R ventricle, causing R ventricular hypoplasia
  - –With or without murmur; reduced PVM; reduced R-sided forces with L-axis deviation
- Truncus arteriosus
  - –Single outlet to ventricles divides into aorta and pulmonary arteries
  - –VSD always present
  - –PE normal; possibly increased PVM; ECG normal
- Total anomalous pulmonary venous return
  - –Cardiac cause of cyanosis that mimics respiratory disease with respiratory distress and "white-out" of lungs
  - –Consider for patients who appear to have bad respiratory disease
  - –With or without murmur; increased PVM; ECG normal
- Ebstein anomaly
  - –The tricuspid valve is displaced down into the R ventricle, usually with severe tricuspid regurgitation with R-to-L atrial level shunting
  - –Murmur; huge heart; R atrial enlargement (tall P waves)
- Other: Respiratory most common, polycythemia, hypoglycemia

Workup and Diagnosis

- History
  - –Sometimes a family history of congenital heart disease
  - –Usually presents on second day of life rather than in the delivery room
- Physical exam
  - –Almost all patients with cyanotic heart disease have single S_2, however, splitting of S_2 difficult to appreciate in babies due to fast heart rate
  - –See Differential Diagnosis for findings by lesion
- Hyperoxia test
  - –Used to differentiate cardiac from respiratory causes
  - –Administration of 100% O_2 for 10 minutes
  - –PaO_2 improves with respiratory causes of cyanosis, but not cardiac causes, because oxygenated blood in the lungs is not transported systemically
  - –Arterial blood gas PaO_2 >200 is more indicative of respiratory disease; <100 consistent with cyanotic heart disease or very severe respiratory disease
- Chest X-ray shows PVM, cardiac silhouette
- Electrocardiogram
  - –Evaluates the presence/absence of R ventricle
  - –Normal newborns have a dominant R wave in lead V1 with a QRS axis of 60–180
- Echocardiogram
  - –Definitive test for cardiac anatomy and function
- Cardiac catheterization is rarely needed except in some instances with very complicated anatomy

Treatment

- NICU admission with cardiac monitor, pulse oximetry
- Supplemental O_2 rarely helps with cardiac cyanosis, because the blood does not get to the lungs
- Prostaglandin E1 used to open the ductus arteriosus and increase blood flow to the lungs
  - –Side effects: Apnea (more common at higher doses)
  - –Must be prepared to intubate (advisable before transport to a referral center)
  - –Fever and hypotension (via vasodilation)
- Blalock-Taussig shunt
  - –Gore-Tex tube graft surgically placed from the innominate artery to the pulmonary artery
  - –Improves pulmonary blood flow
- Balloon atrial septostomy
  - –In TGV, improves cyanosis by atrial mixing
  - –Catheter placed into L atrium, balloon inflated, and pulled back to R atrium to enlarge the atrial foramen
- Anatomy determines further surgical repair or palliation

138. Edema

Edema is defined as the accumulation of excessive amounts of fluid in the cells and tissues of the body and is relatively rare in children. It is usually generalized and dependent (i.e., fluid tends to accumulate in the most dependent areas, such as the lower extremities).

Differential Diagnosis

- Kidney disease (nephrotic syndrome)
  - –Insidious onset, periorbital and lower extremity edema, abdominal distension
  - –Various types include minimal change disease (MCNS), focal segmental glomerulosclerosis, acute and chronic glomerulonephritis
- Chronic renal failure from any cause may result in impaired fluid excretion
- Liver disease from any cause resulting in impaired production of albumin
- Congestive heart failure (CHF)
- Protein losing enteropathy
  - –Menetrier disease (typically CMV), inflammatory bowel disease, neuroblastoma, intestinal lymphangiectasia, trypsinogen deficiency
- Celiac disease
- Sepsis, with capillary leak (movement of fluid out of the blood vessels into the interstitium)
- Hereditary angioneurotic edema
  - –Intermittent swelling of extremities
  - –Often preceded by trauma
  - –Decreased C4 and C1 esterase inhibitor
- Rocky Mountain spotted fever
- Stevens-Johnson syndrome
- Vitamin E deficiency
- Hypothyroidism
- Severe malnutrition
  - –Marasmus (calorie deficiency)
  - –Kwashiorkor (protein deficiency)
- Zinc deficiency
- Hydrops fetalis
- Impaired lymphatic drainage
  - –Milroy disease
  - –Meigs syndrome
  - –Yellow nail syndrome
  - –Lymphedema praecox
- Filariasis (nematode infection resulting in elephantiasis)
- Immobility including placement of body casts and paralysis

Workup and Diagnosis

- History
  - –Onset, duration, severity
  - –History of heart, kidney, or liver disease; GI bleeding, hypertension, weight gain, feeding intolerance
  - –Chest pain, shortness of breath, orthopnea (cardiac disease), jaundice, acholic stools, abdominal distension, GI bleeding (liver disease), oliguria, facial edema, headache or vision changes (hypertension), diarrhea, fever
- Physical exam
  - –Blood pressure (hypo- or hypertension), cardiac exam (JVD, murmur)
  - –Hepatomegaly, splenomegaly, ascites, scleral icterus
  - –Periorbital, lower extremity or presacral edema, abdominal distension, poor peripheral perfusion
- Labs
  - –Urinalysis (no proteinuria excludes renal protein loss)
  - –Serum chemistries: Albumin, triglycerides, liver transaminases
  - –Stool for α-1 antitrypsin for protein-losing enteropathy
  - –Prothrombin time (impaired hepatic function)
- Abdominal ultrasound (for liver or kidney disease)
- Studies depending on clinical situation
  - –Echocardiogram/ECG for cardiac failure
  - –Renal biopsy (if kidney disease other than MCNS is suspected)
  - –GI imaging or endoscopy

Treatment

- Nephrotic syndrome
  - –Younger children treat with empiric corticosteroid
  - –Older children or those with atypical features of MCNS: Renal biopsy with treatment based on results
- Edema related to chronic renal failure
  - –Treat with loop diuretics (e.g., furosemide)
  - –Other diuretics are ineffective due to renal impairment
- Severe symptomatic edema
  - –Treat with IV albumin/furosemide (or other diuretics)
  - –Use with caution in patients with oliguria or renal insufficiency, because pulmonary edema could result
- Edema related to liver disease
  - –Aldosterone inhibitors (spironolactone) may help
- Sepsis
  - –Antibiotics/antivirals
  - –Blood pressure support with IVF and/or pressors
  - –Additional intensive care support

139. Hand & Foot Rashes

Hand and foot rashes are generally nonspecific, but their presence or absence might help in establishing the diagnosis in a wide variety of conditions. The palms and soles are covered with squamous epiderma that is thicker than in other parts of the body (1.5 mm) and hairless; the innervation is abundant and contains specialized receptors, such as Meissner and Ruffini corpuscles. On hands and feet, edema is likely to be noticeable early (along with the eyelids/face and the genitalia) due to a relative skin excess.

Differential Diagnosis

Infectious

- Enterovirus infection (hand-foot-and-mouth disease, Coxsakie virus, other nonpolio enteroviruses)
- Kawasaki disease (one of the five criteria)
- Scabies
- Tinea
- Candidal skin infection
- Ricketsial rash: Rocky Mountain spotted fever (RMSF), murine typhus
- Mononucleosis (EBV)
- Measles: Atypical forms start on hands/feet
- Scarlet fever, post-streptococcal infection desquamation rash
- Infectious endocarditis: Janeway lesions, Osler nodules
- Spirochete infection: Secondary syphilis, Lyme disease (acrodermatitis chronica atrophicans)
- Congenital toxoplasmosis
- Rat-bite fever (*Streptobacillus moniliformis, Spirillum minus*)

Immune-mediated

- Urticaria: Hands and feet involved in 85% of the cases
- Juvenile rheumatoid arthritis
- Systemic lupus erythematosus
- Raynaud phenomenon (acrocyanosis)
- Acute graft-vs-host disease

Skin disorders

- Atopic dermatitis (infantile)
- Dyshydrotic eczema, pompholyx
- Chronic allergic contact dermatitis
- Psoriasis
- Lichen simplex
- Papillon-Lefèvre syndrome
- Olmsted syndrome
- Acrodermatitis enteropathica (zinc deficiency) can be presenting sign of cystic fibrosis
- Toxic shock syndrome: Desquamation during the recovery phase; major criteria for staphyloccocal TSS
- Drugs: Ampicillin, especially in patients with infectious mononucleosis
- Chronic liver disease: Cirrhosis, hepatoma
- Metabolic disease: Gangliosidosis
- Malignancy: Acute leukemia, lymphoma

Workup and Diagnosis

- History
  - –Season of onset (can be a clue for various infectious etiologies)
  - –Patient's age
  - –Presence of fever, pruritus (typical of urticaria)
  - –Tick/rat/bat bites (e.g., rat bite fever or Lyme disease)
  - –Travel (to endemic areas for Lyme, RMSF)
  - –Sick contacts
  - –Contact allergen
- Physical exam
  - –Rash pattern and distribution, desquamation (interdigital, periungal), edema, involvement of other areas of the body
  - –Other signs and symptoms associated (oral lesions, URI symptoms, arthritis, genital chancre)
  - –Verify criteria for disease such as Kawasaki, Lyme, juvenile rheumatoid arthritis
- Labs
  - –CBC, ESR/CRP
  - –Serologic testing for RMSF, Lyme, syphilis, toxoplasmosis, SLE
  - –Throat swabs and stool culture for enterovirus serotype (no therapeutic significance)
  - –KOH prep for hyphae
- ECG, echocardiography, and cardiology consult if Kawasaki disease or endocarditis is suspected

Treatment

- Directed toward the causative condition
- Skin disorders: Topical steroids, wet dressings, and antibiotics for secondary infections; psoriasis requires UV light and topical applications of tar products
- Viral infections: Generally self-limited and do not require supportive treatment; acyclovir may have a role in treating HFMD
- Kawasaki disease: Treat with IVIG, high-dose aspirin
- Bacterial infections require antibiotics (RMSF, Lyme disease, syphilis, streptococcal infections, TSS, rat-bite fever)
- Fungal infections require topical antifungal treatment
- Parasitic infections: Topical permethrin or lindane for scabies
  - –Pyrimethamine and sulfadiazine for congenital toxoplasmosis (regardless of symptoms)
- Acrodermatitis enteropathica: Lifelong oral zinc supplements

140. Hirsutism

The etiology and significance of hirsutism depend on whether the patient is hirsute only (excessive hair), or if he/she is also virilized (increased weight, clitoromegaly, acne, deep voice). Polycystic ovarian syndrome (PCOS) is a very common cause; the incidence may be as high as 10–15% of women.

Differential Diagnosis

- Drug-induced
  - –Cyclosporin, steroids, oral contraceptives, Dilantin, some diuretics (acetazolamide, hydrochlorothiazide), Minoxidil, penicillamines
- Syndrome-associated
  - –Cornelia de Lange syndrome
  - –Trisomy 18
  - –Hurler syndrome
  - –Bloom syndrome
  - –Seckel syndrome
  - –Marshall-Smith syndrome
  - –Rubinstein-Taybi syndrome
  - –Leprechaunism
- Ovarian
  - –PCOS
  - –Gonadal dysgenesis
  - –Ovarian tumors
- Adrenal
  - –CAH
  - –Cushing syndrome
  - –17α-hydroxylase deficiency
  - –21-hydroxylase deficiency
  - –Adrenal tumor
- Other causes
  - –Idiopathic
  - –5 α-reductase deficiency
  - –Hyperprolactinemia
  - –HAIR-AN syndrome (hirsutism, androgenization, insulin resistance, and acanthosis nigricans)
  - –Achard-Thiers syndrome: Obesity and facial hirsutism develop by 15–30 years of age; hypertension and obesity occur later
  - –Porphyria: Congenital erythropoietic porphyria have increased body hair, red urine, photosensitivity with bullae, and red to pink teeth (werewolves of old)

Workup and Diagnosis

- History
  - –Age of onset (PCOS presents in teen years, CAH can present in infancy or adulthood)
  - –GU development and menstrual history
  - –Associated symptoms such as stress, weight changes, acne, voice changes
  - –Medications
  - –Family history of hair growth patterns or endocrine abnormalities
- Physical exam
  - –Vital signs and complete exam of all systems to evaluate for signs of androgen excess
  - –Breast exam and detailed GU exam
  - –Abdominal exam to rule out pelvic or adrenal mass
- Labs
  - –If virilization is present, check serum testosterone level, 17-hydroxyprogesterone and dehydroepiandrosterone
  - –If patient is not pregnant, progesterone challenge test may be performed; patient should have withdrawal bleeding after cessation of progesterone
  - –If no withdrawal bleeding occurs after challenge, check levels of estradiol, FSH, LH, and prolactin
  - –LH:FSH ratio >2.5:1 in PCOS (low relative FSH does not allow androstenedione to be converted to estradiol in the ovary, resulting in androgen buildup and anovulation)
- Newborn screen for CAH

Treatment

- PCOS and idiopathic
  - –Estrogen-predominant oral contraceptives decrease plasma androgens
  - –Depo-Provera may also be used
  - –Spironolactone works by competing for androgen receptors
  - –Cimetidine has a side effect of decreasing testosterone and increasing estrogen levels
  - –GnRH agonist to facilitate better function of the hypothalamic-pituitary axis
- Drug-induced: Eliminate causative medication if possible and hirsutism may resolve spontaneously
- Hyperprolactinemia: Bromocriptine (prolactin antagonist)

141. Hyperhidrosis (Excessive Sweating)

The common causes of excessive sweating are benign and are the body's natural cooling response or the response to emotional stimuli. The most important cause to keep in mind is congestive heart failure, especially when accompanied by poor feeding in an infant, as well as night sweats which may be an ominous sign.

Differential Diagnosis

- Fever
- Emotional stimuli
  - –Sweaty palms and soles is referred to as volar hyperhidrosis
- Exercise
- Increased ambient temperature (heat)
- Spicy foods
- Obesity
- Atopy
- Congestive heart failure
  - –May also be accompanied by poor feeding, pallor, cyanosis, tachypnea, lethargy, exercise intolerance
  - –Causes include congenital heart disease, cardiomyopathies and viral myocarditis
- Shock, respiratory failure
- Hypoglycemia
- Syncope
  - –Vasovagal syncope is commonly preceded by sweating
- Medications/drugs
  - –Withdrawal (e.g., alcohol, opioids)
  - –Overdose of salicylates, organophosphates
  - –Insulin, emetics
- Cluster headaches
- Hyperthyroidism
- Pheochromocytoma
  - –An adrenal tumor associated with hypertension and symptoms of excessive catecholamines
- Familial dysautonomia (Riley-Day syndrome)
  - –An autosomal-dominant sensory neuropathy
  - –Characterized by hypotonia, feeding problems, and poor autonomic control
- Spinal cord injury
- Juvenile rheumatoid arthritis
- Lymphoma
- Raynaud phenomenon
  - –Sweating often accompanies the extremity color changes
- Night sweats
  - –Most commonly associated with TB and malignancy (see also "Night Sweats" entry)

Workup and Diagnosis

- History
  - –Precipitating factors, including emotional stimuli, exercise, heat, spicy foods
  - –Fever, associated symptoms
  - –Current medications
  - –Possibility of ingestions
  - –Any problems with feeding or exercise
  - –Past medical history including chronic illnesses
  - –Family history of any cardiac or sweating problems
- Physical exam
  - –Vital signs, including temperature, pulse, respiratory rate, and blood pressure
  - –Assessment of airway, breathing, and circulation
  - –Cardiac and lung exam, paying special attention to any murmurs, abnormal heart sounds, pulses, irregular rhythms
  - –Skin for capillary refill, rashes, pallor, or cyanosis
  - –Signs of systemic illness
- Labs
  - –Since most causes of excessive sweating are benign, laboratory evaluation is not usually needed
  - –Consider obtaining glucose, drug screen, thyroid function tests
  - –Based on history and physical exam, consider an electrocardiogram or echocardiogram

Treatment

- If the patient is critically ill, stabilize the patient's airway, breathing, and circulation
- Remove precipitating factors
  - –Put patient in cool environment, remove excessive clothing, and offer cool fluids
- Treat fever with antipyretics
  - –The patient may sweat more with defervescence
- Treat infections with appropriate medications
- Address congestive heart failure
  - –Consult cardiology
  - –Initially, diuretics are used
  - –Digoxin, an antiarrhythmic and inotrope, is also used
  - –Corrective surgery or cardiac transplantation
- For excessive sweating that is bothersome to the patient, topical aluminum chloride may be used; anticholinergics work, but have many side effects
- Surgery, including removal of axillary sweat glands and cervicothoracic sympathectomy, is rarely used

142. Hypopigmented Lesions

Hypopigmented lesions are extremely variable in etiology. A careful history and physical examination by an experienced clinician are usually sufficient to make the diagnosis. Hypopigmentation may be of significant cosmetic concern, particularly patchy lesions in exposed areas on dark-skinned individuals. Unfortunately, some hypopigmentation conditions are difficult to treat.

Differential Diagnosis

- Tinea versicolor
  - –Infection of the skin by *Trichophyton*
  - –Manifests as patchy hypopigmentation and sometimes hyperpigmentation
  - –Commonly found on the trunk
- Vitiligo
  - –Progressive patchy depigmentation
  - –Common on hands, arms, face, neck
  - –Associated with thyroid disease
- Congenital nevus depigmentosus
  - –Areas of depigmentation exist at birth
  - –Individual lesions may enlarge; however, new ones do not generally form
- Pityriasis alba
  - –Related to eczema
  - –Hypopigmented patches on the face
- Postinflammatory hypopigmentation
  - –May occur after any type of cutaneous inflammation
  - –More obvious in dark-skinned individuals
  - –Duration is weeks to months
- Post-topical steroid hypopigmentation
  - –Topical steroids, particularly fluorinated, may cause thinning, atrophy, and hypopigmentation with prolonged use
  - –More common on the face and perineum
- Tuberous sclerosis (TS)
  - –A neurocutaneous disorder affecting the brain, eyes, kidney, skin, and heart
  - –Systemic symptoms are preceded by ash-leaf macules, which are usually present in affected infants
  - –Other skin findings are shagreen patches, adenoma sebaceum, periungual fibromas
  - –Mental retardation, seizures are common
- Congenital oculocutaneous albinism
  - –May involve the hair, skin, or eyes
  - –Inherited in autosomal recessive, autosomal dominant, and X-linked forms
  - –Variable degree of hypopigmentation
  - –Photophobia is a frequent finding
  - –Patients are prone to skin cancer
- Partial albinism (piebaldism)
  - –White forelock, nonpigmentad patches on the face, trunk, elbows, and knees
- Waardenburg syndrome
  - Facial dysmorphism, a white forelock, and hypopigmentation
  - –May be accompanied by hearing deficit

Workup and Diagnosis

- History
  - –Onset, duration, progression of lesions
  - –Past medical history including medication use
  - –Family history of hypopigmentation, neurocutaneous disorders
- Physical exam
  - –Size, distribution, number of lesions
  - –Wood lamp examination for fungus
  - –Ash-leaf macules are pale, leaf-shaped patches; adenoma sebaceum smooth, round flesh-colored papules on the face; shagreen patches have an orange-peel texture
  - –Consider developmental, IQ testing
  - –Test hearing if Waardenburg is suspected
- Labs
  - –Albinism: Assay for tyrosinase (an enzyme necessary for melanin production) activity
- Radiology
  - –Echo for rhabdomyomas (TS)
- Studies
  - –Biopsy for presense or absence of melanocytes (present but defective in albinism, absent in vitiligous regions)
  - –Genetic testing for known albinism mutations as well as piebaldism and Waardenburg syndrome
  - –Hair bulb incubation test for albinism (helps distinguish type by evaluating tyrosinase activity)
  - –EEG if seizures may be occurring (TS)

Treatment

- Tinea versicolor: Selenium sulfide shampoo
- Vitiligo: Avoid trauma, as lesions tend to advance in areas of trauma; monitor for endocrine abnormalities, especially DM, adrenal insufficiency, and thyroid disease; oral or topical psoralens and UV light may result in cosmetic improvement
- Pityriasis alba: Usually self-limiting, topical steroids may help
- Postinflammatory: Self-limiting
- Post-topical steroid: Discontinue use of steroid
- Tuberous sclerosis: Control of seizures, developmental support, periodic Echo for rhabdomyosarcoma
- Albinism: Scrupulous use of protective clothing, hats, sunglasses, and sunscreen to prevent actinic keratosis and carcinoma
- Waardenburg syndrome: Hearing aids, developmental support

143. Jaundice in Infants – Direct

Jaundice refers to the presence of a yellow hue of the skin, sclerae, or mucous membranes. Direct, or more specifically, conjugated hyperbilirubinemia represents a pathologic condition of cholestasis. It is defined as a direct bilirubin fraction greater than 2 mg/dL, or greater than 15% of the total serum bilirubin. Because the outcome of treatment varies greatly with the rapiditiy of diagnosis, prompt recognition and evaluation are critical in the neonatal period.

Differential Diagnosis

- Bile duct obstruction
  - –Biliary atresia: Represents the most frequent cause for liver transplantation in the pediatric patient; prompt diagnosis is crucial, as patient outcome is better if intervention comes before 60 days of life
  - –Choledochal cyst
  - –Common bile duct gallstone
  - –Choledochocele
  - –Bile duct stricture
  - –Alagille syndrome
  - –Caroli disease
  - –Congenital hepatic fibrosis
- Neonatal hepatitis
  - –Idiopathic hepatitis: Diagnosis of exclusion that should be made only when other causes are excluded; accounts for 60% of patients with neonatal cholestasis
  - –Infections: TORCH, hepatitis B, HIV, *E. coli*, adenovirus, enterovirus, parvovirus B16, tuberculosis, listeriosis, malaria
- Metabolic disorders
  - –α-1 antitrypsin deficiency
  - –Cystic fibrosis
  - –Hypothyroidism
  - –Neonatal iron storage disease
  - –Amino acids: tyrosinemia
  - –Carbohydrates: Galactosemia, fructosemia
  - –Lipids: Niemann-Pick, Gaucher, Wolman, cholesterol ester storage disease
  - –Mitochondropathies
  - –Bile acid synthetic disorders
  - –Peroxisomal: Zellweger syndrome
  - –Urea cycle defects
- Toxins
  - –Total parenteral nutrition
  - –Drugs: Trimethaprim-sulfamethoxazole, anticonvulsants
- Miscellaneous
  - –Sepsis/hypoperfusion
  - –Erythrophagocytic lymphohistiocytosis
  - –Extracorporeal membrane oxygenation
  - –Trisomy 17, 18, 21
  - –Neonatal lupus erythematosus
  - –Donohue syndrome
  - –Rotor syndrome
  - –Dubin-Johnson syndrome
  - –Byler disease (PFIC type 1)
  - –Cholestasis of North-American Indians
  - –Nielsen syndrome

Workup and Diagnosis

- History
  - –Prenatal/perinatal history: Infections, gestational age, birth weight, miscarriages, newborn screen
  - –Age of onset, activity level, oral intake, urine output, stool color, emesis, hematemesis, hematochezia, melena, bruising, bleeding, fever, developmental milestones, medications, formula type
- Physical exam: Weight/length, icteris, dysmorphic features, cardiac murmur, ascites, abdominal distension, hepatosplenomegaly, edema, bruising, tone, reflexes
- Labs (initial): Fractionated bilirubin (total, indirect, direct), AST, ALT, GGT, alkaline phosphatase, total protein, albumin, CBC, electrolytes including glucose, PT, PTT, blood/urine culture, U/A
- Labs (directed): Thyroid function tests, serum α-1 antitrypsin level, urine for reducing sugars, serum and urine amino acids, urine organic acids including succinylacetone, infectious serologies, serum iron levels, sweat test, consider Alagille genetic testing
- Ultrasound provides best initial radiographic study for obstruction, hepatosplenomegaly
- Hepatobiliary scintigraphy (HIDA scan)
- Percutaneous liver biopsy
  - –Histology, virology, electron microscopy for bile duct expansion/paucity, storage disorders
- Exploratory laparotomy and intraoperative cholangiogram to rule out biliary atresia
- Consider X-ray for butterfly vertebrae (for Alagille)

Treatment

- Varies by specific disorder
- General medication principles of cholestasis include
  - –Promoting bile flow with ursodeoxycholic acid
  - –Consider phenobarbital (increases bile excretion)
  - –Fat-soluble vitamins including K, D, E
  - –Vitamin A is a relative contraindication given hepatotoxicity at high levels
- Consider formula with medium chain triglycerides as fat source (does not require bile acids to be absorbed)
- Treat underlying disorder
  - –Kasai portoenterostomy for biliary atresia
  - –Surgical repair of choledochal cyst
  - –Special formulas for tyrosinemia
  - –Lactose free formula for galactosemia (e.g., soy based)
  - –Remove toxic exposures
  - –Treat infections
  - –Treat hypothyroidism

144. Jaundice in Infants – Indirect

Jaundice is the presence of a yellow hue of the skin, sclerae, or mucous membranes due to elevation of serum bilirubin; it usually becomes apparent at a total serum bilirubin level of 5 mg/dL. It is present in approximately 60% of term infants and 80% of premature infants during the first week of life. Although the indirect form is neurotoxic, differentiating the nonpolar, lipid-soluble, indirect form from the potentially more serious polar, water-soluble direct form represents the most important first step.

Differential Diagnosis

- Icterus neonatorum (physiologic jaundice)
  - The most common form of indirect jaundice in infants under 14 days of age
  - Caused by increased bilirubin production with transient limited conjugation abilities
- Breast-feeding jaundice
  - Occurs in first week of life in 13% of breast-fed infants
  - Secondary to poor volume intake
- Breast-milk jaundice
  - Occurs in about 2% of breast-fed infants after day 7 of life
  - Secondary to glucuronidase in breast milk
- Hematologic: Hemolysis increases bili load
  - Rh incompatability
  - ABO incompatability
  - Glucose-6-phosphate dehydrogenase (G6PD) deficiency
  - Pyruvate kinase deficiency
  - Hereditary spherocytosis
  - Elliptocytosis
  - Thalassemia
  - Polycythemia
- Extravascular blood
  - Cephalohematoma
  - Trauma
  - Swallowed maternal blood
- Endocrinologic
  - Hypothyroidism
  - Maternal diabetes
- Sepsis
- Metabolic
  - Crigler-Najjar I
  - Crigler-Najjar II (Arias syndrome)
  - Crigler-Najjar III
- Cardiopulmonary
  - Congestive heart failure
  - Patent ductus arteriosus
  - Portal vein thrombosis
- Anatomic
  - Pyloric stenosis
  - Duodenal atresia/stenosis
  - Duodenal web
- Drugs
  - Oxytocin
  - Sulfonamides
  - Ceftriaxone
  - Chuen-Lin
- Lucey-Driscoll syndrome

Workup and Diagnosis

- History
  - Prenatal/perinatal: Pregnancy complications, gestational age, maternal blood type/Rh, drug use, infections, delivery method, delivery intervention, birth weight, newborn screen results, previous miscarriages
  - HPI: Onset of jaundice, feeding tolerance, appropriate weight gain, trauma, evidence of bleeding/bruising, urine output, stool output/diarrhea, emesis, lethargy, drug exposure
  - Diet history: Breast- and/or formula-fed, length of time on each breast, latch strength
  - Family history: Bleeding disorders, perinatal deaths, endocrinopathies
- Physical exam
  - Weight, overall appearance, level of jaundice, fontanelle size, cranial abnormalities, scleral icteris, mucous membranes, cardiac murmurs, hepatosplenomegaly, bruising, bleeding, reflexes, tone, seizures
- Labs: Fractionated bilirubin (total, indirect, direct), CBC with smear, reticulocyte count
- Hemolysis: Blood type/Rh, Coombs, hemoglobin electrophoresis
- Thyroid function tests (check state newborn screen)
- Limited value of imaging unless looking for obstruction or bleeding
- Hearing evaluation if kernicterus likely

Treatment

- Treatment options vary based on level of bilirubin, age of presentation, and cause
  - Goal is prevent levels high enough to cause kernicterus
- Phototherapy involves the use of photon energy to change the structure of bilirubin and permit excretion without glucuronidation
  - Decisions for use are age-based
  - Considered when serum level above 14 mg/dL
- Exchange transfusion should be considered with serum levels above 25 mg/dL
- IVF or breast-feed more frequently to increase volume
- Correct endocrine abnormality
- Improve perfusion if cardiac problem
- Correct anatomic abnormality
- Consider enteral binding agents
  - Cholestyramine, charcoal, calcium phosphate
- Crigler-Najjar: Phenobarbital, may need liver transplantation

145. Morbilliform Rashes

The term morbilliform means "measles-like." Approximately 80% of all cutaneous drug reactions are morbilliform in nature, and many nonspecific viruses cause a morbilliform rash. True measles is rare in the developed nations because the measles vaccine is very effective.

Differential Diagnosis

- Measles
  - –Also called rubeola, a highly contagious (>90% exposed patients acquire the disease), moderately severe viral illness
  - –Characterized by fever and malaise in prodrome, cough, conjunctivitis, Koplick spots on buccal mucosa, and an exanthem on day 3–4
  - –The exanthem of measles is blotchy, blanching, erythematous maculopapules beginning at the head and spreading distally
  - –Severe complications, such as pneumonia, DIC, encephalitis, can occur
- Viral exanthems
  - –Adenovirus: Many types can cause a morbilliform rash that is usually generalized when first identified, often accompanied by upper respiratory symptoms
  - –Rubella (German measles): Without a prodrome in young children, the exanthem is pinkish, fine maculopapules with a distribution similar to that of measles
  - –Other viruses may also cause this rash
- Drug eruptions
  - –Erythematous, maculopapular rash that may be blanching or fine in nature
  - –May be generalized, or begin on the trunk or face then spread to the extremities
  - –Rash usually begins 1–2 weeks into therapy
  - –May be pruritic
  - –Drugs commonly resulting in morbilliform reactions are anticonvulsants, cephalosporins, pencillins, and sulfonamides

Workup and Diagnosis

- History
  - –Presence of prodrome such as fever, upper respiratory symptoms
  - –Onset and duration of rash, distribution and spread of the rash over time
  - –Sick contacts, especially daycare or school
  - –Immunization history, past medical history, medications
- Physical exam
  - –Vital signs
  - –General exam of systems with special attention to mucous membranes and HEENT exam
  - –Evaluation of the characteristics of the rash such as distribution, type, confluence, blanching, and other skin findings
- Diagnostic testing is not usually needed; however, viral cultures or titers for measles can be sent if necessary to confirm diagnosis

Treatment

- Viral exanthems will resolve spontaneously in most cases
- Morbilliform drug reactions are common and resolve within a week of stopping the offending medication
- Measles
  - –Isolation precautions
  - –Notification of health department and infectious disease authorities
  - –Supportive care including ICU when necessary; there is no specific antiviral therapy

146. Pallor

Pallor describes reduced coloring of the skin and/or mucous membranes and is very subjective. How easily pallor is diagnosed varies with skin color and the thickness and vascularity of the subcutaneous tissue. Sometimes it is only a subtle lightening of skin color. It may be very difficult to detect in a dark-skinned person. It may be only apparent by examining the conjuctiva or oral mucous membranes. Anemia of any cause is the most common reason for pallor, but it lacks sensitivity and specificity as an exam finding.

Differential Diagnosis

- Anemia
- Hypoglycemia
- Circulatory failure: Acute reduction in blood flow to the skin or mucous membranes
  - –Vasovagal event
  - –Shock
  - –Hypotension
  - –Asphyxia (including birth asphyxia)
  - –Hypothermia
  - –Congenital or acquired heart disease
  - –Sepsis (viral or bacterial)
  - –Severe dehydration
- Adrenal failure
  - –Recent or long-term use of steroids
  - –Addison disease
- Malaria
- Hypopituitarism
- Congenital/familial
- Malnutrition (e.g., anorexia nervosa)
- Generalized edema
- Increased thickness of the skin
  - –Myxedema
  - –Acromegaly
- Ingestion (e.g., diethylene glycol)
- Localized loss of pigment (vitiligo)
- Cystic fibrosis
- Chronic inflammatory condition
  - –Juvenile rheumatoid arthritis
  - –Inflammatory bowel disease
  - –Systemic lupus erythematosus
  - –Diabetes mellitus
  - –Chronic renal disease
- Lack of sun exposure
- Atopy
- Migraine
- Breath-holding spell
- Infantile spasms
- Intussusception

Workup and Diagnosis

- History
  - –Onset, constant or fluctuating
  - –Fever and fever pattern, exposure to illness
  - –Fatigue, lethargy, cough, generalized aches
  - –Dehydration (vomiting, diarrhea, decreased intake)
  - –Travel to malaria-endemic regions
  - –Heat or cold intolerance, weight gain or loss
  - –Symptoms of anemia, jaundice, previous transfusion, ethnic and cultural background
  - –Abnormal sweating
  - –Familial red blood cell, heart, or thyroid disease
- Physical exam
  - –Ill, vital signs, alertness, sensory exam
  - –Pupil size, conjunctival pallor
  - –Work of breathing, pulse oximetry
  - –Murmur, decreased perfusion, gallop (S_3)
  - –Palmar pallor, acrocyanosis, bronzed discoloration
  - –Patchy depigmentation, tenting or doughy consistency, abnormal skin thickness, lanugo
- Labs/studies
  - –CBC with differential and smear
  - –Electrolytes (especially glucose)
  - –BUN, Cr, albumin, LFT
  - –Blood culture and urine culture
  - –Thyroid functions and/or cortisol level
  - –Specific infection titers, exam for *Plasmodium*
  - –Chest X-ray, ECG, and echocardiogram
  - –Toxicology screen

Treatment

- Immediate respiratory and cardiovascular stabilization
- Cardiovascular collapse or hypoglycemia should be treated appropriately
- Suspected sepsis or infection should be promptly treated with broad-spectrum antimicrobial therapy and supportive treatment
- Stress-dose steroid therapy if insufficiency suspected
- Children with acute blood loss may not manifest anemia until the blood has had a chance to equilibrate
  - –Any suspected severe blood loss needs to be managed aggressively
- For children who are stable at presentation
  - –First ascertain whether pallor is true or relative
  - –Most pallor is due to anemia, so treatment should be directed at underlying cause of decreased hemoglobin production and concentration

147. Petechiae

Idiopathic thrombocytic purpura (ITP) is the most common cause of petechiae in an otherwise well child. It is an autoimmune process which typically occurs about 4 weeks after a viral infection. The child will have sudden onset of generalized petechiae. Most cases resolve spontaneously, although 10–20% children with ITP may develop chronic ITP.

Differential Diagnosis

- Antibody-mediated
  - –ITP
  - –Immunologic disorders
  - –Infection
- Coagulopathy
  - –Disseminated intravascular coagulopathy
  - –Sepsis
  - –Necrotizing enterocolitis
  - –Cavernous hemangioma (Kasabach-Merritt syndrome)
- Congenital
  - –Fanconi anemia: Pancytopenia usually does not occur until after age 5. Associated with short stature, hyperpigmentation, thumb anomalies, renal problems, and microcephaly; autosomal recessive
  - –Wiskott-Aldrich syndrome: Immune defects with increased IgE and IgA, and decreased IgM; associated with eczema and thrombocytopenia; X-linked
  - –Thrombocytopenia absent radii: Thrombocytopenia is most marked during the first year of life; autosomal recessive
  - –May-Heglin anomaly: Giant platelets and leukocyte inclusions
  - –Bernard-Soulier disease: Giant platelets
  - –Glanzmann thrombocytopenia
  - –Metabolic disorders
  - –Osteopetrosis
- Acquired decreased production
  - –Leukemia or other malignancy
  - –Aplastic anemia
  - –Folate or vitamin B12 deficiency
- Other causes
  - –Hemolytic uremic syndrome
  - –Thrombotic thrombocytopenic purpura
  - –Drug-induced
  - –Hypersplenism
  - –Respiratory distress syndrome
  - –Uremia
  - –Progressive pigmentary dermatosis (Schamberg disease): Petechiae typically over the lower extremities

Workup and Diagnosis

- History
  - –Age of the patient, recent state of health
  - –Past medical history, medications, family history
  - –Onset sudden or gradual, bleeding from mucous membranes, preceding viral infection, weight loss, appetite, night sweats, frequent emesis, tight tourniquet or blood pressure cuff
- Physical exam
  - –Vital signs, stability, temperature, blood pressure
  - –General appearance (well- or ill-appearing)
  - –Examine gums, nose, ears for signs of bleeding
  - –Evaluate presence and location of petechiae, purpura, hemangiomas, and other skin findings such as eczema
  - –Note lung sounds, presence or absence of cardiovascular hyperdynamic state; palpate spleen
- Labs
  - –CBC with differential to discover thrombocytopenia and determine whether other cell lines are involved
  - –Bone marrow aspirate if thrombocytopenia cannot be explained by history or physical or if there is a worrisome history or involvement of other cell lines
- Additional tests: Blood culture, peripheral smear, radiographic studies, U/A, ANA, HIV all may be useful depending on the history/physical

Treatment

- Idiopathic thrombocytic purpura
  - –Most cases resolve spontaneously without treatment
  - –IVIG or steroids are needed in the more severe cases where there is significant bleeding or platelet count is <10,000
  - –RhoGam can be given to Rh+ patients as an option for patients who don't respond to other therapies
- Platelet transfusion is indicated for patients with low platelets where production is limited, destruction is not rapid, and platelet count is dangerously low, such as leukemia
- Splenectomy may be an option if platelets are sequestered chronically

148. Pigmented Lesions

Pigmented lesions are very common in children. Most lesions are benign but can be a sign of a genetic syndrome. Malignant melanoma (MM) in children is commonly associated with giant congenital melanocytic nevi (CMN), so early detection and prevention is crucial. MM comprises 1–3% of pediatric malignancies; 10% of familial atypical multiple mole melanoma (FAMMM) patients develop MM before 20 years of age.

Differential Diagnosis

- Mongolian spots ("dermal melanosis")
  - –Present at birth; incidence 90% in black children, 80% in Asian, 65% in Latin-American, 5% in white; disappears in childhood, may persist on distal extremities
- Postinflammatory hyperpigmentation
  - –Most common pigmentation disorder, follows skin inflammation, resolves within months, more common on dark skin
- Acquired melanocytic nevi (AMN, "moles")
  - –Begin in early childhood, darken and increase in size, can become raised during puberty, by late adolescence most people have 20–30; regress and disappear with age
- Dysplastic nevi ("atypical moles")
  - –Sporadic or familial (autosomal dominant, FAMMM), incidence 2–5% (adults), usually develop in puberty, risk of malignant change (MM) is 5–10%
- Congenital melanocytic nevi
  - –1–2% of newborns
  - –Small CMN: Malignancy risk uncertain
  - –Giant CMN: 2–15% lifetime malignancy risk, <1/20,000 births, 3% of MM arise in giant CMNs
  - –LMM: Seen in 30% of giant CMN
- Malignant melanoma (MM) may arise in acquired, dysplastic or congenital nevi, on normal skin or extracutaneous; rarely congenital MM (transplacental); risk factors are fair skin, >50–100 nevi, multiple dysplastic nevi, excessive sun exposure, FAMMM, scleroderma pigmentosum, immunosuppression
- Freckles
- Lentigines
- Tinea versicolor (fungus *Malassezia furfur*)
- Urticaria pigmentosa: Most common form of mastocytosis; juvenile-onset 7% risk of malignancy and adult-onset 30% risk
- Incontinentia pigmenti: Streaks/whorls
- Café au lait macules: Incidence 10% of children, >5 lesions of >1.5 cm diameter after puberty indicates neurofibromatosis, also in McCune-Albright, tuberous sclerosis, Bloom
- Other nevi: Ito/Ota, Blue, Spitz, Becker, halo, zosteriform, lentiginous, nevus spilus

Workup and Diagnosis

- Mongolian spots: Poorly defined, several cm diameter, blue/grey macules, mostly on buttocks, back, arms, and legs; not on palms, soles, face, mucosal surfaces
- AMN: pink/brown/black macules or papules, <5 mm diameter, 90% flat (junctional), 10% raised, may have hair; sun-exposed skin; not on palms, soles, genitals, mucosal surfaces
- Dysplastic nevi: Pink/brown/black macules or papules, >5 mm diameter, irregular border, on sun-exposed skin
- CMNs: Brown/black/blue, flat/nodular, leathery
  - –Small CMN: <1 cm, on trunk and proximal limbs
  - –Giant CMN: >20 cm diameter, may grow hair, midline of back, often satellite nevi
- LMM: May show CNS symptoms (e.g., seizures, hydrocephalus, motor deficits)
- Freckles: Light brown, jagged borders, darken in sun
- Lentigines: Dark brown, any part of skin/mucosa, may be seen with syndromes (Peutz-Jeghers)
- Nevi of Ito/Ota: Shoulder/fronto-periorbital areas
- Urticaria pigmentosa: Darier sign (pruritus/erythema upon stroking), symptoms from mast cell degranulation
- Tinea versicolor: Guttate pattern, can be hypopigmented
- Excisional biopsy: Dysplastic nevi, CMM, MM, and other lesions; distinctive histologic/cytologic features
- MRI of brain and spinal fluid exam: Indicated in giant CMN located on head or paraspinal to rule out LMM

Treatment

- Early detection
  - –Acquired melanocytic nevi: Regular exams to detect atypical changes
  - –Dysplastic nevi: Exam every 6–12 months with comparative photographs
  - –CMN: Small/intermediate need regular exams with careful palpation (MM may arise deep within nevus without surface change)
- Excision
  - –Malignant melanoma
  - –Dysplastic and acquired melanocytic nevi: If tender, ulcerating, pruritus, erythema, satellite lesions, regional lymphadenopathy or change in color, size, shape, borders, or texture
  - –Giant CMN: Early excision if amenable to surgery
  - –After excision, close follow-up is indicated
- Tinea versicolor: Topical antifungal
- Prevention: Protection from excessive sun exposure

149. Pruritus

Pruritus is the desire to scratch that is induced by unpleasant cutaneous sensations caused by histamines and other endogenous substances. Atopic dermatitis is one of the most common childhood skin diseases; emergencies include severe angioedema/anaphylaxis and Stevens-Johnson syndrome. Topical preparations are common allergens.

Differential Diagnosis

- Urticaria
  - –Hypersensitivity reaction causing edema via mast cell/basophil release of histamine, kinins, prostaglandins, and serotonin, mostly IgE-mediated
  - –Hives; subcutaneous and mucous membranes
  - –Angioedema: Most cases acute (resolving within 48 hours); chronic > 6 weeks
  - –Anaphylaxis: May be life-threatening
- Atopic dermatitis
  - –Incidence 2–10%; often begins in infancy
  - –Most cases improve with age
  - –Frequent remissions/exacerbations
  - –Increased risk of infection (herpes, eczema herpeticum; staph, strep)
  - –Can be exercise-induced
- Xerosis (dry skin)
  - –Idiopathic or due to excessive bathing, low humidity, etc.
- Tinea (dermatophytoses, "ringworm")
  - –Fungal infection (*Trichophyton, Microsporum, Epidermophyton*)
  - –Scalp (tinea capitis), face, trunk, extremities (t. corporis), feet (t. pedis)
  - –complications: superinfection and kerion
- Contact dermatitis
  - –Allergens (poison ivy, cosmetics, dyes, drugs, foods, jewelry/nickel, animals)
  - –Irritants (soap, chemicals, wool, fiberglass)
- Scarlet fever (group A strep): "Sandpaper rash," incubation period 1–7 days; age 5–15 years, 15–20% colonized (oropharyngeal)
- Herpes: Varicella, zoster, herpes simplex
- Lice (pediculosis): Head or pubic area
- Mites (scabies [*Sarcoptes scabiei*])
- Pinworms (*Enterobius vermicularis*)
- Cholestasis (TPN, biliary atresia)
- Erythema multiforme ("bull's eye rash"): Stevens-Johnson syndrome
- Drug-induced: Opiates, barbiturates, isoniazid, phenothiazines, erythromycin
- Systemic diseases: Malignancies, renal failure, mastocytosis, SLE, JRA, hypo- and hyperthyroidism, DM
- Prurigo gestationis
- Parasites ("swimmer itch," trematodes)
- Chronic skin diseases (psoriasis)

Workup and Diagnosis

- History and physical exam
  - –Location, duration, rash, exposure, chronic illness, associated symptoms, ill contacts
  - –Urticaria: Exposure to foods, drugs, bacteria, viruses, insect bites, etc.; wheals (erythematous, raised, well-circumscribed lesions) usually self-limited; may also have angioedema, wheezing, stridor, hoarseness, anaphylaxis, hypotension
  - –Atopic dermatitis: Family history; ill-defined, erythematous, scaly plaques; in infant, head, extensor surfaces, and trunk; in child, antecubital/popliteal fossae, neck, wrist/ankle; may also have Morgan folds (lines under lower eyelids)
  - –Tinea: Erythematous, scaly, circular plaque with central clearing; kerion is inflammatory, painful mass with sterile pustules and regional lymphadenopathy
  - –Poison ivy: Linear streaks of vesicles, may last several weeks; exposure to poison ivy, oak, or sumac
  - –Lice: Nits on hair shafts
  - –Mites: 1–2 mm papules and burrows on palm, sole, interdigital web, axilla, genitalia, wrist, ankle
  - –Pinworm: Nocturnal anal pruritus
  - –Scarlet fever: Erythematous, finely granular rash, most prominent in axilla and groin, circumoral pallor
- Pinworm: Apply tape to anus, see microscopic egg
- Scarlet fever: Throat culture or antigen detection
- Tinea: KOH preparation, culture, or Wood lamp to confirm diagnosis (usually diagnosed clinically)

Treatment

- Urticaria: Antihistamine; if nonresponsive, corticosteroid, avoid triggers
- Severe angioedema/anaphylaxis
  - –Epinephrine 1:1,000, 0.01 mg/kg SC every 15 minutes
  - –Maximum dose 0.3 mg, IV fluids for hypotension
  - –Give epinephrine kits to patient for self-administration
- Atopic dermatitis: Topical corticosteroid or nonsteroidal immunosuppressant (e.g., pimecrolimus), oral antihistamine, moisturizing agent, room humidifier; avoid heat, stress, wool
- Tinea: Topical antifungals, oral for tinea capitis
- Poison ivy: Topical or systemic corticosteroid
- Scarlet fever: Penicillin (to prevent rheumatic fever)
- Lice/mites: Topical permethrin
  - –Consider sexual abuse if pubic lice
- Pinworm: Mebendazole or pyrantel pamoate
- Avoid scratching/heat/tight clothing
- Tepid water bath, moisturizer, topical anesthetic

150. Purpura

Purpura represents leakage of blood from vessels into skin/mucous membranes; thus, it is nonblanching on pressure; petechiae are <3 mm, ecchymosis >3 mm in diameter. Idiopathic thrombocytopenic purpura (ITP) is the most common cause of thrombocytopenic and Henoch-Schönlein purpura (HSP) the most common form of non-thrombocytopenic purpura in children; von Willebrand disease (vWD) is the most common bleeding disorder.

Differential Diagnosis

- Vasculitis (palpable purpura)
  - HSP: Most common vasculitis, incidence: 0.01%, in 50% follows URI; other triggers are bacterial infection, drugs, vaccines, food, insect bites; lasts 1–2 weeks, age 2–8 (mean 4 years), M > F, IgA-mediated, small vessels
  - Polyarteritis nodosa (PAN), Wegener granulomatosis (WG): Rare in children
- Hematologic
  - ITP: Age 1–5 years; autoantibodies against platelets (platelets destroyed by splenic macrophages); usually 1–6 weeks after viral infection; 70–80% acute self-limited; 10–20% chronic recurrent; <1% associated with intracranial hemorrhage
  - Other causes of thrombocytopenia: Wiscott-Aldrich syndrome, aplastic anemia, leukemia, disseminated intravascular coagulation (DIC), thrombocytopenia absent radius (TAR)
- Coagulation factor deficiencies:
  - Hemophilia A/B (factors VIII/XI): A (1/7,500 male births) four times more common than B; X-linked recessive
  - vWD: Prevalence 1%, autosomal dominant, vW factor deficiency or decreased function
  - Liver disease: Decreased production of coagulation factors
  - Hemorrhagic disease of the newborn: Decreased vitamin K-dependent coagulation factors (II, VII, IX, X)
- Infections
  - Bacterial/rickettsial: Meningococcemia (MC), Group A strep (scarlet fever), *Streptococcus viridans/Staphylococcus aureus* (endocarditis), Gonococcus (disseminated), *Leptospirosis, Rickettsia rickettsii* (Rocky Mountain spotted fever), *R. prowazekii* (epidemic typhus), *Ehrlichiosis*
  - Viral: Hepatitis B, Dengue hemorrhagic fever, atypical measles
- Drugs: Coumadin, heparin, aspirin, thiazide, corticosteroids, penicillins, sulfonamides
- Others: Trauma/abuse, scurvy (vitamin C deficiency)

Workup and Diagnosis

- Determine location, duration, associated/preceding symptoms, family history of bleeding disorders, social history (for abuse), insect bites, travel history, drugs, easy bruising; meningeal signs; purpura fulminans
- HSP: Purpura mostly on buttocks and legs; arthritis, abdominal pain, +/− GI hemorrhage, renal disease, self-limited; complications: intussusception, end-stage renal disease <1%; increased platelet/ESR/WBC/IgA
- ITP: Sudden petechiae/ecchymoses, epistaxis, or menorrhagia; rare splenomegaly; platelet count usually <20,000; bone marrow exam if other marrow disease is suspected
- MC: Septic shock, +/− meningitis; culture and Gram stain (blood and CSF)
- Hemophilia A/B: Easy bruising, intramuscular hematomas, hemarthroses, B milder than A; mild: 5–30%, moderate: 1–5%, severe: <1% of normal factor level
- vWD: Petechiae/ecchymoses, epistaxis, menorrhagia
- Endocarditis: Janeway lesions, splinter hemorrhages
- PAN/WG: Painful skin nodules, any organ (PAN); skin, kidneys (glomerulonephritis), pulmonary hemorrhage (WG); biopsy; angiography in WG (for aneurysms)
- Atypical measles: clinical diagnosis, history of killed vaccine + exposure
- DIC: Increased PT/PTT, decreased platelets, increased FDP/D-dimers, hemolysis

Treatment

- HSP: Analgesia, hydration, treat complications
  - Corticosteroid use is controversial
- ITP with platelet count < 20,000
  - IV immunoglobulin to block macrophage receptors
  - Anti-Rh immunoglobulin binds to RBCs so the spleen destroys RBCs instead of platelets, corticosteroids
  - Treat to raise platelet count and decrease risk of intracranial hemorrhage
  - Emergency: Platelet transfusion
  - Chronic: Immunosuppressant or splenectomy
- Hemophilia A: Recombinant F VIII
  - IV or intranasal DDAVP (desmopressin) releases F VIII and vWF from endothelial cells
- Hemophilia B: Recombinant or plasma-derived F IX
- DIC: Treat cause; transfuse platelets, cryoprecipitate, or fresh frozen plasma
- vWD: DDAVP or plasma-derived vWF
- PAN: Oral or IV corticosteroid

151. Urticaria

Drug-induced urticaria is the most common form of urticaria in children; anaphylaxis and hereditary angioedema are life-threatening conditions; remember ABCs of resuscitation (airway, breathing, circulation); best treatment is prevention; that is, avoidance of causative agents.

Differential Diagnosis

- Urticaria
  - –Epidemiology: Lifetime incidence 20%; most cases resolve within 48 hours; chronic >6 weeks
  - –Pathophysiology: Hypersensitivity reaction: allergens (IgE-mediated, prior sensitization), complement, and other cytokines activate mast cells and basophils to release histamine (also kinins, prostaglandins, serotonin) with plasma extravasation; wheals/hives: dermis edema
  - –Triggers: Most cases are idiopathic
  - –IgE-mediated: Insects (bees, wasps, scorpions, spiders, jellyfish), foods (eggs, shellfish, tree nuts, peanuts, tomatoes), drugs (penicillins, cephalosporins, NSAIDs, barbiturates, amphetamines, insulin, blood products), pollen, danders, food additives
  - –Non-IgE-mediated: Infections (strep, EBV; hepatitis A, B, and C; adenovirus, enterovirus; fleas, mites), drugs (opiates, acetylsalicylic acid, local anesthetics), physical (exercise, cold/heat, UV light, water, pressure), contrast dyes, latex
- Chronic urticaria: Associated with collagen vascular diseases (SLE, cryoglobulinemia), inflammatory bowel disease, malignancy, thyroiditis, hyperthyroidism, Behçet disease, vasculitis
- Angioedema: 50% of urticaria cases; subcutaneous and mucous membrane edema
- Anaphylaxis (IgE-mediated)
  - –Most potent foods: Peanuts, fish
  - –Mortality: 100–500 deaths/year in U.S.
  - –Associated shock has a poor prognosis
- Hereditary angioedema
  - –High mortality
  - –Most cases are autosomal dominant
  - –C1 esterase inhibitor deficiency
  - –Recurrent episodes of edema (face, upper airway, extremities)
  - –Triggers: Trauma, surgery
  - –Unresponsive to epinephrine, antihistamines
- Others: Erythema multiforme, mastocytosis, guttate psoriasis, flushing, cellulitis

Workup and Diagnosis

- History: Exposure to triggers, associated symptoms, symptoms of hypo-/hyperthyroidism, "feeling of impending doom" (anaphylaxis), history of atopy, family history of systemic diseases
- Physical exam
  - –Wheals/hives: Transient, elevated, erythematous, severely pruritic plaques, sudden onset; each wheal lasts 30 minutes to 3 hours, reappearing in other areas
  - –Papular uritcaria: 2–3 mm red papules surrounded by 10–20 mm wheals, most common in toddlers, due to fleas and mites (e.g., scabies)
  - –Physical urticaria: 10–20 mm erythematous macules with central wheal
  - –Angioedema: Edema of face, hands, feet, genitalia
  - –Anaphylaxis: Irritability, wheals, broncho- or laryngospasm (wheezing/stridor), angioedema, hypotension (late finding in children), vomiting, bloody diarrhea, mental status change; develops over minutes to hours; may develop DIC
  - –Hereditary angioedema: Nonpruritic edema
- Labs/studies
  - –Urticaria/anaphylaxis: IgE antibody skin test or radioallergosorbent test for IgE-mediated causes; culture, microscopy (ova and parasites)
  - –Angioedema: C1 esterase inhibitor, C3, C4
  - –Chronic urticaria: ANA, urinalysis, CBC, CRP, ESR, thyroid antibodies

Treatment

- Urticaria: Antihistamine; if nonresponsive to antihistamine or chronic uritcaria, then use corticosteroids
- Severe angioedema/anaphylaxis: ABCs of resuscitation
  - –Epinephrine: 1:1,000, 0.01 mg/kg SC (1:10,000 IV/IO if in shock), every 15 minutes up to three doses, maximum cumulative dose: 0.3 mg (child), 0.5 mg (adult)
  - –IV fluids if hypotension
  - –Nebulized Albuterol; antihistamine; corticosteroid (for late phase)
  - –Observation: Mild, 2–4 hrs; severe, 12–24 hours
  - –Consult pediatric allergist
  - –Give patient EpiPen for self-administration
- Hereditary angioedema
  - –C1 esterase inhibitor concentrate; adults, danazol
- Avoid exposure to causative agents
- Desensitization to insect venoms
- Treat underlying disorders

152. Vesicular Rashes

A vesicle is <5 mm and a bulla is >5 mm in diameter (epidermal is flaccid; sub-epidermal is tense), a pustule is a pus-filled vesicle or bulla. The most common causes are benign lesions of the newborn (e.g., miliaria, erythema toxicum), infections, and hypersensitivity reactions. Bullous diseases resemble burns and can become emergencies.

Differential Diagnosis

- Infection
  - –HSV: Primary infection followed by latent infection in sensory ganglia; recurrences triggered by cold, UV light, stress, fever; HSV-2 (genital herpes) in child suspect sexual abuse; transmission by direct contact
  - –Varicella (chickenpox) and herpes zoster (VZV): Shingles, reactivation of latent virus in sensory ganglia
  - –Coxsackie virus (CV): Herpangina, "hand-foot-and-mouth disease"
  - –Tinea ("ringworm"): Fungal infection
  - –Bullous impetigo (BI): Staph, strep
  - –Scabies (mites)
  - –Staphylococcal scalded skin syndrome (SSSS): Tender skin, generalized exfoliation
- Contact dermatitis (CD): Poison ivy, drugs, foods, jewelry, chemicals
- Erythema multiforme (EM)/Stevens-Johnson syndrome (SJS):
  - –EM: "Bull's eye rash," central vesicle, bulla or urticaria
  - –SJS: More severe, two or more mucous membranes involved
  - –Triggers: Drugs (sulfonamides, NSAIDs, phenytoin), infection (herpes, EM; mycoplasma, SJS), chemicals, malignancies
- Toxic epidermal necrolysis (TEN, a.k.a. Lyell syndrome): Sudden-onset erythema, bullae, tender skin; same triggers as EM/SJS
- Neonatal
  - –Erythema toxicum: In up to 60% of newborns, disappears after 1 week
  - –Miliaria: Obstructed sweat ducts
  - –Pustular melanosis: Pustule then macule
  - –Neonatal acne
  - –Sucking blisters (bullae on hand)
  - –Acropustulosis
  - –Eosinophilic pustular folliculitis
  - –Congenital candidiasis
- Folliculitis: Staph and strep infections
- Autoimmune: Dermatitis herpetiformis (DH), pemphigus vulgaris (PV), linear IgA disease, bullous pemphigoid (BP)
- Hereditary: Incontinentia pigmenti, epidermolysis bullosa (EB)
- Others: Mastocytosis, friction, burns

Workup and Diagnosis

- History and physical exam
  - –Location, exposure, associated symptoms, social history
- HSV: Tingling/burning, vesicle on red base, 7–10 days, no scar
  - –HSV-1: Mouth (ulcers, vesicles), skin, cerebral (80% asymptomatic); "herpetic whitlow" (fingers); "herpetic gladiatorum" (contact sports)
  - –HSV-2: Genital, congenital; encephalitis (temporal lobe), dissemination, superinfection, keratitis
- Varicella: Red pruritic macule/papule on face, trunk; then vesicle/pustule on red macule; then noncontagious crust/scab; can get superinfection, pneumonia, encephalitis, hemorrhagic varicella
- H. zoster: Face/trunk, single dermatome, coalescing and grouped vesicles, crust after 7 days, common in immunocompromised patients, rare in children
- CV: Red macule/papule/vesicle on posterior oropharynx, hands, feet; may result in myocarditis
- Tinea: Can have kerion, a fluctuant mass with pustules
- BI: Erosion, honey-colored crust with adjacent bulla
- SSSS: Nikolsky sign, skin rubbing leads to bulla/peeling
- EB: Trauma, warm weather results in bulla
- Labs/Studies
  - –HSV/VZV: PCR, culture of lesions/fluids; Tzanck test: scrape from vesicle base shows multinucleated giant cells/nuclear inclusions; brain MRI/EEG (HSV)
  - –Tinea: KOH preparation, culture, or Wood lamp
  - –DH: Test for celiac disease (tissue transglutaminase)
  - –Biopsy when diagnosis unclear

Treatment

- HSV/VZV: Topical or systemic antivirals (e.g., acyclovir), topical anesthetics
- BI: Antibiotic for staph, strep
- EM/SJS/TEN: Symptomatic (TEN is similar to burn; use fluid therapy, emollient, antihistamine, topical anesthetic, Burow solution compresses), remove/treat cause, treat superinfection
- Tinea: Topical or oral (t. capitis) antifungal
- Scabies: Permethrin cream
- SSSS: Treat as TEN plus systemic antibiotic
- CD: Topical/systemic corticosteroid, antihistamine
- Folliculitis: Mild, topical; severe, systemic antibiotic
- DH/linear IgA disease: Oral sulfapyridine or dapsone
- PV/BP: Systemic corticosteroid, immunosuppressant
- Prevention: Varicella vaccine, VZIG (immunoglobulin) to prevent varicella after exposure; avoid exposure to causative agents

Section 17

Mental Status

KATHLEEN O. DeANTONIS, MD
MUSTAFA SAHIN, MD, PhD
JONATHAN E. TEITELBAUM, MD

153. Coma

Coma is a state of total unawareness of the self and the environment. There is no eye opening or response to voice or painful stimuli. Coma can be due to dysfunction of either bilateral cerebral cortex or the reticular activating system in the brainstem or both combined. Locating the lesion is very helpful in determining the etiology and thus the management.

Differential Diagnosis

- Infection
  - –Meningitis/encephalitis
  - –Bacteria, virus, fungi, spirochete
- Increased intracranial pressure
  - –Tumor, abscess, hydrocephalus
- Vascular
  - –Intracranial hemorrhage, stroke
  - –Hypoxic ischemic injury (hypotension, cardiac arrest, arrhythmia, near-drowning)
  - –Vasculitis
- Toxins
  - –Uremia, ethanol, atropine, opiates, lead, substance abuse
- Trauma: Concussion, contusion
- Seizure
  - –Nonconvulsive status epilepticus
  - –Postconvulsive state (postictal state)
- Electrolyte imbalance
  - –Hyponatremia, hypernatremia
  - –Hypomagnesimia
  - –Hypoglycemia, hyperglycemia
  - –Hypercalcemia, hypocalcemia
- Postinfectious
  - –Acute disseminated encephalomyelitis (ADEM)
- Endocrine disorders
  - –Adrenal insufficiency
  - –Thyroid disorders
- Degenerative and metabolic diseases
  - –Urea cycle disorders
  - –Reye syndrome
  - –Mitochondrial disease
- Systemic infection and sepsis
- Hepatic encephalopathy
- Psychogenic

The mnemonic **AEIOU-TIPS** has been used to recall portions of the differential diagnosis:

Alcohol ingestion and acidosis
Epilepsy and encephalopathy
Infection
Opiates
Uremia
Trauma
Insulin overdose or inflammatory disorders
Poisoning and psychogenic causes
Shock

Workup and Diagnosis

- History
  - –Trauma, seizures, diabetes; cardiac, liver, renal disease
  - –Presence of delirium before the onset of coma
  - –Fever, neck stiffness, headache
  - –Possible toxins at home
- Physical exam
  - –Vital signs, temperature
  - –Pattern of breathing (Cheyne-Stokes, apneustic, ataxic)
  - –Retinal hemorrhages, otorrhea, spinal fluid rhinorrhea
  - –Thyroid, cardiac rhythm, murmur
  - –Skin (cyanosis, petechiae, splinter hemorrhages)
  - –Hepatosplenomegaly, meningismus
- Neuro exam: Response to voice and noxious stimulation
  - –Papilledema, pupillary size, and light reflex
  - –Eye movements (spontaneous, doll's, calorics), corneals
  - –Gag, motor response to pain, DTRs, Babinski
  - –Decerebrate or decorticate posturing, muscle tone
- Labs
  - –Toxicology screen, glucose, electrolyes
  - –CBC, ABG, LFT, ammonia
  - –BUN, creatinine, TSH, blood culture
- Studies
  - –Neuroimaging: CT or MRI
  - –Lumbar puncture (after herniation has been ruled out)
    - –If subarachnoid hemorrhage or infection is suspected
  - –EEG to rule out nonconvulsive status epilepticus, gives clues to a metabolic process (triphasic waves)

Treatment

- First assess airway, breathing, and circulation (ABCs)
  - –Obtain intravenous access
  - –Treat for hypoglycemia
  - –Look for signs of herniation and increased ICP
- Reverse toxins if possible: Naloxone for opioids
- Treat with antibiotics for possible infectious agents
  - –Cephalosporins (for bacteria), acyclovir (for herpes)
- Increased intracranial pressure (ICP)
  - –Keep head of the bed up
  - –Intubate and hyperventilate
  - –Give mannitol (an osmotic agent)
- Seizures: Treat with benzodiazepines and fosphenytoin
- Treat the underlying systemic illness
- Observe in the intensive care unit with frequent neurologic examinations
  - –Closely observe fluid status, changes in temperature
  - –Prevent iatrogenic problems (e.g., DVT, corneal abrasions, decubitus ulcers)

154. Delirium

Delirium is an alteration in consciousness that can be associated with hallucinations, disorientation, and delusions. Normal thought processes are altered, including judgment, and rational behavior may be lost. Causes are typically metabolic derangements, acute infections, or drug use.

Differential Diagnosis

- Acute systemic infection
  - –May be viral or bacterial cause
  - –Often associated with high fever
- Hypoglycemia, diabetic ketoacidosis
- Central nervous system infection
  - –Meningitis, encephalitis, brain abscess
- Drugs
  - –Alcohol: Acute intoxication
  - –Amphetamines: Also tremors, dry mouth, tachycardia, hyperactivity
  - –Hallucinogens (LSD, mescaline, PCB) also tremors, dilated pupils, nausea, and abdominal pain
  - –Phencyclidine (a.k.a. Angel Dust) with atxia, nystagmus, hyperreflexia, and hypertension
  - –Opiates: Also with pinpoint pupils
  - –Antihistamines
  - –Phenothiazines
  - –Organic solvents
  - –Salicylates
  - –Glucocorticoids
- Head injury
- Rocky Mountain spotted fever (RMSF)
  - –Delirium and hallucinations may precede rash; fever, headache, myalgias, chills
- Malaria
- Rabies
- Syphilis
  - –Tertiary syphilis is rare in children
- Hyponatremia
- Uremia
- Migraine
- Hypoxia
- Heat stroke
- Hepatic failure
- Systemic lupus erythematosus
  - –Delirium is due to cerebral vasculitis
- Pellagra
  - –Due to niacin deficiency
  - –Also with diarrhea, dermatitis, dementia
- Hartnup disease
  - –Rash, ataxia, psychological disturbance
  - –Symptoms may be intermittent
- Porphyria
  - –Attacks of abnormal behavior do not begin until late adolescence

Workup and Diagnosis

- History
  - –Duration of delirium
  - –Exposure to excessive heat
  - –Ingestion of drugs
  - –Associated signs and symptoms (fever, diarrhea, vomiting, rashes, sweating)
  - –Recent head trauma
  - –Unusual or fad diets (diets that are mainly corn-based can lead to pellagra)
- Physical exam
  - –Vital signs
  - –Pupil size and reactivity
  - –Nuchal ridgidity, Kernig and Brudzinski sign
  - –Head exam for signs of trauma
  - –Scaling rashes (pellagra), petechiae of palms and soles (RMSF), sun sensitivity scars (porphyria)
  - –Ataxia, asterixis (flapping at wrists with uremia)
- Labs
  - –All patients should have a glucose measurement
  - –Strongly consider toxicology evaluation for all patients (typically do both blood and urine)
  - –Serum electrolytes, BUN, creatinine
  - –Liver testing (ALT, AST, bilirubin, PT/PTT)
  - –Specific testing of enzyme levels (porphyries), urinary amino acids (Hartnup disease), niacin levels (pellagra)
- Studies
  - –Consider LP and head imaging (CT or MRI)

Treatment

- Correction of any metabolic derangements, including alterations of glucose and sodium
- Drug ingestion
  - –Discuss with poison control center
- Infectious causes
  - –Use of appropriate antibiotics based on likely organisms
- Psychological disturbance
  - –Antipsychotics if appropriate
- Heat stroke
  - –Aggressive rehydration
- Hepatic failure
  - –Supportive therapy
  - –Lactulose may help to improve mental state/cognition
- Hartnup
  - –Supplemental nicotinamide
- Pellagra
  - –Supplemental niacin

155. Hallucinations

Hallucinations are defined as perceptual experiences that do not occur in reality. They may be auditory (most common), visual, tactile, or olfactory.

Differential Diagnosis

- Hallucinogenic drugs
  - LSD, "mushrooms," mescaline, and PCP are primarily hallucinogens
  - Amphetamines, cocaine, inhalants, and marijuana may also produce hallucinations
- CNS acute events
  - Trauma
  - CNS infection
  - Hypoxic events
- Psychosis
  - Defined as a mental state with significant impairment in cognition, interpersonal relations, and reality testing
  - Hallucinations may be a major or minor component
  - Psychosis may be psychiatric or organic (secondary to CNS insult)
- Schizophrenia
  - A disorder of impaired perception, cognition, interpersonal relations, and behavior with illogical and disordered thought content
  - Hallucinations (most often auditory) and delusions are common findings
  - Onset is frequently in adolescence
  - Frequently a positive family history
- Seizure disorders
  - Prominent auras may manifest as perceptual disturbances; visual and olfactory are the most common; tactile may also occur
- Narcolepsy
  - Hypnagogic hallucinations are hallucinations that occur while falling asleep; they may be visual or auditory
- Medications
  - Antipsychotics, anticholinergics, and corticosteroids can rarely cause hallucinations

Workup and Diagnosis

- History
  - History of mental illness
  - Recent behavioral patterns including relationships, self-care, and school performance
  - Medication and illicit drug use
  - Trauma, CNS infection, hypoxic episodes
  - Family history of mental illness
- Physical exam
  - Vital signs: Hallucinogens, amphetamines, and cocaine may cause tachycardia, hypertension, and hyperthermia
  - Hallucinogens, amphetamines, and cocaine may also cause pupillary changes, tremor, ataxia, arrhythmia, and hyperreflexia
- Mental status exam
  - Orientation and general appearance
  - Long- and short-term memory
  - Affect and behavior
  - Thought processing and content
  - Speech and language
- Labs
  - Urine and serum toxicologic screen
- Studies
  - Cranial imaging is most useful when there is a history of head trauma
  - EEG for patients in whom a seizure is suspected

Treatment

- Hallucinogens and other drugs of abuse
  - May require intensive outpatient or inpatient management for successful cessation
  - Cessation of the drug usually results in cessation of hallucination; however, for some hallucinogens such as LSD, flashbacks may occur for years
- CNS insults generally require neurologic and multisystem intensive care
- Schizophrenia is generally treated with antipsychotics; compliance is frequently problematic
- Narcolepsy is treated with daytime stimulants and night-time sleep aids or tricyclic antidepressants
- Medications: Discontinue the causative drug

Blood/ Laboratory Anomalies

Section 18

KATHERINE MACRAE DELL, MD
SARAH FRIEBERT, MD
ADDA GRIMBERG, MD
MARIA HENWOOD, MD
FRANCIS HOE, MD

156. Anemia

Anemia is decreased concentration of red cells or hemoglobin in the peripheral blood, resulting in decreased oxygen-carrying capacity of blood. It results from blood loss, decreased or failed production of red blood cells, or increased destruction/utilization in the peripheral blood. The clinical impact of anemia depends on degree, rate of development, and cardiopulmonary status of the patient. Common time points for anemia to arise are during the physiologic nadir of development (at about age 2 months) and during growth spurts.

Differential Diagnosis

- Often multifactorial

Hypochromic, microcytic

- Common
  - Iron deficiency
  - Thalassemias
  - Lead poisoning
- Less common: Acute infection or chronic disease, renal disease (decreased erythropoietin), sideroblastic anemia, protein-calorie malnutrition/anorexia, metabolic defects of iron metabolism

Normocytic, Normochromic

- Blood loss (acute blood loss due to trauma, occult blood loss such as GI, periodic blood loss such as occurs with menstruation)
- Marrow failure
  - Diamond-Blackfan anemia
  - Fanconi anemia
  - Transient erythroblastopenia of childhood
- Increased destruction of RBCs
  - Sickle cell disease
  - Membrane abnormalities
  - Enzyme deficiencies (G6PD, pyruvate kinase)
- Hemolysis: Drug-induced, immune
- Microangiopathic hemolytic anemia
- Hormone deficiencies (e.g., thyroid, growth)
- Acquired pure red cell aplasia
- Pregnancy/obstetric accident
- Marrow invasion or dysfunction
- Early iron deficiency

Macrocytic

- Common
  - Vitamin B12 and/or folate deficiency
- Less common: Drug-induced, Diamond-Blackfan anemia, Fanconi anemia, congenital heart disease, Down syndrome, myelodysplastic syndromes, erythroleukemia, reticulocytosis (hemolysis, blood loss, marrow recovery), pure red cell aplasia, hypothyroidism, liver disease, metabolic disease, asplenia, spurious

Workup and Diagnosis

- Symptoms are rare unless severe and vary by age
  - Younger: Pallor, irritability, sleepiness, failure to thrive
  - Older: Shortness of breath, exercise intolerance, pallor, palpitations, syncope, headache
- History: Age, gender, race/ethnicity, gestation, blood group; strenuous exercise, previous anemia, travel, jaundice; diet history (especially high milk intake); pica, age of home (older homes used lead-based paint); dark urine, transfusions; symptoms of malignancy (fever, weight loss, night sweats, bone pain), menorrhagia
- Family history: Anemia, cholecystectomy, splenectomy
- Physical exam: Vital signs, growth; nodes, murmur, edema, liver/spleen ascites, masses; spoon nails, frontal bossing, triphalangeal thumbs, hypoplasia of thenar eminence; vibratory and position sense (for B12 deficiency); hyperpigmentation, petechiae, purpura, jaundice
- Labs: CBC, peripheral smear, RBC indices (MCV, RDW, RBC, Mentzer index); reticulocyte count, hemoglobin electrophoresis; stool for occult blood; lead level in younger children; Coombs test and haptoglobin if suspicious of blood loss; iron studies (serum iron, ferritin, total iron binding capacity, % saturation)
- Less often: Urinalysis, G6PD screen, folic acid and vitamin B12 levels, ESR, osmotic fragility
- Bone marrow exam

Treatment

- Dependent upon etiology; if secondary, treat underlying cause or remove offending drug/agent
- Iron deficiency
  - Iron (6 mg/kg/day elemental iron) for 3 months
  - Decrease milk and tannic acid intake
  - Increase vitamin C intake (helps iron absorbtion)
  - Response to therapy is diagnostic
- Thalassemias, hemoglobinopathies, and membrane abnormalities: Referral to pediatric hematologist, may require chronic transfusions
- Folic acid/vitamin B12 deficiency
  - Identify cause (pernicious anemia, drugs, malnutrition, malabsorption, alcoholism, hemolysis, pregnancy)
  - Provide repletion
  - Treat B12 deficiency early to prevent neurologic damage

157. Hypercalcemia

Hypercalcemia is defined as total calcium >10.5 mg/dL. Hypercalcemia occurs when the resorption rate of bone mineral or the absorption of intestinal calcium exceeds the renal excretory capacity for calcium or when there is increased renal tubular absorption of calcium. Symptoms are nonspecific and do not usually develop until calcium is >14 mg/dL.

Differential Diagnosis

- Hyperparathyroidism
  - Primary
    - Sporadic
    - Familial (MEN types 1 and 2A)
    - Most common endocrinopathy in children with MEN 1
    - PTH-secreting adenoma
    - PTH gland hyperplasia
  - Secondary/tertiary
    - Following renal transplantation
    - Chronic hyperphosphatemia
- Familial hypocalciuric hypercalcemia (FHH)
- Vitamin D excess
  - Nutritional excess
  - Inflammatory/granulomatous diseases
    - Sarcoidosis
    - Eosinophilic granulomas
    - Tuberculosis
    - Coccidioidomycosis
    - Histoplasmosis
    - Lymphoma
- Immobilization
  - Bone resorption exceeds bone mineral accretion
- Malignancy
  - Neoplasms (leukemia, rhabdomyosarcoma, ovarian tumor, brain tumor)
  - Bony metastases
  - Synthesis of parathyroid-related protein (PTHrP)
- Drugs
  - Thiazide diuretics
  - Lithium
  - Vitamin A analogs
  - Calcium supplements
  - Alkali
- Hypophosphatemia
- Hyperthyroidism
- Adrenal insufficiency
- Pheochromocytoma
- Renal failure
- Williams syndrome
- Juvenile rheumatoid arthritis

Workup and Diagnosis

- History
  - Infant/young child: Constipation, anorexia, poor weight gain and/or poor linear growth
  - Older child/adolescent: Anorexia, nausea, vomiting, abdominal pain, dyspepsia, constipation; polyuria, polydipsia; weakness; impaired ability to concentrate, altered consciousness (irritability, confusion, depressive symptoms, lethargy)
  - All ages: Dietary intake, medications/supplements, family history of calcium disorders or neoplasms
- Physical exam: Usually normal
- Labs
  - Total and ionized calcium, urinary calcium excretion
  - Phosphorus
  - Intact PTH, PTHrP
  - T4, TSH
  - Complete metabolic panel
  - Vitamin D levels: 25-OH-vitamin D and 1,25-$(OH)_2$-vitamin D
  - Evaluation of associated endocrine tumors (for MEN)
- Studies
  - ECG: Shortened QT interval
  - Abdominal ultrasound: Nephrocalcinosis, renal calculi

Treatment

- Treatment depends on severity and etiology
- Keep well hydrated (orally) to prevent renal damage
- FHH: No therapy required
- If Ca <12 mg/dL and patient is asymptomatic: May delay treatment until cause is identified
- If Ca 10.5–12 mg/dL patient is symptomatic: Begin treatment; if Ca >12 mg/dL: Treat immediately
- Elements of therapy
  - Hydration: IV 0.9% saline (2× maintenance)
  - Calciuresis: IV Lasix (1 mg/kg/dose)
  - Antiresorptive agents if hydration and diuretics are ineffective
- PTH gland adenoma/hyperplasia
  - Parathyroidectomy
- Immobilization
  - Low-calcium diet, avoidance of vitamin D, hydration
- Discontinue drugs that increase serum calcium
- Treatment of endocrine disorders

158. Hyperglycemia

Diabetes mellitus is the most common endocrine disorder of childhood, affecting about 2/1,000 school-age children in the U.S. The absolute or relative lack of insulin results in an abnormal metabolic state, including hyperglycemia. Children with diabetes are at risk for the acute complications of dehydration and diabetic ketoacidosis (DKA), and for the long-term complications of retinopathy, nephropathy, neuropathy, atherosclerosis, and ischemic heart disease.

Differential Diagnosis

- Type I diabetes mellitus
  - –Most common form of diabetes in children
  - –Prevalence: 1.9/1,000
  - –Autoimmune-mediated destruction of pancreatic islets (β-cells)
  - –Absolute insulin deficiency
  - –Often presents with ketosis and DKA
- Type II diabetes mellitus
  - –Increasing prevalence in children, especially among obese
  - –In children, onset usually in mid-puberty
  - –More frequent in blacks, Hispanics, Pacific Islanders, Asians, and Native Americans (Pima Indians)
  - –Strong association with family history of type II diabetes
  - –Insulin resistance and inadequate insulin secretion results in relative insulin deficiency
- Maturity-onset diabetes of the young (MODY)
  - –Infrequent
  - –Autosomal dominant disease
  - –Onset usually between 9 and 25 years old
  - –Genetic defects in enzymes or nuclear transcription factors involved in islet cell development or the regulation of insulin secretion
- Drug- or chemical-induced diabetes
  - –Glucocorticoids, β-adrenergic agonists, phenytoin, asparaginase, cyclosporine, tacrolimus, vacor, pentamidine, diazoxide, nicotinic acid, thyroid hormone, thiazides
- Other endocrinopathies: Cushing disease, acromegaly, pheochromocytoma
- Exocrine pancreatic diseases
  - –Cystic fibrosis
  - –Hemochromatosis
- Pancreatectomy
- Physiological stress (trauma, infection)
- Infections
  - –CMV
  - –Congenital rubella
- Genetic syndromes: Prader-Willi syndrome, Down syndrome, Turner syndrome, Klinefelter syndrome, Wolfram syndrome

Workup and Diagnosis

- History
  - –Classic symptoms: Polyuria, polydipsia, weight loss
  - –Also polyphagia, nocturia, secondary enuresis, intermittent blurry vision
  - –Nausea, vomiting, abdominal pain with ketoacidosis
  - –Mental status changes with severe acidosis and dehydration
  - –Family history of DM, autoimmune, endocrinopathy
- Physical exam
  - –Vital signs, weight, body mass index
  - –Ketoacidosis: Funduscopic exam (blurred optic discs with cerebral edema), Kussmaul respirations, fruity odor to breath, tachycardia/hypotension/poor perfusion, severe dehydration, mental status changes
  - –Type II diabetes: Obesity and acanthosis nigricans
- Diagnostic criteria for diabetes
  - –Random plasma glucose >200 mg/dL
  - –Fasting plasma glucose >126 mg/dL
  - –Or 2-hour plasma glucose during the oral glucose tolerance test >200 mg/dL
  - –Lab abnormalities must be present on two different days or in the presence of symptoms of diabetes (polyuria, polydipsia, weight loss)
- Other tests
  - –Hb_{A1c}, urinalysis for glucose and ketones
  - –If suspect DKA, check electrolytes and blood gas
  - –To help distinguish type I from type II diabetes, check fasting insulin, C-peptide, and β-cell autoantibodies

Treatment

- Initial management
  - –Fluid to correct dehydration
  - –Insulin to correct hyperglycemia and acidosis
  - –Intravenous therapy required if patient in DKA
- Long-term management: Goal is to normalize blood glucose and HbA1c to decrease risk of acute and chronic complications
- Type II diabetes
  - –Absolute daily insulin requirement
  - –Monitor blood glucose (metabolic control)
  - –Attention to dietary intake (carbohydrate counting)
- Type II diabetes
  - –Weight management via diet changes and exercise
  - –Most require medication (insulin and/or metformin)
- Prognosis
  - –Chronic hyperglycemia increases long-term risk of microvascular (retinopathy, nephropathy, neuropathy) and macrovascular (atherosclerosis and ischemic heart disease) complications

159. Hyperkalemia

Hyperkalemia is defined as a serum potassium concentration ($[K^+]$) >5.5 mmol/L. The normal response to a potassium "load" and increased plasma $[K^+]$ includes an immediate response (K^+ moves into cells, H^+ out), without an effect on net total body potassium, and a delayed response (increased renal excretion via increased aldosterone). Potassium is removed from the body by secretion primarily in the collecting tubule, under the influence of aldosterone. This process requires sufficient delivery of sodium and water to the distal tubule.

Differential Diagnosis

- Laboratory artifact
  - –Due to hemolyzed specimen; very common seen with heel-stick blood collection or difficult phlebotomy
  - –Thrombocytosis
  - –Leukocytosis
- Impaired renal excretion
  - –Renal failure
  - –Volume depletion or decreased effective circulating volume (e.g., congestive heart failure), leading to decreased sodium delivery to the distal tubule and impaired potassium excretion
  - –Hypoaldosteronism (Addison disease, congenital adrenal hyperplasia)
  - –Type IV RTA/aldosterone resistance
  - –Potassium-sparing diuretics
  - –Medications (trimethoprim, pentamidine)
- Increased potassium load
  - –Overly rapid administration of IV potassium
  - –Use of aged banked blood
  - –Increased cell breakdown (rhabdomyolysis, tumor lysis syndrome, burns, starvation)
  - –Geophagia
- Transcellular shifts
  - –Hypoaldosteronism
  - –Adrenal insufficiency
  - –Medications (NSAIDs, ACE inhibitors, cyclosporine, FK506, β-blockers, digitalis)
  - –Metabolic acidosis from any cause
  - –Hyperglycemia/insulin deficiency

Workup and Diagnosis

- History
  - –Symptoms including oliguria, edema, dizziness, arrhythmias, flaccid paralysis, paresthesias
  - –Renal disease, heart disease, diabetes, cancer
  - –Medications, IV potassium administration
  - –Heavy exercise
  - –Family history including recurrent rhabdomyolysis (rare metabolic condition)
- Physical exam
  - –Blood pressure (hypertension suggests renal disease, hypotension could suggest adrenal insufficiency)
  - –Cardiac findings (gallop, JVD)
  - –Muscle tenderness (rhabdomyolysis)
  - –Lymphadenopathy (potential malignancy)
- Labs
  - –Serum chemistries obtained by venipuncture
  - –Urinalysis
  - –CBC and differential
- Studies
  - –CXR: If cardiac disease or volume overload suspected
  - –ECG: Early findings include peaked T-waves; late findings include widened QRS and ventricular fibrillation

Treatment

- Immediately remove all sources of potassium administration (including IVF and dietary)
- If significant ECG changes are present, immediate lowering of potassium and cardiac stabilization are achieved temporarily by agents that induce rapid transcellular movement of potassium into cells without net removal from the blood
  - –Calcium (stabilizes cardiac rhythm)
  - –Insulin (with glucose to prevent hypoglycemia)
  - –Bicarbonate (promotes metabolic alkalosis)
- More definitive measures to remove total body potassium (delayed effect 6–8 hours)
  - –Cation exchange resins
  - –Diuretics (especially loop diuretics)
- In cases of severe, life-threatening hyperkalemia, acute dialysis may be required

160. Hypernatremia

Hypernatremia is defined as a serum sodium concentration ($[Na^+]$) >147 meq/L (some texts use >150 meq/L). In the normal state, the response to increased serum osmolarity is stimulation of thirst (promotes fluid intake) and an increase in ADH (increases water uptake in the renal collecting tubule). Severe hypernatremic dehydration can be associated with a high mortality, particularly in young infants.

Differential Diagnosis

- Dehydration
  - –GI losses, especially watery diarrhea or profuse vomiting (very common)
  - –Impaired oral intake and inability to respond to normal thirst mechanisms (e.g., young infants, altered mental status, or iatrogenic administration of IV fluids)
- Central diabetes insipidus (DI)
  - –Decreased or absent production of ADH
  - –Idiopathic
  - –Head trauma
  - –Suprasellar or infrasellar tumors
  - –Langerhans cell histiocytosis
  - –Granulomatous disease (including tuberculosis, Wegener granulomatosis and sarcoidosis)
  - –Infection
  - –Cerebral hemorrhage
- Nephrogenic DI (NDI)
  - –Inability to respond to ADH
  - –Primary (congenital abnormality)
  - –Secondary (acquired renal tubular dysfunction, e.g., progressive renal insufficiency; medications, e.g., lithium)
- Severe skin or other insensible losses
  - –Excessive sweating
  - –Persistent rapid breathing
  - –Burns
- Increased total body sodium (rare in children)
  - –Salt intoxication from
    - –Sodium chloride tablets
    - –IV NaCl or $NaHCO_3$
    - –Breast milk after significant maternal sodium load
    - –Concentrated formula
  - –Primary hyperaldosteronism

Workup and Diagnosis

- History
  - –Vomiting, diarrhea
  - –Poor oral intake, recurrent dehydration
  - –Medications or salt supplementation
  - –Bicarbonate administration
  - –Burns
  - –Renal disease
- Symptoms
  - –Lethargy, seizures, coma
  - –Polyuria, polydipsia
  - –Headache, vision changes
- Family history
  - –Recurrent dehydration or early infant death (NDI)
- Physical exam
  - –Blood pressure
  - –Assessment of hydration status (pulse, perfusion)
  - –Midline defects (suggests presence of pituitary/hypothalamic defects/central DI)
  - –Funduscopic exam
- Labs
  - –Chemistry panel
  - –Serum osmolarity
  - –Urinalysis
  - –Urine osmolarity
- Additional evaluation based on the clinical situation
  - –Water deprivation test (to evaluate for central vs nephrogenic DI)
  - –CT or MRI of the head

Treatment

- If dehydration is present
  - –Fluid resuscitation with normal saline (20 cc/kg bolus)
  - –Water deficit = $0.6 \times \text{weight} \times (1 - 140/[Na^+])$
  - –Administer hypotonic IV solutions to correct sodium and rehydrate over 48 hours
- Too rapid correction can result in water shift into brain cells (due to the presence of "idiogenic" osmoles produced in response to the hypernatremia) resulting in cerebral edema
- Central DI
  - –Treat with exogenous vasopressin (DDAVP)
- Nephrogenic DI
  - –Treat with infusions of hypotonic saline or D5W (depending on the clinical situation and hydration status)
  - –Allow free access to water

161. Hypocalcemia

Hypocalcemia is defined as total calcium <7.5 mg/dL. Causes include inadequate inflow of calcium from the GI tract, bone, or kidney, or excessive loss of calcium into urine, stool, and bone. Calcium level is affected by pH: Systemic acidosis decreases total calcium and increases the ionized form (Ca^{++}), whereas systemic alkalosis increases total calcium and lowers Ca^{++}.

Differential Diagnosis

- Hypoparathyroidism
  - –Congenital: Transient neonatal vs heritable forms
  - –Acquired: Autoimmune, postsurgical, radioablation, infiltrative
  - –DiGeorge Syndrome
  - –Polyglandular autoimmune disease type 1 (Blizzard syndrome)
  - –Pseudohypoparathyroidism (PHP) or PTH resistance
    - –PHP type IA (Albright dereditary osteodystrophy)
    - –PHP type IB, type II
- Vitamin D deficiency
  - –Nutritional deprivation
    - –Most common cause of rickets
    - –Seen in breast-fed and black children
  - –Malabsorption/steatorrhea/liver disease
  - –1-α hydroxylase deficiency
  - –Chronic renal disease
- Calcium deficiency
  - –Nutritional deprivation
  - –Malabsorption
  - –Hypercalciuria
- Hypomagnesemia
  - –Impairs secretion of, and end-organ responsiveness to, PTH
  - –Inherited forms
  - –Intestinal losses
  - –Renal wasting: RTA, drugs
- Hyperphosphatemia
- Hypoproteinemia
  - –Total calcium is a measure of calcium bound to albumin
- Drugs
  - –Loop diuretics (furosemide) promote renal calcium excretion
  - –Anticonvulsants interfere with GI vitamin D absorption
  - –Antacids impair GI calcium absorption
  - –Antineoplastic agents
  - –Citrated blood products
- Critical illness
  - –Rhabdomyolysis
  - –Toxic shock syndrome
  - –Pancreatitis
- Organic acidemia
- Infant of a diabetic mother

Workup and Diagnosis

- History
  - –Age at onset, age developmental milestones reached
  - –Dietary intake, recurrent infections, medications
  - –Paresthesias, jitteriness, seizures
  - –Muscle cramping, tetany, carpal-pedal spasm
  - –Cardiac disease, neck surgery
  - –Autoimmune disorders, liver disease, renal disease
- Physical exam
  - –Vital signs, growth parameters
  - –Facial dysmorphism (DiGeorge syndrome, PHP IA)
  - –Skeletal deformities (bowed legs, widened wrists/ankles, rachitic rosary, frontal bossing)
  - –Cardiac exam (heart murmur with DiGeorge)
  - –DTRs for hyperreflexia, carpal-pedal spasm
  - –Chvostek sign (twitching of circumoral muscles after tapping on facial nerve in front of the ear)
  - –Trousseau sign (carpal-pedal spasm after maintaining arm BP cuff 20 mmHg above systolic BP for 3 minutes)
  - –Thrush, vitiligo, alopecia, nail fungal infection (for Blizzard)
- Labs: PTH, total and ionized calcium, vitamin D levels, alkaline phosphatase, LFT, BUN, Cr, magnesium, phosphorus, albumin; urine calcium and Cr
- ECG: Prolonged QT interval
- CXR: Absent thymus in DiGeorge
- Long bone films: Rachitic changes
- CT brain: Evaluate for calcification of basal ganglia

Treatment

- Acute correction of hypocalcemia: IV calcium gluconate (bolus or infusion) until Ca >7 mg/dL
- Hypoparathyroidism
  - –Oral calcium supplement (dose as elemental calcium)
  - –1,25-$(OH)_2$-vitamin D analog (calcitriol)
- Vitamin D deficiency (nutritional rickets)
  - –25-OH-vitamin D analog (ergocalciferol) 2,000–4,000 IU/day
  - –Oral calcium supplement (dose as elemental calcium) to prevent "hungry bone syndrome"
- Hypomagnesemia
  - –Treat with magnesium supplementation
- Drugs
  - –Discontinue offending agents if possible
- Goals of management
  - –Hypoparathyroidism: Maintain calcium at 8–9 mg/dL to avoid nephrocalcinosis
  - –Vitamin D deficiency: Maintain normal calcium range

162. Hypoglycemia

Hypoglycemia is defined by venous plasma glucose below 60 mg/dL. Normally, the body has several mechanisms that prevent hypoglycemia during fasting. Recurrent hypoglycemia suggests a defect in one of these fasting systems. The brain relies on glucose as an energy source; in infancy and childhood, hypoglycemia can injure the developing brain and result in permanent neurodevelopmental sequelae.

Differential Diagnosis

- Normal neonates (in first 24 hours of life)
- Ketotic hypoglycemia
- Insulin excess
  - Exogenous insulin
  - Sulfonylurea ingestion
  - Infant of a diabetic mother
  - Perinatal stress-induced hyperinsulinism
  - Congenital hyperinsulinism
  - Beckwith-Wiedemann syndrome
- Hormone deficiency
  - Panhypopituitarism
  - Growth hormone deficiency
  - ACTH or cortisol deficiency
  - Defects of glycogenolysis
  - Glycogen storage diseases
- Defects of gluconeogenesis
  - Glycogen storage disease type 1
  - Fructose-1,6-diphosphatase deficiency
  - Pyruvate carboxylase deficiency
  - PEPCK deficiency
- Fatty oxidation and ketogenesis defects
  - Medium-chain acyl-CoA dehydrogenase deficiency (most commonly)
  - Carnitine transport and metabolism
  - Electron transfer
  - HMG CoA synthase deficiency
  - HMG CoA lyase deficiency
- Liver disease
- Galactosemia
- Hereditary fructose intolerance
- Disorders of amino acid metabolism
  - Maple syrup urine disease
  - Methylmalonic acidemia
  - Tyrosinemia
- Dumping syndrome
  - Associated with Nissen fundoplication
- Reye syndrome
- Ethanol intoxication
  - Impaired gluconeogensis
- Salicylate intoxication
- Diarrhea and malnutrition
- Malaria
- Jamaican vomiting sickness
- Measurement error
  - Glucometer measurements are inaccurate in low range
  - Plasma glucose levels gradually fall if samples are not immediately tested

Workup and Diagnosis

- History
  - Classic symptoms associated with hypoglycemia that resolve with glucose ingestion
  - Symptoms of hypoglycemia: Anxiety, irritability, hunger, diaphoresis, tachycardia, shakiness, nausea/vomiting, weakness, headache, visual changes, poor speech, poor concentration, confusion, lethargy, somnolence, loss of consciousness, coma, hypothermia, seizure, personality changes
  - Fasting duration or frequency of feeding
  - Intercurrent illness, medications in the home
  - Birth history: Gestational diabetes, birth weight, stress
  - Developmental history: Delayed milestones
- Physical exam
  - Weight and height
  - Dysmorphism consistent with known genetic syndrome
  - Hyperpigmentation (in primary adrenal insufficiency)
  - Funduscopic exam (e.g., cataracts in galactosemia)
  - Midline defects (cleft palate, central incisor, microphallus) in hypopituitarism
  - Hepatomegaly (in glycogen storage and liver disease)
  - Neurologic exam for signs of CNS disease
- Critical labs during hypoglycemia: Electrolytes, HCO_3, insulin, C-peptide, cortisol, GH, free fatty acids, lactate, ammonia, β-hydroxybutyrate, acetoacetate, total and free carnitine, acyl carnitine profile, urine organic acids
  - Glycemic response to glucagon during hypoglycemia suggests hyperinsulinism or hypopituitarism

Treatment

- If awake and alert, give glucose/feed orally
- If impaired consciousness, D_{10} or D_{25} 2-4 cc/kg IV/NG
- For hyperinsulinism:
  - Glucagon injection acutely
  - Supranormal glucose intake chronically
  - Dietary manipulation (increased feeding frequency, some are protein sensitive)
  - Medical options: Diazoxide, octreotide
  - Surgical option: Subtotal pancreatectomy
- For defects in fasting adaptation (including defects in glycogenolysis, gluconeogenesis, fatty acid oxidation, and ketogenesis): Frequent or continuous feeding, night-time cornstarch helpful for some
- For hormone deficiencies: Hormone replacement (i.e., growth hormone and/or hydrocortisone)
- Goals of therapy: Prevent recurrent hypoglycemia, prevent catabolic state, promote growth and development

163. Hypokalemia

Hypokalemia is defined as serum potassium concentration ($[K^+]$) <3.5 mmol/L. The normal response to decreased plasma $[K^+]$ includes an immediate response (K^+ moves out of cells, H^+ moves in) and a delayed response (decreased renal excretion by suppression of aldosterone). Factors that affect K^+ distribution and transcellular shifts include acid-base status, insulin, catecholamines, aldosterone, and dietary intake.

Differential Diagnosis

- Diarrhea (very common)
  - –May be related to infection
  - –Other GI losses (e.g., ostomies)
  - –Patients with eating disorders
  - –Laxative abuse
- Vomiting (very common)
  - –Potassium losses are primarily from the kidney, not the stomach
  - –Loss of hydrogen ions and fluids leads to metabolic alkalosis, which causes movement of potassium into cells and aldosterone upregulation, which worsens hypokalemia and alkalosis
- Medications (causing renal K^+ wasting)
  - –Diuretics
    - –Loop diuretics (e.g., furosemide)
    - –Thiazides (e.g., hydrochlorothiazide)
    - –Diuretic abuse (eating disorder)
  - –Aminoglycosides
  - –Amphotericin
  - –Cisplatin
- Metabolic alkalosis from any cause stimulates potassium movement into cells in exchange for hydrogen ions
- Medications that cause transcellular shifts
  - –β-agonists (e.g., albuterol)
  - –Insulin
  - –Caffeine
  - –Theophylline
- Renal tubular acidosis
  - –Type I, distal
  - –Type II, proximal
- Inherited tubular disorders (very rare)
  - –Bartter/Gitelman syndromes
  - –Liddle syndrome
- Mineralcorticoid excess; hyperaldosteronism
  - –Adrenal adenoma
  - –Patients with hepatic dysfunction and decreased aldosterone metabolism
- Familial periodic paralysis (very rare)
- Impaired dietary intake (rare)
- Hypomagnesemia
- Fanconi syndrome
- Cystic fibrosis (due to chloride depletion)
- Licorice ingestion

Workup and Diagnosis

- History
  - –Symptoms include weakness, fatigue, constipation, muscle cramps, hypertension, polyuria, enuresis (sign of tubular dysfunction)
  - –GI losses (vomiting, diarrhea)
  - –Past medical history including growth
  - –History of eating disorder, laxative or diuretic use
  - –History of hypertension
  - –Medications
  - –Family history: Kidney disease, recurrent weakness
- Physical exam
  - –Vital signs: Blood pressure, pulse
  - –Assessment of hydration status (including pulse, blood pressure, skin turgor, mental status)
  - –Growth parameters
  - –Parotid enlargement (chronic vomiting/bulimia)
  - –Abdominal masses, striae (glucocorticoid excess)
- Labs
  - –Serum chemistries, magnesium
  - –Urinalysis
  - –For patients with metabolic acidosis, urine chloride to distinguish GI (urine Cl^- <10 meq/L) from renal (urine Cl^- >10 meq/L) potassium losses
  - –Diuretic screen
  - –AM cortisol level
- ECG
  - –Findings include ST depression, flattened T waves, increased U waves

Treatment

- Dehydration: Rehydrate with potassium-containing IV fluids (or oral rehydration solutions)
- Mild-moderate hypokalemia ($[K^+]$ >2.5 mmol/L)
  - –Oral rather than IV repletion is preferred, unless patient is symptomatic or taking digoxin
- Severe hypokalemia ($[K^+]$ <2.5 mmol/L)
  - –IV repletion should be considered
  - –Given by slow infusion at no more than 1 meq/kg over 4 hours; may require repeated infusions
  - –Rapid infusion can cause life-threatening hyperkalemia
- Adjust medications, if possible
- Treat underlying endocrine disorders, if identified
- Encourage consumption of high-potassium foods (bananas, tomatoes, oranges)
- Replete magnesium if low
  - –Hypokalemia may not be correctable until magnesium level is normal

164. Hyponatremia

Hyponatremia is defined as a serum sodium concentration ($[Na^+]$) <135 mEq/L (some texts use <130). Sodium concentration does not give any information about sodium content or volume status. Assessing the patient's volume status is essential to understanding the etiology and appropriate treatment of hyponatremia. In general, the severity of symptoms relates to how rapidly the hyponatremia develops as well as how fast the correction occurs.

Differential Diagnosis

- Hyponatremic dehydration
  - Etiologies include GI losses (very common), burns, diuretics, renal disease with tubular salt wasting
  - Secretion of ADH is stimulated, inhibits the normal suppression of ADH that should occur with low osmolarity
  - Causes both sodium losses and an inability to excrete a "free water" load (e.g., very hypotonic fluids)
- Hyponatremia with volume expansion
  - Etiologies include congestive heart failure, liver disease, nephrotic syndrome
  - Perceived (not actual) decreased effective circulating blood volume causes impaired free water excretion by the same mechanisms outlined above
- Syndrome of inappropriate ADH secretion (SIADH)
- "Pseudohyponatremia"
  - Hyperlipidemia: Lab artifact due to apparent dilution of serum sodium with an exogenous substance (e.g., lipids)
- Hyperglycemia
  - Osmotic force of increased glucose tends to draw water out of the interstitium and cells, and into the plasma
  - Serum osmolarity is normal or high but [Na+] is low
  - Hyponatremia resolves as the hyperosmolarity is corrected
- Psychogenic polydipsia
  - Psychiatric condition causing compulsive consumption of large amounts of fluid (>20 L/day has been reported in some patients)
  - Rare in children
- Cerebral salt wasting (rare)
  - Poorly understood disease
  - Typically presents after significant CNS insult (e.g., head trauma)
  - Normal to increased urine output
  - Rapid decline in serum sodium
  - High urinary sodium
- Endocrine disorders
  - Adrenal insufficiency
  - Glucocorticoid deficiency
  - Hypothyroidism
- Cystic fibrosis
- Medications (e.g., diuretics)

Workup and Diagnosis

- History
  - Vomiting, diarrhea, abdominal pain, nausea
  - Headache, confusion
  - Decreased urine output, and edema (suggest renal, cardiac, or liver disease)
  - Oral intake (particularly the consumption of water or other non-sodium-containing fluids)
  - Increased thirst and urine output (diabetes mellitus)
  - Medications (e.g., diuretics)
  - Lung or CNS disease/trauma
  - Family history of DM or kidney disease
- Physical exam
  - BP, hydration status (weight, pulse rate, perfusion)
  - Cardiac murmur, gallop, JVD, rales, hepatomegaly
  - Stigmata of liver disease, edema
  - Neurologic exam
- Labs
  - Chemistry panel, serum albumin, transaminases, urinalysis, urine specific gravity
  - Urinary sodium measurement/osmolarity (suspected SIADH or cerebral salt wasting)
- Radiology
  - CT scan if altered mental status or history of trauma
- For hyperglycemia, correct for increased glucose
  - Add 1.6 to $[Na^+]$ for every 100 mg/dL glucose >100
  - If corrected value is normal, there is no actual sodium deficit and therapy is directed at normalizing the serum glucose level

Treatment

- If evidence of volume depletion
  - Calculate Na^+ deficit: $(140 - [Na^+]) \times \text{Weight} \times 0.6$
  - Treat with IV infusion of D5 half-normal saline
  - Correct serum sodium over 24 hours
  - Include maintenance sodium and water
  - Correct no faster than 1–2 mEq/hour unless patient symptomatic (e.g., seizures); too rapid correction leads to central pontine myelinolysis
  - If seizures or significant neurologic symptoms are present (seen with serum Na <120 or rapid decline in sodium over a few hours), correct sodium with 3% NaCl (serum sodium concentration = 513 mEq/L) to >120 mmol/L (or until symptoms subside)
- If evidence of volume overload/SIADH
  - Restrict fluids to approximately 2/3 "maintenance"
  - Consider diuretics if nephrotic syndrome, liver disease or CHF

165. Leukocytosis

Normal white blood cell (WBC) counts fluctuate with age, so determination of leukocytosis should be based on the absolute number of cells per microliter of blood (not on the percentage of cells in the differential count) and compared with normal values for age. Often the specific diagnosis can readily be determined by knowing the specific class of white cell that is elevated and the duration of the elevation.

Differential Diagnosis

- Neutrophilia
  - –Increased production: Chronic infection or inflammation, tumor, drug-related, myeloproliferative disorders, chronic idiopathic neutrophilia, leukemoid reaction (Down syndrome, sepsis), chronic blood loss
  - –Increased release from marrow/ demargination: Corticosteroids, stress, exercise, hypoxia, endotoxin, acute infection
  - –Decreased removal from circulation due to splenectomy/asplenia, corticosteroids, leukocyte adhesion deficiency
  - –Others: Hemolysis, infarction, diabetic ketoacidosis, renal failure, hepatic failure, thyrotoxicosis
- Lymphocytosis
  - –Infection: EBV, CMV
  - –Heme/onc: Leukemia, neutropenia
  - –Endocrine: Thyrotoxicosis, Addison
- Basophilia
  - –Infection: Sinusitis, Varicella, smallpox
  - –Endocrine: Hypothyroidism, ovulation, pregnancy, stress
  - –Drugs
  - –Heme/onc: Hemolytic anemia, Hodgkin disease, CML, polycythemia vera
  - –Inflammatory/collagen vascular disease
- Monocytosis
  - –Infection: Syphilis, tuberculosis, subacute bacterial endocarditis, malaria, typhoid fever, Rocky Mountain spotted fever
  - –Heme/onc: Recovering marrow, hemolysis/hemolytic anemia, leukemias, Hodgkin disease, non-Hodgkin lymphoma, postsplenectomy, myeloproliferative disorders, congenital and acquired neutropenia, metastatic solid tumors
  - –Chronic inflammatory, collagen vascular
- Eosinophilia: Can be inherited
  - –Allergy/asthma; parasitic infection
  - –Heme/onc: Hodgkin disease, leukemias, immunodeficiency, postsplenectomy, solid tumors, pernicious anemia
  - –Chronic inflammatory/collagen vascular/
- Other: Rheumatoid arthritis, periarteritis nodosa, cirrhosis, Loeffler syndrome, sarcoid, dialysis

Workup and Diagnosis

- History: Duration of leukocytosis; fever, frequent infections, cough, acute illness; symptoms associated with malignancy (malaise, lethargy, night sweats, bruising, weight loss, bone pain, epistaxis, bleeding gums, hematochezia, petechiae); known allergies/sensitivities; joint symptoms; bowel habits (diarrhea with parasites), travel; steroid use; radiation therapy; failure to thrive, delayed puberty
- Family history: Myeloproliferative disease, hematologic malignancies, sarcoid, hepatosplenomegaly, early infant death
- Physical exam: General appearance, growth parameters; iritis, uveitis, mucositis, allergic shiners, pharyngeal cobblestoning; rash, purpura, petechiae, ecchymoses, striae; lymph nodes; hepatomegaly, splenomegaly; thryoid exam; joint swelling, decreased range of motion
- Labs
  - –CBC with differential and peripheral smear, ESR
  - –Leukocyte alkaline phosphatase
  - –Liver and renal function
  - –Stool hemoccult
  - –Specific infectious titers
  - –Specific autoimmune or rheumatologic tests
- Studies (as indicated by history and physical exam)
  - –CXR
  - –Bone marrow exam

Treatment

- Dependent upon diagnosis
- If malignancy is suspected, prompt multimodal treatment, based upon specific diagnosis, should be obtained at a tertiary pediatric oncology center
- If likely cause is evident (trauma/stress, acute infection, drugs) removal of the offending agent and watchful waiting is often sufficient
- Leukopheresis is prudent for extremely elevated WBCs to prevent pulmonary and cerebrovascular congestion/infarction

166. Metabolic Acidosis

Metabolic acidosis (defined as a serum bicarbonate <20 mEq/L) can be due to a primary metabolic cause, or it can represent a secondary metabolic compensation for a primary respiratory process. These processes can be distinguished by evaluation of a venous (or arterial) blood gas. An acidotic pH suggests a primary metabolic acidosis; alkalotic pH suggests secondary (since the body cannot completely compensate to a normal value).

Differential Diagnosis

- Increased anion gap (AG) metabolic acidosis, due to production of exogenous acid
"MUDPILES"
  - **M**ethanol
  - **U**remia
  - **D**KA
  - **P**araldehyde
  - **I**ngestions/inborn errors of metabolism
  - **L**actic acidosis
  - **E**thylene glycol
  - **S**alicylates
- Normal anion gap metabolic acidosis, due to bicarbonate loss in the GI tract or kidneys or impaired acid secretion by the kidney
  - –Diarrhea, other GI losses (very common)
  - –Type I (distal) renal tubular acidosis (RTA): Inability to excrete hydrogen ion, urine pH always high (>6.5), caused by a variety of medications, inherited forms, or renal insufficiency; often associated with low potassium and hypercalciuria
  - –Type II (proximal) RTA: Impaired reabsorption of bicarbonate from the proximal tubule, usually associated with other evidence of proximal tubule dysfunction (Fanconi syndrome), such as phosphaturia or glycosuria
  - –Type IV (hyperkalemic) RTA: Inadequate aldosterone production or inability to respond appropriately to aldosterone; commonly seen in patients with a history of obstructive uropathy or as a transient occurrence in patients with acute pyelonephritis

Workup and Diagnosis

- History
  - –Symptoms of fever, flank pain and vomiting (pyelonephritis), lethargy/altered mental status (intoxication or metabolic disease)
  - – GI losses (diarrhea), ingestions, poor growth, increased or decreased urine output, history of urinary tract abnormalities (e.g., congenital obstructive uropathy)
  - –Family history of kidney disease, kidney stones, metabolic disease, early infant deaths
- Physical exam: Assessment of hydration status (heart rate, blood pressure, mucous membranes, skin perfusion), growth parameters, respiratory status (tachypnea suggests either primary respiratory process or respiratory compensation for severe metabolic acidosis) abdominal exam, complete neurologic exam
- Labs
  - –Chemistry panel
  - –Calculation of AG $=[Na^+] - [HCO_3^- + Cl^-]$; normal = 10–12; when increased anion gap is due to exogenous acid, AG is often ≥20
  - –Venous blood gas, if the etiology of the acidosis is unclear (i.e., primary vs secondary); urinalysis (to help distinguish proximal vs distal RTA)
- Additional evaluation based on the clinical situation, e.g., toxicology, metabolic screens (increased AG acidosis), renal ultrasound (nephrocalcinosis with type I RTA)

Treatment

- If primary respiratory process identified, then treat the cause and the acidosis will resolve over time
- Dehydration: Oral or IV fluid replacement; even with normalization of fluid status, improvement in serum bicarbonate may not occur for 2–3 days
- For primary metabolic process
  - –Estimate deficit $= 20 - [HCO_3] \times$ Weight (kg) $\times 0.5$
  - –Replace over 24–48 hours with oral bicarbonate (e.g. bicitra solution 1 cc = 1 meq) or IV bicarbonate added to IV fluids; IV sodium bicarbonate "boluses" should be avoided unless acidosis is severe or symptomatic
- Increased AG acidosis: Identify and treat cause
- Distal or proximal RTA: Usually requires bicarbonate supplementation
- Hyperkalemic RTA: Correct serum bicarbonate, increase fluids to improve sodium delivery to distal tubule to enhance potassium secretion

167. Neutropenia

Neutropenia is based on absolute neutrophil count (ANC), calculated from the percentage of total white blood cell count made up by neutrophils and band forms. Norms are age-dependent and race-dependent. An ANC <1,500 cells/μl is mild neutropenia, <1,000 is moderate, and <500 is severe. The most common cause of neutropenia is viral infection, which is generally self-limited. The risk of serious infection rises exponentially when the ANC is <500.

Differential Diagnosis

<u>Extrinsic to bone marrow</u>

- Acute infection
  - –Viral (HAV, HBV, VZV, RSV, EBV)
  - –Bacterial (group B strep, typhoid, TB, tularemia), fungal
  - –Rickettsial (typhus, RMSF)
  - –Protozoal (malaria, toxoplasmosis)
- Drug-induced
  - –Penicillin, sulfonamides
  - –Ibuprofen, indomethacin
  - –Ranitidine, cimetidine
  - –Penicillamine
  - –Barbiturates, benzodiazepines
  - –Phenothiazines
  - –Antithyroid medications
  - –Anticonvulsants
- Environmental toxins (arsenic, benzene)
- Autoimmune
- Isoimmune neonatal
- Splenic or hepatic sequestration
  - –Especially with concomitant mild thrombocytopenia or anemia
- Metabolic disorders
  - –Glycogen storage diseases Ib

<u>Intrinsic to bone marrow or myeloid cell progenitors</u>

- Chronic benign or idiopathic neutropenia
- Cyclic neutropenia (autosomal dominant)
- Marrow replacement with leukemia, lymphoma, or metastatic solid tumors
- Kostmann syndrome
  - –Severe congenital neutropenia
- Hypo- or dysgammaglobulinemia
- Myelodysplastic syndrome
- Myelofibrosis
- Schwachman syndrome
- Fanconi anemia
  - –May involve neutropenia, anemia, thrombocytopenia, or pancytopenia
  - –Associated with absent radius, thumb abnormalities, short stature
- Cartilage-hair hypoplasia
- Dyskeratosis congenita
- Chédiak-Higashi
- Reticular dysgenesis
- Myelokathexis

Workup and Diagnosis

- History
  - –Duration (acute or chronic)
  - –History and pattern of fever, chronic cough, wheezing
  - –Mucositis, aphthous ulcers, "cold sores"
  - –Adenitis, signs of malignancy
  - –Malabsorption
  - –Family history (leukopenia, unusual infections, immunodeficiencies, unexplained early death)
  - –Type and frequency of infections
  - –Exposure to toxins or drugs
  - –Delayed separation of umbilical cord
- Physical exam: Growth, vital signs, pallor, toxic, phenotypic anomalies, scarred tympanic membranes, allergic shiners, pharyngeal cobblestoning, gingivitis, mucositis/ulcers, lymph nodes, wheeze, chest deformity, splenomegaly, hepatomegaly, rectal abscess, clubbing, cyanosis, skin/nail dystrophies, abnormal thumbs
- Labs
  - –CBC with differential and smear
  - –Immunoglobulin levels
  - –Cultures (blood, urine, sputum, throat, oral, or skin)
  - –Lymphocyte subsets, specific antibody responses
  - –Folate level, vitamin B12, metabolic screening
  - –HIV, specific infection serologies
  - –Exocrine pancreatic function
- Radiology: Chest X-ray, bone survey
- Studies: Bone marrow biopsy (neutrophil production), liver biopsy (definitive for glycogen storage diseases)

Treatment

- If a self-limited viral infection is suspected, repeat CBC in 3–4 weeks
- If cyclic neutropenia suspected, repeat three times per week for 4 weeks
- If febrile (≥100.4°F [38.0°C]) and/or presenting with acute illness
  - –Cultures of blood, urine, sputum if applicable, throat if symptomatic
  - –Appropriate broad-spectrum empiric antibiotic therapy
- Chronic neutropenia
  - –May be cyclic or idiopathic (not associated with specific etiology or infection)
  - –Granulocyte colony stimulating factor (GCSF) may be helpful
- Drug-induced neutropenia usually resolves with removal of the offending agent

168. Thrombocytopenia

Thrombocytopenia is defined as a platelet count of <150,000. Mild (100,000–150,000) and moderate (50,000–100,000) thrombocytopenia are rarely associated with significant bleeding. In contrast to the deep muscle and joint bleeds seen with coagulation factor deficiencies, clinical manifestations of bleeding due to thrombocytopenia involve skin or mucous membrane, GI tract, and menstrual bleeding. A rare but devastating consequence of a low platelet count is intracranial hemorrhage.

Differential Diagnosis

Disorders of increased destruction

- Immunologic platelet consumption
  - –Immune thrombocytopenic purpura (ITP)
  - –Drug-induced (antiepileptics, septra)
  - –Infection (EBV, CMV, malaria, Parvovirus, HIV, other viral illnesses)
  - –Autoimmune disease (SLE)
  - –Evans syndrome: ITP with immune hemolytic anemia
  - –Allergy or anaphylaxis
  - –Posttransplant
- Nonimmunologic
  - –Chronic microangiopathic hemolytic anemia
  - –Hemolytic-uremic syndrome (HUS)
  - –Thrombotic thrombocytopenic purpura
  - –Shear (catheters, cardiopulmonary bypass, congenital or acquired heart disease)

Disorders of decreased production

- Bone marrow infiltration: Leukemia, neuroblastoma, histiocytosis, osteopetrosis
- Marrow failure: Aplastic anemia, congenital microangiopathic anemia, thrombocytopenia with absent radii (TAR), Fanconi anemia, myelodysplasia, amegakaryocytic thrombocytopenia
- Abnormal platelet size or morphology
  - –Bernard-Soulier
  - –May-Hegglin
  - –Gray platelet
  - –Wiskott-Aldrich
- Severe nutritional deficiency
  - –B12, folate

Combined disorders

- DIC, Kasabach-Merritt syndrome, storage diseases, renal disease, pre-eclampsia

Sequestration

- Hypersplenism/portal hypertension, thrombosis, cavernous transformation of portal vein, hypothermia

Neonatal

- Congenital anomalies (trisomy 13 or 18)
- Maternal causes: ITP, SLE, HELLP syndrome, DIC, hyperthyroidism, viral illness, drug use
- NEC

Workup and Diagnosis

- History: Recent illness, diet history; bleeding (nose, gum, stool, urine, skin, duration, amount); bone pain, fever, lethargy or crankiness, limp; HIV risk factors, diet history; exposure to toxins or radiation
- Medical history: Congenital anomalies; bleeding with previous surgery or trauma, menorrhagia; frequent infections, congenital cyanotic heart disease
- Family history: Thrombocytopenia; autoimmune or collagen vascular diseases; blood dyscrasias, hematologic malignancies; storage diseases
- Physical exam
  - –General appearance, growth
  - –Petechiae, purpura, ecchymoses, eczema, pallor
  - –Jaundice, nail dystrophy
  - –Lymph node chains
  - –Splenomegaly, hepatomegaly, bruit, masses
  - –Caput medusae or spider hemangiomas
  - –Palatal petechiae, gum bleeding, leukoplakia
  - –Absent radii, thumb anomalies, joint abnormalities
- Studies
  - –Bone marrow exam
  - –Abdominal ultrasound; chest X-ray
- Labs
  - –All patients: CBC/diff with peripheral smear
  - –Selected patients: direct and indirect Coombs, LDH, DIC panel (PT/PTT, fibrinogen, D-dimers), blood culture, HIV, ANA, urinalysis, renal function, CMV and EBV titers, hepatitis B and C serologies

Treatment

- Dependent upon etiology, severity, and presence of acute bleeding
- ITP
  - –Bone marrow exam before treatment with steroids
  - –Treatment with IVIG or WinRho does not need bone marrow exam
  - –Platelet transfusion is ineffective in ITP but should be considered at counts <20,000 in the neonate or with life-threatening hemorrhage
  - –Severe injury is unlikely if count >10,000
  - –Treatment does not hasten resolution of ITP
  - –About 90% of children have resolution in 3–6 months
  - –Older girls more likely to become chronic
- Acute, isolated thrombocytopenia is almost never malignancy
  - –Marrow exam should be done in children with chronic or complex illness or with no response to therapy

Index

Index

Index

Index

Index

Index

Index

Index

Index

Index

Index

Index

Index

Index

Index

Index

Index

Index

Index

Index

Index

Index

Index

Index

Index

Index

Index

Index

Index

Index

Index

Index

Index

Index

Index

Index

Index

Index

Index

Index

Index

Index

Index

Index

Index

Index

Index

Index

Index

Index